Primary Care Sleep Medicine

CURRENT ◇ CLINICAL ◇ PRACTICE

NEIL S. SKOLNIK, MD • SERIES EDITOR

Primary Care Sleep Medicine: *A Practical Guide,* **edited by** *JAMES F. PAGEL AND S. R. PANDI-PERUMAL,* **2007**

Practical CPT Coding: *A Four-Step Guide for Physicians,* **by** *CHRISTOPHER L. TAYLOR, 2007*

Essential Practice Guidelines in Primary Care, **edited by** *NEIL S. SKOLNIK,* **2007**

Sexually Transmitted Diseases: *A Practical Guide for Primary Care,* **edited by** *ANITA NELSON AND JOANN WOODWARD,* **2007**

Allergic Diseases: *Diagnosis and Treatment, Third Edition,* **edited by** *PHIL LIEBERMAN AND JOHN A. ANDERSON,* **2007**

Headache and Chronic Pain Syndromes: *The Case-Based Guide to Targeted Assessment and Treatment, DAWN A. MARCUS,* **2007**

Bone Densitometry in Growing Patients: *Guidelines for Clinical Practice,* **edited by** *AENOR J. SAWYER, LAURA K. BACHRACH, AND ELLEN B. FUNG,* **2007**

The Handbook of Contraception: *A Guide for Practical Management,* **edited by** *DONNA SHOUPE AND SIRI L. KJOS,* **2006**

Obstetrics in Family Medicine: *A Practical Guide, PAUL LYONS,* **2006**

Psychiatric Disorders in Pregnancy and the Postpartum: *Principles and Treatment,* **edited by** *VICTORIA HENDRICK,* **2006**

Disorders of the Respiratory Tract: *Common Challenges in Primary Care,* **edited by** *MATTHEW L. MINTZ,* **2006**

Cardiology in Family Practice: *A Practical Guide, STEVEN M. HOLLENBERG AND TRACY WALKER,* **2006**

Bronchial Asthma: *A Guide for Practical Understanding and Treatment, Fifth Edition,* **edited by** *M. ERIC GERSHWIN AND TIMOTHY E. ALBERTSON,* **2006**

Dermatology Skills for Primary Care: *An Illustrated Guide, DANIEL J. TROZAK, DAN J. TENNENHOUSE, AND JOHN J. RUSSELL,* **2006**

Thyroid Disease: *A Case-Based and Practical Guide for Primary Care, EMANUEL O. BRAMS,* **2005**

Primary Care Sleep Medicine

A Practical Guide

Edited by

James F. Pagel, MS, MD

Department of Family Practice
University of Colorado School of Medicine
Southern Colorado Family Medicine Residency
Pueblo, CO

and

S. R. Pandi-Perumal, MSc

Comprehensive Center for Sleep Medicine
Department of Pulmonary, Critical Care, and Sleep Medicine
Mount Sinai School of Medicine
New York, NY

HUMANA PRESS TOTOWA, NEW JERSEY

Softcover reprint of the hardcover 1st edition 2007
999 Riverview Drive, Suite 208
Totowa, New Jersey 07512

humanapress.com

This publication is printed on acid-free paper. ∞
ANSI Z39.48-1984 (American Standards Institute) Permanence of Paper for Printed Library Materials.

Cover design by Donna Niethe

Production Editor: Amy Thau

For additional copies, pricing for bulk purchases, and/or information about other Humana titles, contact Humana at the above address or at any of the following numbers: Tel.: 973-256-1699; Fax: 973-256-8314; E-mail: orders@humanapr.com, or visit our Website: http://humanapress.com

10 9 8 7 6 5 4 3 2 1
eISBN: 978-1-59745-421-6
Library of Congress Cataloging in Publication Data

Primary care sleep medicine : a practical guide / edited by James F. Pagel and S.R. Pandi-Perumal.
p. ; cm. — (Current clinical practice)
Includes bibliographical references and index.
ISBN 978-1-61737-871-3
1. Sleep disorders—Treatment. 2. Primary care (Medicine) I. Pagel, James F. II. Pandi-Perumal, S. R. III. Series.
[DNLM: 1. Sleep Disorders. 2. Primary Health Care. 3. Sleep Disorders—therapy. WM 188 P952 2007]
RC547.P7558 2007
616.8'498—dc22

2007004654

Dedication

To the primary care practitioner of medicine, who deemphasizes ego and income while facilitating the distribution of knowledge, the best in patient care, and the highest quality of life.

Two are better than one,
Because they have a good reward for their labor.
For if they fall, one will lift up his companion.
But, woe to him who is alone when he falls,
For he has no one to help him up.

—*Ecclesiastes 4:9*

Series Editor Introduction

Primary Care in Sleep Medicine: A Practical Guide, edited by James F. Pagel and S. R. Pandi-Perumal, is an important book coming at an important time for the increasing number of patients with sleep disorders who are seen in primary care practices. The importance of primary care physicians having more in-depth education and training in sleep medicine has been emphasized in the Institute of Medicine report, "Sleep Disorders and Sleep Deprivation—An Unmet Public Health Problem," issued in April 2006. This landmark report estimates that 50 to 70 million Americans chronically suffer from a sleep disorder that interferes with their daily function and has long-term adverse effects on their health and quality of life. Lack of sleep can lead to increased rates of hypertension, diabetes, obesity, depression, heart attack, and stroke. In addition, one-fifth of all serious car accidents are associated with driver sleepiness. The Institute of Medicine report, after carefully examining and reporting on the evidence, concluded that increased awareness and training in the field of sleep disorders for primary care physicians is urgently needed to help address the increasing unmet needs of large numbers of patients with sleep disorders. *Primary Care in Sleep Medicine: A Practical Guide* is an excellent book that should help to meet this important need.

Neil Skolnik, MD
Professor of Family and Community Medicine
Temple University School of Medicine
Associate Director of the Family Medicine Residency Program
Abington Memorial Hospital

Preface

Most patients with sleep disturbances receive their medical care in the primary care setting. The spectrum of sleep disorders mirrors the clinical population of patients in a broad-based practice of primary care, with those chronic diseases that result in physical or mental discomfort for the patient inducing disturbances in the state of sleep. Evidence exists documenting the importance of the diagnosis and treatment of sleep disorders in the primary care practice in reducing morbidity and mortality, improving comorbid disease processes, and improving patient quality of life. However, the overwhelming majority of individuals that suffer from disorders of sleep and wakefulness are undiagnosed and untreated.

This field is relatively new, with few physicians having expertise or training in the area because sleep medicine is irregularly taught in medical schools or in physician training programs. The result is that few practicing physicians complete training with a clear understanding of the morbidity and mortality associated with sleep-related disease. There are few, if any, texts on sleep medicine oriented to the primary care physician. Those that exist emphasize the office evaluation and treatment of sleep-associated diagnoses, such as insomnia, that do not require sleep laboratory evaluation for diagnosis and treatment. Sleep laboratory polysomnographic testing provides a wealth of useful information for the primary care physician involved in the treatment of a patient's sleep disorder. The management of diabetes, hypertension, and congestive heart failure are core aspects of primary care medicine. Sleep laboratory testing can be utilized as an objective insight into the patient's pulmonary, cardiac, neurological, endocrine, cognitive, and psychiatric status. *Primary Care Sleep Medicine: A Practical Guide*, based on the sleep medicine syllabus utilized to train pulmonologists in sleep medicine, provides a high-quality, up-to-date background to support the primary care physician in appropriately utilizing sleep diagnostic testing in his or her clinical practice.

Primary Care Sleep Medicine: A Practical Guide is a clinical text geared toward the practicing primary care physician. This is the first text in which evidence-based practice recommendations are presented, as available, based primarily on practice parameter papers developed by the American Academy of Sleep Medicine. Both physicians in training and those in practice can utilize this text to obtain an understanding of appropriate sleep medicine diagnosis and treatment utilizing current evidence-based knowledge in the field to provide high-quality sleep medicine in the primary care practice.

Primary care physicians have training and experience in the full extent of medical and psychiatric illness affecting patients with sleep disorders. The close relationships that primary care physicians have with their patients provide an awareness and understanding of the bio–psycho–social context in which their patients live. These are advantages that the primary care physician has over the specialist in the diagnosis and management patients with sleep disorders.

Inasmuch as we envision continuing updates of this volume, readers are encouraged to contact us with any thoughts and suggestions for topics to be included in future editions.

James F. Pagel
S.R. Pandi-Perumal

Acknowledgments

The conceptual framework for *Primary Care Sleep Medicine: Practical Guide* came out of discussions between members of the Primary Care Task Force for Sleep Medicine convened in the spring of 2006 by the American Association of Chest Physicians (AACP). Members of that task force include Lee Brown, MD, Dick Simon, MD, Barbara Phillips, MD, James Pagel, MD, Susan Harding, MD, Richard Castriotta, MD, Mike Borisaw, and Jennifer Pitts. Mike Borisaw of the AACP was instrumental in obtaining the kind permission of that organization to utilize the already developed Sleep Medicine Syllabus 2005 as the core text on which this volume was based. The outstanding authors of individual chapters of that syllabus are thanked for the permission they were willing to give for utilization of their work in a primary care format.

Richard Lansing, Executive Editor at Humana Press, was instrumental in bringing this process to fruition on a short time line. We also would like to acknowledge our debt to the staff at Humana Press whose caring manner, commitment to quality, and professionalism was consistently upheld throughout the entire process of putting this volume together on a tight schedule. We are profoundly grateful for their sound advice and help.

Our greatest gratitude goes to our families for their wisdom, creativity, patience, and support, and we owe everything to our wonderful wives and families. You are the source of joy and inspiration for us. We are thankful for the love, support, and encouragement of our families who sacrificed many evenings and weekends of family time—Thank you!

One of the editors (JFP) also would like to thank the Garangi tribe of central Australia. If he would have accepted the invitation and been there as planned to celebrate the fourtieth anniversary of their walk-out and the dawn of aboriginal rights, this text would never have been completed.

To all these people goes our sincere gratitude.

Contents

Contributors

CHARLES W. ATWOOD, JR., MD, FCCP • Division of Pulmonary, Allergy, and Critical Care Medicine, VA Pittsburgh Healthcare System, Sleep Disorders Program, University of Pittsburgh Medical Center, Sleep Medicine Center, Pittsburgh, PA

FIONA C. BAKER, PhD • Human Sleep Laboratory, SRI International, Menlo Park, CA and Brain Function Research Unit, School of Physiology, University of the Witwatersrand, Johannesburg, South Africa

RUTH M. BENCA, MD, PhD • Department of Psychiatry, University of Wisconsin/ Madison, Madison, WI

BRIAN A. BOEHLECKE, MD, MPSH, FCCP • Department of Medicine, Division of Pulmonary Diseases and Critical Care Medicine, University of North Carolina School of Medicine, Chapel Hill, NC

BASHIR A. CHAUDHARY, MD, FCCP, FACP, FAASM • Georgia Sleep Center, Emeritus Professor of Medicine Medical College of Georgia, and Sleep Institute of Augusta, Augusta, GA

DONALD A. FALACE, DMD • University of Kentucky College of Dentistry, Department of Oral Medicine, Lexington, KY

NEIL S. FREEDMAN, MD, FCCP • The Sleep and Behavioral Medicine Institute, Bannockburn, IL and The Sleep Center at Lake Forest Hospital, Lake Forest, IL

LAUREN HALE, PhD • Department of Preventive Medicine, State University of New York, Stony Brook, Stony Brook, NY

SUSAN M. HARDING, MD, FCCP • Department of Medicine, Division of Pulmonary, Allergy, and Critical Care Medicine, Medical Director, UAB Sleep/Wake Disorders Center, University of Alabama at Birmingham, Birmingham, AL

DAVID M. HIESTAND, MD, PhD • Department of Pulmonary and Critical Care Medicine, Departments of Internal Medicine and Pediatrics, University of Kentucky, Lexington, KY

LOIS E. KRAHN, MD • Associate Professor of Psychiatry, Chair, Department of Psychiatry and Psychology, Mayo Clinic, Scottsdale, AZ

KATHRYN A. LEE, RN, PhD, FAAN • Department of Family Health Care Nursing, N411Y School of Nursing, University of California, San Francisco, CA

R. MANBER, RN, PhD, FAAN • Department of Psychiatry and Behavioral Sciences, Stanford University, Palo Alto, CA

JAMES F. PAGEL, MS, MD • Department of Family Practice, University of Colorado School of Medicine, Southern Colorado Family Medicine Residency, Pueblo, CO

S. R. PANDI-PERUMAL, MSc • Department of Pulmonary, Critical Care, and Sleep Medicine, Comprehensive Center for Sleep Medicine, Mount Sinai School of Medicine, New York, NY

JAMES M. PARISH, MD, FCCP • Sleep Disorders Center, Division of Pulmonary and Critical Care Medicine, Mayo Clinic, Scottsdale, AZ

BARBARA A. PHILLIPS, MD, MSPH, FCCP • Department of Internal Medicine, Division of Pulmonary and Critical Care Medicine, University of Kentucky College of Medicine, Lexington, KY

VIREND K. SOMERS, MD, PhD • Department of Internal Medicine, Division of Hypertension and Cardiology, Mayo Clinic, Rochester, MN
EDWARD J. STEPANSKI, PhD • Supportive Oncology Services, Inc. Accelerated Community Oncology Research Network, Memphis, TN
MICHAEL J. THORPY, MD • Sleep/Wake Disorders Center, Montefiore Hospital, New York, NY

1 Sleep Disorders in Primary Care

Evidence-Based Clinical Practice

James F. Pagel, MS, MD

Contents

INTRODUCTION

Each of us spend one-third of our lives asleep. Dysfunctions in this basic state lead to declines in quality of life, diminished waking performance, more frequent illness, and increases in both morbidity and mortality. Recent epidemiological data have emphasized the significant contribution of obstructive sleep apnea (OSA), one of the most physiological disruptive and dangerous sleep-related diagnosis, to pulmonary, cardiac, endocrine, and cognitive diseases *(1–4)*. Yet sleep medicine is not just a pulmonary subspecialty. The spectrum of sleep disorders mirrors the clinical population of patients in a broad-based practice of primary care *(5)* (Table 1). Almost all chronic diseases result in physical or mental discomfort for the patient and consistently induce disturbances in the state of sleep.

In clinical practice, sleep disorders are often only rarely addressed or treated. Despite the high prevalence of sleep disorders in the population and primary care setting, several studies suggest that sleep complains are under addressed by physicians. Only one-third of patients with insomnia mention it to their physicians and only 5% seek treatment *(6,7)*. Sleep problems are even more rarely addressed in the pediatric age population.

From: *Current Clinical Practice: Primary Care Sleep Medicine: A Practical Guide*
Edited by: J. F. Pagel and S. R. Pandi-Perumal © Humana Press Inc., Totowa, NJ

Table 1
Sleep Disorder Diagnoses[a]

Circadian-rhythm sleep disorder	*Current diagnostic code*
Delayed sleep phase type	327.31
Advanced sleep phase type	327.32
Irregular sleep-wake type	327.33
Nonentrained type (free running)	327.34
Jet lag type	327.35
Shift work type	327.36
Owing to medical condition	327.37
Other	327.39
Owing to drug or substance (alcohol)	292.85 (291.82)
Insomnia	
Adjustment insomnia	307.41
Psychophysiological insomnia	307.42
Paradoxical insomnia	307.42
Idiopathic insomnia	307.42
Insomnia as a result of mental disorder	327.02
Inadequate sleep hygiene	V69.80
Behavioral insomnia of childhood	V69.50
Insomnia as a result of drug or substance (alcohol)	292.85 (291.82)
Insomnia as a result of medical condition	327.01
Parasomnia	
Confusional arousals	327.41
Sleepwalking	307.46
Sleep terrors	307.46
REMS behavior disorder	327.42
Recurrent isolated sleep paralysis	327.43
Nightmare disorder	307.47
Sleep-related dissociative disorders	300.15
Sleep enuresis	788.36
Sleep-related groaning (catathrenia)	327.49
Exploding head syndrome	327.49
Sleep-related hallucinations	368.16
Sleep-related eating disorder	327.49
Parasomnia, unspecified	327.40
Parasomnias as a result of drug or substance (alcohol)	292.85 (291.82)
Parasomnias as a result of medical condition	327.44
Insomnia not owing to substance or known physiological condition, unspecified	780.52
Physiological insomnia, unspecified	327
Sleep-related breathing disorders	
Primary central sleep apnea	327.21
Central sleep apnea as a result of cheyne stokes breathing pattern	786.04
Central sleep apnea as a result of high-altitude periodic breathing	327.22
Central sleep apnea as a result of medical condition not cheyne stokes	327.28
Central sleep apnea as a result of drug or substance	327.29
Primary sleep apnea of infancy	770.81
OSA	327.23
Sleep-related nonobstructive alveolar hypoventilation, idiopathic	327.24

(Continued)

Table 1 *(Continued)*

Sleep-related hypoventilation/hypoxemia as a result of	*Current diagnostic code*
Congenital central alveolar hypoventilation syndrome	327.25
Lower airways obstruction	327.27
Neuromuscular and chest wall disorders	327.27
Sleep-related movement disorder	
Restless legs syndrome	333.99
Periodic limb movement disorder	327.52
Sleep-related leg cramps	327.53
Sleep-related bruxism	327.54
Sleep-related rhythmic movement disorder	327.59
Sleep-related movement disorder, unspecified	327.59
Sleep-related movement disorder as a result of drug or substance	327.59
Sleep-related movement disorder as a result of medical condition	327.59
Other sleep disorder	
Physiological sleep disorder, unspecified	327.80
Environmental sleep disorder	307.48
Fatal familial insomnia	046.80
Pulmonary parenchymal or vascular pathology	327.27
Sleep apnea/sleep-related breathing disorder, unspecified	327.20
Hypersomnia: Narcolepsy	
With cataplexy	347.01
Without cataplexy	347
Owing to medical condition with cataplexy	347.11
Owing to medical condition without cataplexy	347.10
Unspecified	347
Kleine–Levin syndrome	327.13
Menstrual-related hypersomnia	327.13
Idiopathic hypersomnia with long sleep time	327.11
Idiopathic hypersomnia without long sleep time	327.12
Behavioral-induced insufficient sleep syndrome	307.44
Hypersomnia owing to medical condition	327.14
Hypersomnia as a result of drug or substance (alcohol)	292.85 (291.82)
Hypersomnia not as a result of substance or known physiological condition	327.15
Physiological hypersomnia, unspecified	327.10

[a]From ref. *5*.

In a review of 50,000 physician patient contacts in family practice and general pediatric clinics, notes mentioning sleep were found in only 123 *(8)*.

These findings are in part a result of the fact that the field of sleep medicine is relatively new with few physicians having expertise or training in the area. Sleep medicine has not been regularly taught in medical schools or in physician training programs. Few practicing physicians complete training with a clear understanding of the morbidity and mortality associated with sleep-related disease. Most patients with sleep disturbance receive their medical care in the primary care setting. The evidence exists documenting the importance of the diagnosis and treatment of sleep disorders in primary care practice in reducing morbidity and mortality, improving comorbid disease processes, and improving patient quality of life. This book presents the argument for an evidence-based practice of sleep medicine in primary care.

SLEEP DISORDERS: THE CLINICAL SPECTRUM

Sleep diagnoses have been variably classified. Sleep quality worsens with age and stress. Sleep disruption occurs in association with psychiatric disorders and is often a component of DSM-IV-based diagnostic criteria. Pregnancy and menopause induce insomnia and sleep disruption. Pediatric sleep disorders are common. The most recent diagnostic classification (International Classification for Sleep Disorders, 2nd Edition) presents a framework for classification based on complaint, organ system, and etiology utilizing both medical and psychiatric diagnostic codes *(5)* (Table 1). Sleep diagnoses are divided into six primary categories: insomnias, sleep-related breathing disorders, hypersomnias not otherwise classified, circadian-rhythm sleep disturbance, parasomnias, and sleep-related movement disorders. Sleep disorders that cannot otherwise be classified are included as isolated symptoms, normal variants, and as alternative/other diagnosis.

THE INSOMNIAS

Insomnia is a primary care problem. The specialty of sleep medicine is new with few physicians boarded and trained in the area. Yet in the medical care setting sleep disorders are common. Whereas 30% of the general population report symptoms of sleep disruption, more than 50% of primary care patients have sleep complaints *(9)*. Diagnostically, about 75 million adults have occasional insomnia, whereas 25 million (11–14% of the population) have an ongoing problem with chronic insomnia *(6,10)*. At least 40% of American adults struggle with occasional insomnia. Those most at risk include women, sometimes because biological changes such as menstrual periods, pregnancy, or menopause may contribute to bouts of insomnia. Older adults report disruptions to their sleep as a result of medical conditions, sleep disorders, or discomfort. They are also more sensitive to environmental stimuli *(11,12)*.

The insomnias share the complaint of difficulty with sleep initiatiation, duration, consolidation, or quality associated with daytime functional impairment. The daytime functional impairment in insomnia can be fatigue, impaired memory or concentration, mood disturbance, daytime sleepiness, reduced motivation or energy, tension, headaches, or gastrointestinal symptoms as well as concerns and worries about sleep. In adults, chronic insomnia is associated with impaired social and vocational function and reduced quality of life, and in severe cases may be associated with an increased risk of traffic and work site accidents as well as psychiatric disorders. In children chronic insomnia is associated with poor school performance.

There is no question that insomnia is a quality-of-life issue. Individuals with chronic insomnia consistently report lower values of quality of life particularly on somatic/physical scales. Chronic insomnia is also associated with higher levels of reported cognitive impairment, increased job absenteeism, psychiatric illness, increased accident risks, and higher health care costs *(13)*. There is a strong association between insomnia and other illness. Chronic insomniacs have an increased risk of depression and anxiety *(14)*. Recent data have pointed out the association between insomnia and obesity. Sleepless individuals are much more likely to be obese *(15)*. Chronic insomnia is also associated with increased pain in rheumatic disease with the degree of insomnia on any given night being a predictor of pain intensity the following day *(16)*. Chronic insomniacs also report a 4.5 times higher incidence of serious accidents and injuries *(17)*. The American Academy of Sleep Medicine has developed a series of evidence-based criteria for the evaluation and treatment of insomnia *(18–20)*.

Table 2
Evidenced-Based Recommendations for the Diagnosis and Treatment of Insomnia

The evaluation of chronic insomnia does not require polysomnographic evaluation except when associated with other sleep-associated diseases such as OSA or PLMD	B	Consensus guidelines, usual practice, disease-oriented evidence, prospective diagnostic cohort study
Drug treatment of chronic insomnia leads to improvements in associated sleep states and daytime performance	B	Retrospective cohort and case–control studies with good follow-up
Behavioral treatment of chronic insomnia leads to improvements in associated sleep states and daytime performance	C	Consensus guidelines, usual practice

From refs. *11–13,17–22.*

The cost and health-care utilization data have been calculated for the common sleep disorders including insomnia and OSA. The annual direct costs of Insomnia in the United States include $1.97 billion for medications and 11.96 billion for health-care services. Indirect costs include decreased productivity, higher accident rate, increased absenteeism, and increased comorbidity with total annual cost estimates ranging from $30 to $107.5 billion *(10,21)*.

Insomnia as a symptom often arises secondary to underlying medical conditions, mental disorders, and other sleep diagnosis. Diagnosing insomnia can be a complex task as the origin of a patient's insomnia is often multifactorial. Life stressors, concomitant illness, family and social structure can precipitate symptomatic insomnia. The primary care physician often has a more complete knowledge of these factors than the polysomnographic-oriented subspecialist. Healthy sleep is under assault by the stressful culture in which we live. The primary care physician is in the ideal position to define the cause of the sleep–wake disturbance in a patient with insomnia. Like diet and exercise, sleep disruption and insomnia are lifestyle issues for which primary care physician are best suited to address. Evidence-based criteria for the evaluation and treatment of insomnia are addressed in Tables 2 and 3 *(18–20,22)*.

THE SLEEP-RELATED BREATHING DISORDERS

The sleep-related breathing disorders include both those occurring secondary to obstruction of the airway resulting in continued breathing effort but inadequate ventilation (OSA), as well as the central sleep apnea syndromes in which respiratory effort is diminished or absent because of central nervous system or cardiac dysfunction. OSA occurs at high frequency in the primary care clinic population. It is one of the most physiological disruptive and dangerous sleep-related diagnosis, affecting at least one of every five adults in some populations *(4)*. As many as 18 million Americans suffer from sleep apnea. It is more common among men, those who snore, are overweight, have high blood pressure, or physical abnormalities in their upper airways *(8)*.

Of the sleep disorders, OSA is the best studied from a cost-effect, epidemiological, and evidence-based perspective. The associated morbidity, mortality, comorbidities, and quality of life effects are well researched and described. Adult OSA has a long-term

Table 3
Evidence-Based Medicine Ratings Based on Strength of Recommendation Taxonomy

Strength of recommendation	*Quality of evidence*	*Consistency of evidence across studies*
A—Recommendation based on consistent good-quality patient-oriented evidence	Good-quality patient-oriented evidence—validated meta-analysis or high quality or prospective cohort studies	Consistent—most studies with similar results or supportive high-quality meta-analysis
B—Recommendation based on inconsistent or limited-quality patient-oriented evidence	Meta-analysis of lower quality, or studies with inconsistent findings, retrospective cohort, and case–control studies with good follow-up	
C—Recommendation based on consensus, usual practice, opinion, disease-oriented evidence, or case studies of diagnosis, prevention, or screening	Consensus guidelines, usual practice, disease oriented evidence, case series of studies	Inconsistent—variation among study findings or lack of coherence of meta-analysis in favor of the recommendation

From ref. *22*.

and clear association with obesity and daytime cognitive impairment (i.e., daytime sleepiness) that has been shown to lead to an increase in motor vehicular accidents in untreated patients. Subjects with apnea–hypopnea index (AHI) of greater than 10 have a 6.3 times odds of having a traffic accident compared with 152 case-matched control with AHI less than 10 *(23)*. Recent epidemiological studies that have cross-matched sleep apnea evaluation with long-term prospective cardiovascular risk studies, have served to point out the consistent and strong association between OSA and essential hypertension. Odds of hypertension increase with increasing severity of apnea in a graded dose response fashion, with an odds ratio of 1.27 for hypertension in group with AHI greater than 30 against the nonapnic grouping with an AHI of less than 5 *(24)*. Research supports the association between OSA and increased mortality, congestive heart failure (both right- and left-sided), myocardial infarction, and cerebral vascular accidents *(25)*. Evidence is slightly less clear or under development for the association of adult OSA with diabetes and metabolic syndrome *(26)*. Cardiac arrhythmias (bradycardia, atrial fibrillation, and ventricular tachycardia) are often seen in polysomnography (PSG) studies of OSA patients; however, the clinical significance and OSA association of these arrhythmias has yet to be fully studied *(27)*.

The pathophysiology and clinical presentation of pediatric OSA differ from that of adult OSA. In pediatric patients OSA is most clearly associated with poor school performance. In first graders performing at the bottom 10% of grade level, more than 20% have OSA. Of the children, all children who had tonsillar-adenectomy (T&A) surgery improved their grades, the others stayed the same *(28)*. Studies also support the association of pediatric OSA with failure to thrive, enuresis, and learning disability. Studies have been contradictory addressing the association of pediatric OSA with obesity and attention deficit/hyperactivity disorder with strong associations occurring in specific patient populations and not in other clinically defined settings *(29)*.

Table 4
Evidence-Based Associations of OSA

Adult OSA	Obesity	A—Consistent systemic meta-analysis
	Cognitive impairment (daytime sleepiness)	A—Consistent systemic meta-analysis
	Motor vehicular accidents	A—Consistent systemic meta-analysis
	Hypertension	A—Prospective diagnostic cohort studies
	Increased mortality	B—Retrospective cohort studies
	Congestive heart failure (right- and left-sided)	B—Inconsistent systemic meta-analysis
	Myocardial infarction	B—Prospective diagnostic cohort study
	Cerebral vascular accidents	B—Prospective cohort study
	Metabolic syndrome	C—Retrospective cohort studies
	Diabetes	C—Retrospective cohort studies
	Cardiac arrhythmias	C—Case series, usual practice
Pediatric OSA	Poor school performance	C—Retrospective cohort studies
	Enuresis	C—Retrospective cohort studies
	Failure to thrive	C—Case series, usual practice
	Learning disability	C—Retrospective cohort studies
	Obesity	C—Retrospective cohort studies
	Attention deficit/hyperactivity disorder	C—Inconsistent retrospective cohort studies

From refs. *1–4,22–34*.

OSA: COST AND HEALTH CARE UTILIZATION

The costs of untreated sleep apnea have been addressed in several studies. In 238 consecutive OSA patients studied in 1999, the mean annual medical cost was $2720 per patient before diagnosis compared with age, body mass index, and gender-matched controls *(30)*. Patients with OSAS use health care resources at higher rates than control subjects for years before diagnosis. Of all comorbid diagnoses, significantly increased utilization is found for cardiovascular disease and hypertension in patients with OSA *(27)*. For the 10 years before OSA diagnosis in 1999, patients with OSA had yearly claims of $3872 per patient compared with matched control claims of $1969 per patient. There was a rise in health care costs each year before diagnosis with initial data suggesting that after diagnosis yearly claims were halved. By the time patients were finally diagnosed for sleep apnea, they had already been heavy users of health services for several years *(31)*. In Canada hospital stays are 1.27 days per patient per year, 1 year before OSA diagnosis and 53 days per patient per year, 1 year after diagnosis. These differences were only seen in those patients adhering to treatment with no difference between patients and controls for nonadherers *(32)*. In pediatric OSA there are also suggestions for increased health care utilization with a 226% increase in health care utilization 1 year before evaluation, more hospital days, more drug use, and more visits to ER with the severity of OSA correlating directly to total annual cost independent of age *(33)* (Table 4).

THE COST-EFFECTIVENESS OF CPAP THERAPY FOR OSA

In OSA patients there is reduced hospitalization with cardiovascular and pulmonary disease in OSA patients on nasal CPAP treatment *(32)*. CPAP treatment reduces the need for acute hospital admission owing to cardiovascular and pulmonary disease in patients with OSAS. For the 2 years before and 2 years after content-positive airway pressure (CPAP) use in CPAP users, 413 hospital days were utilized before treatment and 54 hospital days after treatment. In OSA CPAP nonusers these findings were 137 hospital days before treatment and 188 days after treatment. This reduction of concomitant health care consumption should be taken into consideration when assessing the cost–benefit evaluation of CPAP therapy *(34)*.

HYPERSOMNIAS NOT OTHERWISE CLASSIFIED

In the modern fast-paced world, an adequate level of alertness is required for well being and performance. This diagnostic category includes a group of diagnoses sharing the primary characteristic of inducing significant daytime sleepiness. These diagnoses have significant effects on waking performance and therefore morbidity and mortality. The National Health and safety Administration (NHTSA) in 1999, estimated 1.5% of 100,000 police-reported crashes, and 4% of all traffic crash fatalities involved drowsiness and fatigue as principal causes. Beyond the personal and social loss associated with these accidents, the NHTSA in 1994, estimated cost at $83,000 lifetime per fatality; resulting in a total of $12.5 billion with 85% of cost from workplace loss and loss of productivity *(35)*.

The clinically significant sleep disorders that induce daytime sleepiness occur at lower frequency than OSA in the general population. These diagnoses generally require multiple sleep latency testing (MSLT) for diagnosis, an objective test measuring an individual's tendency to fall asleep in quiet situation *(36)*. Narcolepsy is the most common of the neurological diseases inducing severe daytime sleepiness, present in 1/2000 individuals in the general population.

CIRCADIAN RHYTHM SLEEP DISORDERS

The biological clock for sleeping is based in part on the circadian rhythm of sleep and wake propensity. Chronic sleep disturbance can result from disruptions in this system or from misalignments between an individual's circadian rhythm and the 24-hour social or physical environment. Delayed sleep phase syndrome is symptomatic in 7–16% of adolescents. Shift work disrupts normal sleep patterns for approx 20% of the population. At least 10% of individuals evaluated in sleep laboratories for chronic insomnia have a definite circadian component to their disorder *(8)*.

PARASOMNIAS

Parasomnias are undesirable physical events or experiences that occur during entry into sleep, within sleep, or during arousals from sleep. Parasomnias encompass sleep-related movements, autonomic motor system functioning, behaviors, perceptions, emotions, and dreaming. These are sleep-related behaviors and experiences in which the sleeper has no conscious deliberate control. Parasomnias become clinical diagnoses when associated with sleep disruption, nocturnal injuries, waking psychosocial effects, and adverse health effects. Parasomnias are classified based on sleep stage of origin into the disorders of arousal occurring out of deep sleep (stages 3 and 4), those associated with rapid eye movement sleep (REMS), and a grouping including less well-defined diagnoses with unclear sleep stage association.

Some of the sleep-associated parasomnias are common but of unclear or variable clinical significance. The arousal disorders of somnambulism and night terrors occur in up to

4% of pediatric patients. Enuresis is present in 15–20% of 5-year-old children declining to 1–2% in young adulthood. Recurrent nightmares occur in 15–40% of normal adolescents and may be present in up to 50% of traumatized immigrant communities reflecting a high incidence of post-traumatic stress disorder present in these populations. REMS behavior disorder occurs in 0.38–0.5% of the population *(37)*.

SLEEP-RELATED MOVEMENT DISORDERS

More than 12 million people in this country experience unpleasant, tingling, creeping feelings in their legs during sleep or inactivity as a symptom of a disorder called restless legs syndrome. This neurological movement disorder causes an uncontrollable urge to move and to relieve the sensations in the legs. As a result, sleep is either disrupted and people sleep poorly, become sleep-deprived, and experience daytime sleepiness *(38–40)*.

THE DIAGNOSTIC EVALUATION OF SLEEP DISORDERS

The diagnosis of the insomnias, the circadian-rhythm sleep disturbances, and the movement disorders of sleep are primarily based on a sleep history and physical. However, in order to diagnosis and manage many of the common sleep disorders, sleep physicians routinely utilize diagnostic tests that require the sleep laboratory for evaluation of the patient. The sleep-related breathing disorders and the parasomnias generally require PSG for evaluation. The hypersomnias generally require both PSG and MSLT for diagnostic evaluation and assessment of daytime sleepiness. The results of these tests can provide useful information that the primary care physician can utilize in providing optimal care for patients *(41–43)*.

PSG is the recording of multiple physiological signals during sleep. The standard PSG recording montage includes channels of electroencephalography (EEG), electrooculogram (EOG), and chin electromyelogram (EMG) that are required for sleep staging as well as recordings of respiratory effort, airflow, pulse oximetry, snoring, sleep position, ECG, leg EMG, and video monitoring. Additional channels are sometimes utilized including end-tidal or trans-cutaneous CO_2 and additional EEG channels if potential nocturnal seizure disorders are being evaluated. In evaluating the sleep-related breathing disorders, a split night protocol is often utilized in which a therapeutic treatment or "titration" portion of the PSG is added after at least 120 minutes of diagnostic sleep time. During the titration, C-pap, Bi-pap, and oxygen are utilized in an attempt to eliminate or reduce respiratory events and restore normal sleep. The PSG report is scored by a sleep technologist and interpreted by a sleep medicine physician. The PSG interpretation that you receive should include data as to sleep architecture, respiratory parameters, periodic limb movements, a description of any parasomnia or seizure activity, ECG abnormalities, and the results and appropriate setting of any titration attempted during the night of study (Table 5).

Daytime sleepiness is generally evaluated through MSLT that includes four to five opportunities to nap in the sleep laboratory after a full night PSG under standard conditions with EEG, EOG, and EMG monitored, so that sleep and REMS onset can be determined. MSLT reports should include average or mean latency to sleep, and the number of sleep onset REMS periods recorded (a diagnostic criteria for narcolepsy). The maintenance of wakefulness test is similar to the MSLT. For this procedure, the patient attempts to maintain wakefulness when monitored for appropriate testing periods to assess the patients ability to maintain wakefulness during the day.

Table 5
Polysmnography Report—Required Values That Should be Preset in Any Quality PSG Report and Interpretation

Sleep architecture
Sleep latency—time from lights out to sleep onset
REMS latency—time from lights out to REMS onset
Total recording time
Total sleep time (TST)
Proportion of TST in each sleep stage
Sleep efficiency (TST/total recording time)
Periodic limb movements of sleep
Periodic limb movement index (number per hour)
Periodic limb movement arousal index (number per hour)
Respiratory parameters
Apnea index
Hypopnea index
AHI number of events per hour
Mean and minimum oxyhemoglobin saturation (SaO_2)
Percent or minutes of TST spent below a defined SaO_2 setting (usually 88%)
Detailed report of any parasomnia or seizure activity including video, EEG, and EMG findings
Description of any ECG abnormalities
Titration report if done
Best treatment settings
Respiratory parameters at treatment levels
Pap-interface used (nasal mask, full face mask, nasal pillows, and so on)
Accessories required: chin strap, humidifier, and so on

Sleep laboratory testing can be expensive, and alternative approaches have been attempted. However, at this point in-laboratory full PSG with respiratory titration is the most cost-effective approach to evaluation of sleep disorders when required (Table 6). Limited PSG's including fewer recording channels cannot determine whether the patient is actually asleep during the recording. Full home PSG's are a potential alternative, however, incomplete recordings are obtained in 20% of studies and titration cannot be attempted in the night of study *(44,45)*. Autotitrating pap systems have minimal diagnostic capacity and can report inappropriate settings for misdiagnosed patients, for patients with central apneas, and those with nasal congestion or mouth leaks on pap therapy *(46)*.

Polysomnographic testing provides a wealth of useful information for the physician involved in the treatment of the patient's sleep disorder. The primary care physician able to understand the data and interpretation from a high-quality PSG will find much information useful in patient care. The management of diabetes, hypertension, and congestive heart failure are core aspects of primary care medicine. These disorders as well as the childhood behavioral disorders have significant relationships with the disease processes addressed in sleep medicine. Sleep laboratory testing can be utilized as an objective insight into the patient's pulmonary, cardiac, neurological, endocrine, cognitive, and psychiatric status.

Table 6
Evidence-Based Criteria for Sleep Testing

Full-attended PSG indications		
The diagnosis of sleep-related breathing disorders	A	Standard of care
Positive airway pressure titration	A	Standard of care
Pre- and postoperative evaluation of patients having surgery for OSA	A	Standard of care
Evaluation of patients being treated for OSA with persistent symptoms	A	High-quality cohort studies
Patients with systolic or diastolic heart failure not responding to optimal medical management	A	Prospective diagnostic cohort studies
Diagnosing of narcolepsy (with MSLT)	A	–
Diagnosing nocturnal seizures	C	Standard of care
Diagnosing parasomnias	B	Studies with inconsistent findings
Diagnosing restless leg syndrome/periodic limb movement disorder	C	Standard of care with nocturnal injuries
Diagnosing insomnia in patients not responding to behavioral or medical therapy	C	Disease-oriented evidence Consensus guidelines
Split night attended PSG for the diagnosis and treatment of sleep-related breathing disorders	A	Prospective diagnostic cohort studies
Nonattended PSG for the diagnosis of sleep-related breathing disorders	B	Retrospective cohort and case–control studies with good follow-up
Limited PSG for the diagnosis of sleep-related breathing disorders	–	Opinion and lower initial procedure cost
Autotitrating PAP for treating OSA	B	Case–control studies with good follow-up
MSLT indications		
Diagnosing narcolepsy	A	Standard of care
Assessing daytime sleepiness	B	Meta-analysis, usual practice, usual practice, disease-oriented evidence
Maintenance of wakefulness testing to assess daytime sleepiness	C	Disease-oriented evidence, usual practice

From refs. *11,18–20,22,36–38,40–46*.

CONCLUSION

The field of sleep medicine has shown remarkable growth in the last decades. The number of board-certified sleep physicians have grown from under 500 to more than 3000 in the last 15 years. Yet the overwhelming majority of individuals that suffer from disorders of sleep and wakefulness are undiagnosed and untreated. Primary care physicians have training and experience in the full extent of medical and psychiatric illness affecting patients with sleep disorders. They often have close relationships with their patients and an awareness and understanding of the bio-psycho-social context in which their patients live. These are advantages that the primary care physician has over the specialist in the diagnosis and management of patients with sleep disorders. The physician with training in sleep and an understanding of appropriately utilized testing procedures can utilize current evidence-based knowledge in the field to provide high quality sleep medicine in primary care practice.

REFERENCES

1. Gami AS, Caples SM, Somers VK (2003) Obesity and obstructive sleep apnea. Endocrinol Metab Clin North Am 32(4):869–894.
2. Kenchaiah S, Narula J, Vasan RS (2004) Risk factors for heart failure. Med Clin North Am 88(5):1145–1172.
3. Richert A, Ansarin K, Baran AS (2002) Sleep apnea and hypertension: pathophysiologic mechanisms. Semin Nephrol 22(1):71–77.
4. Young T, Peppard PE, Gottlieb DJ (2002) Epidemiology of obstructive sleep apnea: a population health perspective. Am J Respir Crit Care Med 165(9):1217–1239.
5. American Academy of Sleep Medicine, the International Classification of Sleep Disorders: Diagnostic and Coding Manual—2nd edition, American Academy of Sleep Medicine, Westchester, IL, 2006.
6. Ancoli-Israel S, Roth T (1999) Characteristics of insomnia in the United States: Results of the 1991 National Sleep Foundation Survey. Sleep 22 (Suppl 2):S347–S353.
7. Shochat T, Umphress J, Israel AG, Ancoli-Israel S (1999) Insomnia in primary care patients. Sleep 22 (Suppl 2):S359–S365.
8. Chervin R, Archbold K, Panachi P, Pituch K (2001) Sleep problems seldom addressed at two general pediatric clinics. Pediatrics 107(6):1375–1380.
9. NIH State of the Science conference Statement, Bethesda, MD 2005.
10. Walsh JK, Engelhardt CL (1999) The direct economic costs of insomnia in the United States for 1995. Sleep 22 (Suppl 2):S386–S393.
11. National Center on Sleep Disorders Research, National Heart Lung and Blood Institute, and National Institutes of Health (1999) Insomnia: assessment and management in primary care. Sleep 22 (Suppl 2): S402–S408.
12. Roth T, Roehers TA (2000) Treating Insomnia in the Primary Care Setting: National Sleep Foundation Monograph, Washington, DC.
13. Benca RM (2001) Consequences of insomnia and its therapies. J Clin Psychiatry 62 (Suppl 10): 33–38.
14. Breslau N, Roth T, Rosenthal L, Andreski P (1996) Sleep disturbance and psychiatric disorders: a longitudinal epidemiological study of young adults. Biol Psychiatry 39 (Suppl 6):411–418.
15. Hasler G, Buysse DJ, Klaghofer R, et al. (2004) The association between short sleep duration and obesity in young adults: a 13-year prospective study. Sleep 27:661–666.
16. Roehrs TA, Blaisdell B, Greenwald MK, Roth T (2003) Pain threshold and sleep loss. Sleep 26 (Suppl): A196.
17. Balter MB, Uhlenhuth EH (1992) New epidemiologic findings about insomnia and its treatment. J Clin Psychiatry 53 (Suppl):34–39.
18. Chesson AL Jr, Anderson WM, Littner M, et al. (1999) Practice parameters for the nonpharmacologic treatment of chronic insomnia. An American Academy of Sleep Report. Standards of Practice Committee of the American Academy of Sleep Medicine. Sleep 22:1128–1133.
19. Chesson AL Jr, Hartse K, Anderson WM, et al. (2000) Practice parameters for the evaluation of chronic insomnia. An American Academy of Sleep Medicine Report. Standards of Practice Committee of American Academy of Sleep Medicine. Sleep 23:237–241.
20. Thorpy M, Chesson A, Kader G, et al. (1995) Practice parameters for the use of polysomnography in the evaluation of insomnia. Standards of Practice Committee of the American Sleep Disorders Association. Sleep 18(1):55–57.
21. Stoller MK (1994) Economic effects of insomnia. Clin Ther 16:873–997.
22. Ebell MH, Siwek J, Weiss BD, et al. (2004) Strength of Recommendation Taxonomy (SORT): a patient-centered approach to grading evidence in the medical literature. Am Fam Physician 69:549–557.
23. Teran-Santos J, Jimenez-Gomez A, Cordero-Guevara J (1999) The association between sleep apnea and the risk of traffic accidents. Cooperative Group Burgos-Santander. N Engl J Med 340 (Suppl 11):847–851.
24. Smith R, Ronald J, Delaive K, Walld R, Manfreda J, Kryger M (2002) What are obstructive sleep apnea patients being treated for Prior to this diagnosis? Chest 121:164–172.
25. Wolk R, Shamsuzzaman AS, Somers VK (2003) Obesity, sleep apnea, and hypertension. Hypertension 42(6):1067–1074.
26. Vgontzas AN, Bixler EO (2003) Chrousos GP Metabolic disturbances in obesity versus sleep apnea: the importance of visceral obesity and insulin resistance. J Intern Med 254(1):32–44.

27. Verrier R, Josephson M Cardiac Arrhythmias and Sudden Death During Sleep, in *Sleep: A Comprehensive Handbook* (Lee-Chiong T, ed.) Wiley-Liss, Hoboken, NJ, 2006, pp. 727–732.
28. Gozal D (1998) Sleep-disordered breathing and school performance in children. Pediatrics 102:616–620.
29. Pagel JF, Snyder S, Dawson D (2004) Obstructive Sleep Apnea in Sleepy Pediatric Psychiatry Clinic Patients: Polysomnographic and Clinical Correlates. Sleep Breathing 8(3):125–131.
30. Kapur V, Blough DK, Sandblom RE, et al. (1999) The medical cost of undiagnosed sleep apnea. Sleep 22 (Suppl 6):749–755.
31. Bahammam A, Delaive K, Ronald J, Manfreda J, Roos L, Kryger MH (1999) Health care utilization in males with obstructive sleep apnea syndrome two years after diagnosis and treatment. Sleep 22 (Suppl 6):740–747.
32. Peker Y, Hedner J, Johansson A, Bende M (1997) Reduced hospitalization with cardiovascular and pulmonary disease in obstructive sleep apnea patients on nasal CPAP treatment. Sleep 20:645–653.
33. Tarasiuk A, Simon T, Tal A, Reuveni H (2002) Adenotonsillectomy in children with obstructive sleep apnea syndrome reduces health care utilization. Pediatrics 110:68–72.
34. Ronald J, Delaive K, Roos l, Manfreda J, Bahammam A, Kryger MH (1999) Health care utilization in the 10 years prior to diagnosis in obstructive sleep apnea syndrome patients. Sleep 22(2):225–229.
35. National Highway Traffic Safety Administration. www.nhtsa.dot.gov. Accessed October 2006.
36. Littner MR, Kushida C, Wise M, et al. (2005) Practice parameters for clinical use of the multiple sleep latency test and the maintenance of wakefulness test. Sleep 28(1):113–121.
37. Mahowald M (2000) Parasomnias. in: *Principles and Practice of Sleep Medicine* 3rd editions (Kryger M, Roth T, Dement W, eds.) W. B. Saunders Company, Philadelphia, pp. 693–796.
38. Littner MR, Kushida C, Anderson WM, et al. (2004) Practice parameters for the dopaminergic treatment of restless legs syndrome and periodic limb movement disorder. Sleep 27(3):557–559.
39. Thorpy M, Ehrenberg BL, Hening WA, et al. (2000) Restless Legs Syndrome: Detection and Management in Primary Care. National Heart, Lung, and Blood Institute Working Group on Restless Legs Syndrome. Am Academy Fam Physician 62 (Suppl 1):108–114.
40. Chesson AL Jr, Wise M, Davila D, et al. (1999) Practice parameters for the treatment of restless legs syndrome and periodic limb movement disorder. An American Academy of Sleep Medicine Report. Standards of Practice Committee of the American Academy of Sleep Medicine. Sleep 22(7):961–968.
41. Chesson AL, Ferber RA, Fry JM, et al. (1997) The indications for polysomnography and related procedures. Sleep 20:423–485.
42. Chesson A, Ferber R, Fry J, et al. (1997) Practice parameters for the indications for polysomnography and related procedures. Polysomnography Task Force, American Sleep Disorders Association Standards of Practice Committee. Sleep 20(6):406–422.
43. Kushida CA, Littner MR, Hirshkowitz M, et al. (2006) Practice parameters for the use of continuous and bilevel positive airway pressure devices to treat adult patients with sleep-related breathing disorders. Sleep 29(3):375–380.
44. Ferber R, Millman R, Coppola M, et al. (1994) Portable recording in the assessment of obstructive sleep apnea. ASDA standards of practice. Sleep 17(4):378–379.
45. Thorpy M, Chesson A, Ferber R, et al. (1994) Practice parameters for the use of portable recording in the assessment of obstructive sleep apnea. Standards of Practice Committee of the American Sleep Disorders Association. Sleep 17(4):372–377.
46. Littner M, Hirshkowitz M, Davila D, et al. (2002) Practice parameters for the use of auto-titrating continuous positive airway pressure devices for titrating pressures and treating adult patients with obstructive sleep apnea syndrome. An American Academy of Sleep Medicine report. Sleep 25(2):143–147.

2 Epidemiology of Sleep

Lauren Hale, PhD

CONTENTS

INTRODUCTION

The epidemiology of sleep refers to the study of patterns of sleep and sleep disorders across the population. Under the broad heading of the epidemiology of sleep, there are numerous specific questions to be asked about sleep hygiene practices, sleep architecture, sleep duration, and any one of a set of disorders. This chapter focuses on what is known about patterns of sleep duration, sleep apnea, insomnia, and restless legs syndrome (RLS) in the general US population and how they relate to three important epidemiological categories: sex, race, and age.

SLEEP DURATION

According to self-reported data from the National Sleep Foundation's (NSF) Sleep in America Poll, in 2005, Americans sleep around 6.8 hours per weekday night and 7.4 hours per weekend night *(1)*. Objective data from the coronary artery risk development in young adults study among individuals 38–50 years old, however, indicate that actual sleep time is closer to 6.1 hours, even though self-reports from the same people are around 6.7 and 7.3 hours, respectively *(2)*. Longitudinal data from the NSF polls show that sleep times have been decreasing in recent years. On the one hand, this suggests that the population may experience worse health, as short sleeping is associated with increased hypertension *(3)*, increased obesity *(4)*, reduced emotional and physical well-being *(5,6)*, and increased all-cause mortality *(7–9)*. However, there are also numerous findings showing that long sleeping is associated with increased morbidity and mortality *(7–14)*.

From: *Current Clinical Practice: Primary Care Sleep Medicine: A Practical Guide*
Edited by: J. F. Pagel and S. R. Pandi-Perumal © Humana Press Inc., Totowa, NJ

Sleep Duration and Sex

Several studies indicate that women sleep more than men on average, by around 45 minutes *(1,2,15)*. The objective data from the coronary artery risk development in young adults study also show that women have shorter sleep latency and higher sleep efficiency than men *(2)*. Two studies by Hale *(16,17)* show that women are less likely than men to be short sleepers (<6.5 hours relative to 6.5–8.5 hours), by around 10–20% ($p < 0.01$). And this effect is stronger on the weekends, when women are less likely to be short sleepers (<6.5 hours relative to 6.5–8.5 hours) than men by as much as 40% ($p < 0.01$) *(17)*. Yet these studies do not show differences between men and women in terms of the risk of being a long sleeper (>8.5 hours relative to 6.5–8.5 hours). However, the NSF's Sleep in America Poll *(1)* found that male respondents are more likely than female respondents to report that they get more sleep than they need (49% vs 37%). This may be because male respondents were more likely to report that they needed less sleep than women to function at their best (6.2 vs 6.8 hours). Another study found that whereas women sleep more than men on average, after adjusting for hours in the labor force, men sleep more than women *(18)*.

Sleep Duration and Race

The few studies that have investigated the relationships between race and sleep have revealed only marginal differences in sleep architecture by race *(19)*. However, Lauderdale et al. *(2)* find that black men and women spend less time in bed, get less overall sleep, have increased sleep latency, and reduced sleep efficiency compared with white men and women. Using survey data from the National Health Interview Survey, Hale and Do *(16)* find that black individuals had significantly increased risks of both short (<6.5 hours) and long (>8.5 hours) sleeping relative to whites.

Sleep Duration and Age

In a meta-analysis of the objective sleep parameters across the life-span, Ohayon et al. *(20)* that total sleep time decreases linearly as people age. Sleep efficiency, percentage of slow-wave sleep, percentage of rapid eye movement (REM) sleep, and REM latency all decrease with age, whereas sleep latency, percentage of stage 1 sleep, percentage of stage 2 sleep, and awakenings after sleep onset increased *(20)*. This is consistent with the findings by Hale that long sleeping (>8.5 hours compared with 6.5–8.5 hours) decreases with age *(16,17)*. In the Hale studies, however, short sleeping on the other hand is not associated with age *(16,17)*. In terms of duration alone, this suggests that as people age they move out of the high-risk sleep duration category of sleeping too long. Yet, as the Ohayon analysis shows that slow-wave sleep and REM decrease with age, a decrease in quality of sleep with age might be associated with negative health outcomes. Other studies using self-report data *(15,18)* have found no significant relationships with age and sleep duration.

SLEEP APNEA

Sleep apnea, which is described in more detail in other chapters of this volume, is a relatively common disorder defined by recurring episodes of apnea (breathing pauses) and hypopnea (reduced breathing) events during sleep *(21)*. In the NSF Sleep in America poll, between 5 and 8% of the population report having sleep apnea symptoms at least a few nights a week *(1)*. Other prevalence estimates range from around 1 to 28% of adults in Western countries depending the severity of the sleep apnea *(21–26)*.

Severity of sleep apnea is typically described by the average number of apnea plus hypopnea events per hour of sleep (i.e., the apnea-hypopnea index [AHI]), which can range from 0 to more than 100. There are well-established associations between sleep apnea and multiple harmful health states *(21)* including hypertension *(27,28)*, cardiovascular and cerebrovascular morbidity *(29–31)*, metabolic syndrome and diabetes *(32,33)*, impaired daytime function *(34,35)*, excessive sleepiness, and traffic accidents *(36,37)*, and poor health-related quality of life *(38,39)*. Whereas these associations cannot confirm there is a causal relationship, evidence from recent prospective observational and randomized treatment studies generally support the cross-sectional findings.

Sleep Apnea and Sex

Until the mid-1990s, sleep apnea was considered to be a man's disease. But epidemiological studies show that it is a prevalent condition in women as well *(25)*. Because men are more likely to be referred for evaluation of sleep apnea than women, the ratio of men to women (>5:1) with diagnosed sleep apnea is higher than the ratio (2:1) reported from population-based studies. Understanding the basis for gender differences in both the occurrence and outcomes of sleep apnea could have implications for treatment. On the one hand, several studies have shown that sleep apnea is more severe in men compared with women *(40,41)*. However, other evidence suggests that women may have worse outcomes of sleep apnea *(42–44)*.

In a community based of the Cleveland family study, Patel et al. *(45)* found the AHI to be significantly higher among the men compared with women. For European-American men, the mean was 10.2 events per hour for the men compared with events per hour for the women. The difference between the genders was smaller between African-American men and women at 9.3 and 5.7 events per hour. Cross-sectional results from Wisconsin Sleep Cohort population-based data indicate that men are significantly more likely than are women to have sleep apnea, adjusting for age, education, race, and marital status, body mass index, and smoking habits *(46)*.

Sleep Apnea and Race

In an analysis of the Cleveland family study, Patel *(45)* found significant differences in sleep apnea prevalence by sex, but not by race. On average, the AHI was lower for black men compared with white men, whereas AHI was higher for black women compared with white women. In a different analysis of this same population, Redline et al. *(47)* found that among younger subjects (≤25 years old) blacks are more likely than whites to have sleep apnea after controlling for obesity, race, and familial clustering. Ancoli-Israel et al. *(48)* found that among older adults (≥65 years old), African-Americans are more than twice as likely as Caucasians to have an AHI of 30 events per hour or higher, controlling for BMI and additional confounding factors. Yet in an analysis of the Sleep Heart Health Study sample of 6000 adults, no statistically significant association was found between race and sleep apnea, after controlling for BMI, age, and gender *(49)*. The evidence on race and sleep apnea is thus inconclusive.

Sleep Apnea and Age

Community studies show that sleep apnea prevalence increases with age, with some studies showing extremely high prevalence of sleep apnea in older adults *(21,50)*. However, older patients are not common in sleep clinic settings, so they are more difficult to study *(26)*. A consistent finding among many studies is that sleep apnea prevalence increases steadily with age in midlife *(21,26)*, but some work has shown that the severity decreases with age *(26)*. If clinicians assume that the increasing prevalence of sleep problems in older persons is normal, the prevalence of apnea among older individuals may be underestimated.

INSOMNIA

Chronic insomnia affects between 9 and 24% of the general population *(51–54)*. In the NSF Sleep in America poll, however, more than 50% of the population report having any symptom of insomnia at least a few nights a week (difficulty falling asleep, awake a lot during the night, woke too early and couldn't get back to sleep, and woke up feeling unrefreshed) *(1)*. The discrepancies in the estimates occur because the definition varies—with the lower bound referring to the definition requires that the disturbed sleep affects daytime functioning. Insomnia is associated with a variety of health risks: depressed mood, difficulty with memory and concentration, a variety of comorbidities (e.g., cardiovascular, pulmonary, and gastrointestinal disorders, generalized anxiety, dementia), and, possibly increased mortality *(51)*. However, it is a methodological challenge to separate the effects of insomnia from its comorbidities. Some argue that insomnia *per se* is not directly related to mortality, but rather it is the comorbidities associated with insomnia that affect mortality *(55)*. Whereas these relationships need to be disentangled, the public health burden of insomnia is great. For example, insomnia has large consequences for occupational, physical, and social performance. Overall, scientists have estimated that the economic cost of insomnia in the United States amounts to anywhere from $35 to $77 billion per year *(56,57)*.

Insomnia and Sex

A review of the insomnia literature consistently finds that insomnia is more common among women than among men *(52)*. There are more than 11 studies in which an association between gender and chronic insomnia revealed women are more likely than men to suffer from chronic insomnia *(54,58–68)*, compared with a handful of studies that found no relationship between gender and insomnia *(69–73)*. The Wisconsin Sleep Cohort analysis shows that insomnia, defined as frequently experiencing *any* one of four insomnia symptoms (difficulty falling asleep, difficulty falling back to sleep upon waking during the night, waking repeatedly, or waking too early), is not more common among women than men *(46)*. However, women were significantly more likely than men to have individual insomnia symptoms. The explanation for this discrepancy is that the women tend to have multiple insomnia symptoms, possibly indicating a tendency for more severe, if not more common, insomnia in women.

Insomnia and Race

Research on race and insomnia is limited and the results are mixed. Bixler et al. *(58)* found that chronic insomnia is more common among non-Caucasian minorities, whereas Riedel et al. *(74)* found that the reverse is true. Ancoli-Israel et al. *(75)* and Taylor et al. *(76)* found no significant differences between whites and non-Caucasians regarding insomnia. The Wisconsin Sleep Cohort also found no relationship between race and insomnia, although there was insufficient racial diversity for adequate statistical power *(46)*. Given these varied results, this suggests that if a difference exists it may vary by study sample and may not be prevalent throughout the population.

Insomnia and Age

Many studies reviewed in the literature *(52)* showed an association between age and chronic insomnia *(59–64,66–68,71–73,75,77–81)*, yet other studies found no significant relationship *(58,59,65,74,82–84)*. Of the studies that found a significant relationship between age and chronic insomnia, the direction of this relationship was positive in all, but one of the studies, which found a negative relationship between age and chronic insomnia in female hospital nurses in Japan *(81)*. The Wisconsin Sleep Cohort data demonstrate a varying relationship between insomnia symptoms and age *(1,85)*. Older adults were significantly more likely to report frequent problems with sleep maintenance (difficulty falling back to sleep upon waking during the night or waking repeatedly). Yet younger adults were significantly more likely to report frequent problems initiating sleep. This suggests again that the epidemiology of insomnia depends much on the definition of this disorder.

RESTLESS LEGS SYNDROME

RLS, also known as Ekbom's syndrome, is a sensorimotor disorder identified by leg restlessness and dysethesia during the night. This abnormal sensation to move usually interferes with one's ability to sleep. Self-reported prevalence rates are wide ranging anywhere from 1 to 24% of the population *(85)*. Often RLS is misdiagnosed and or individuals with the symptoms do not seek medical care *(86,87)*. The symptoms used to identify RLS include "repeated urge to move your legs" and "strange and uncomfortable feelings in the legs" when sitting or lying down. Further, the symptoms include that these complaints "get better when you get up and start walking" and that they "disrupt your sleep"*(85)*. There is an association between RLS symptoms and worse self-reported health and a history of cardiovascular disease *(85)*.

RLS and Sex

The NSF Sleep in America Polls do not show a difference in self-reported prevalence rates of RLS by men and women, where both estimates come in at 15% *(1)*. The Wisconsin Sleep Cohort data show that women report monthly rates of RLS symptoms at 17.5% compared with 14.1% men who have prevalence of RLS symptoms at least once a month ($p < 0.05$) *(85)*. Previous published RLS prevalence studies also indicate that it is higher in females than in males *(88,89)*.

RLS and Race

Evidence suggests that RLS complaints are more common in North America and European populations. That is, prevalence rates among African-Americans *(90)* and Asians *(91,92)* are lower than among Caucasians. One concern is that RLS may not be diagnosed as frequently in non-Caucasian communities because of differential health care utilization.

RLS and Age

Wisconsin Sleep Cohort data show that the prevalence of RLS symptoms increases as people get older. The symptoms of RLS rise more steeply for women with age than they do for men *(85)*. Diagnoses of RLS also increase with age in a sample of more than 1.5 million patients in the United Kingdom *(86)*.

CONCLUSIONS

People need healthy sleep not only for their own health, but for their successful functioning in their daily lives. Unfortunately, the high prevalence of sleep disorders (such as sleep apnea, insomnia, and RLS) is a major challenge to the health and well-being of the country, and much of the burden of disease is going undiagnosed. The majority of sleep research is not conducted in epidemiological terms. This is because high-quality sleep studies are difficult to conduct, expensive, and time-consuming. Studies based on diagnoses overlook individuals who do not seek medical care or who are misdiagnosed because of host of other comorbidities. Advances in epidemiological research, survey design, and sleep monitoring technology have allowed more population-based studies to answer questions about sleep patterns in the population. The need for improved research in the epidemiology of sleep is clear. Health care professionals need to better understand the prevalence and severity of various sleep-related conditions. A better understanding of the distribution and determinants of the disorders will enable improvements in prevention and treatment opportunities.

REFERENCES

1. National Sleep Foundation (2005) Sleep in America Poll. Available at: www.sleepfoundation.org/content/hottopic/2005_summary_of_findings.pdf. Accessed Dec. 2006.
2. Lauderdale DS, Knutson KL, Yan LL, et al. (2006) Objectively measured sleep characteristics among early-middle-aged adults: the CARDIA study. Am J Epidemiol 164(1):5–16.
3. Gangwisch JE, Heymsfield SB, Boden-Albala B, et al. (2006) Short sleep duration as a risk factor for hypertension: analyses of the first National Health and Nutrition Examination Survey. Hypertension 47(5):833–839.
4. Gangwisch JE, Malaspina D, Boden-Albala B, Heymsfield SB (2005) Inadequate sleep as a risk factor for obesity: analyses of the NHANES I. Sleep 28(10):1289–1296.
5. Haack M, Mullington JM (2005) Sustained sleep restriction reduces emotional and physical well-being. Pain 119(1–3):56–64.
6. Kaplow R (2005) Sleep deprivation and psychosocial impact in acutely ill cancer patients. Crit Care Nurs Clin North Am 17(3):225–237.
7. Kripke DF, Simons RN, Garfinkel L, Hammond EC (1979) Short and long sleep and sleeping pills. Is increased mortality associated? Arch Gen Psychiatry 36(1):103–116.
8. Tamakoshi A, Ohno Y (2004) Self-reported sleep duration as a predictor of all-cause mortality: results from the JACC study, Japan. Sleep 27(1):51–54.
9. Wingard DL, Berkman LF (1983) Mortality risk associated with sleeping patterns among adults. Sleep 6(2):102–107.
10. Qureshi AI, Giles WH, Croft JB, Bliwise DL (1997) Habitual sleep patterns and risk for stroke and coronary heart disease: a 10-year follow-up from NHANES I. Neurology 48(4):904–911.
11. Patel SR, Ayas NT, Malhotra MR, et al. (2004) A prospective study of sleep duration and mortality risk in women. Sleep 27(3):440–444.
12. Kripke DF, Garfinkel L, Wingard DL, Klauber MR, Marler MR (2002) Mortality associated with sleep duration and insomnia. Arch Gen Psychiatry 59(2):131–136.
13. Ayas NT, White DP, Al-Delaimy WK, et al (2003) A prospective study of self-reported sleep duration and incident diabetes in women. Diabetes Care 26(2):380–384.
14. Ayas NT, White DP, Manson JE, et al. (2003) A prospective study of sleep duration and coronary heart disease in women. Arch Intern Med 163(2):205–209.
15. Jefferson CD, Drake CL, Roehrs T, Roth T (2005) Sleep Habits in Healthy Normals. Sleep 28 (Abstract Suppl): A328–A329.
16. Hale L, Do DP (2006) Sleep and the City: An Analysis of Sleep Duration, Race, and Neighborhood Context in the NHIS. Presented at the Annual Meetings of the Population Association of America.
17. Hale L (2005) Who has time to sleep? J Public Health (Oxf) (2):205–211.

18. Biddle JE (1990) Hamermesh DS. Sleep and the Allocation of Time. The Journal of Political Economy.;98(5):922–943.
19. Rao U, Poland RE, Lutchmansingh P, Ott GE, McCracken JT, Lin KM (1999) Relationship between ethnicity and sleep patterns in normal controls: implications for psychopathology and treatment. J Psychiatr Res 33(5):419–426.
20. Ohayon MM, Carskadon MA, Guilleminault C, Vitiello MV (2004) Meta-analysis of quantitative sleep parameters from childhood to old age in healthy individuals: developing normative sleep values across the human lifespan. Sleep 27(7):1255–1273.
21. Young T, Peppard PE, Gottlieb DJ (2002) Epidemiology of obstructive sleep apnea: a population health perspective. Am J Respir Crit Care Med 165(9):1217–1239.
22. Bearpark H, Elliott L, Grunstein R, et al. (1995) Snoring and sleep apnea. A population study in Australian men. Am J Respir Crit Care Med 151(5):1459–1465.
23. Gislason T, Almqvist M, Eriksson G, Taube A, Boman G (1988) Prevalence of sleep apnea syndrome among Swedish men—an epidemiological study. J Clin Epidemiol 41(6):571–576.
24. Kripke DF, Ancoli-Israel S, Klauber MR, Wingard DL, Mason WJ, Mullaney DJ (1997) Prevalence of sleep-disordered breathing in ages 40-64 years: a population-based survey. Sleep 20(1):65–76.
25. Young T, Palta M, Dempsey J, Skatrud J, Weber S, Badr S (1993) The occurrence of sleep-disordered breathing among middle-aged adults. N Engl J Med 328(17):1230–1235.
26. Bixler EO, Vgontzas AN, Ten Have T, Tyson K, Kales A (1998) Effects of age on sleep apnea in men: I. Prevalence and severity. Am J Respir Crit Care Med 157(1):144–148.
27. Peppard PE, Young T, Palta M, Skatrud J (2000) Prospective study of the association between sleep-disordered breathing and hypertension. N Engl J Med 342(19):1378–1384.
28. Nieto FJ, Young TB, Lind BK, et al. (2000) Association of sleep-disordered breathing, sleep apnea, and hypertension in a large community-based study. Sleep Heart Health Study. JAMA 283(14): 1829–1836.
29. Shahar E, Whitney CW, Redline S, et al. (2001) Sleep-disordered breathing and cardiovascular disease: cross-sectional results of the Sleep Heart Health Study. Am J Respir Crit Care Med 163(1):19–25.
30. Hu FB, Willett WC, Manson JE, et al. (2000) Snoring and risk of cardiovascular disease in women. J Am Coll Cardiol 35(2):308–313.
31. Arzt M, Young T, Finn L, Skatrud JB, Bradley TD (2005) Association of Sleep-Disordered Breathing and the Occurrence of Stroke. Am J Respir Crit Care Med 172 (11):1447–1451.
32. Vgontzas AN, Bixler EO, Chrousos GP (2005) Sleep apnea is a manifestation of the metabolic syndrome. Sleep Med Rev 9(3):211–224.
33. Reichmuth KJ, Austin D, Skatrud JB, Young T (2005) Association of sleep apnea and type II diabetes: a population-based study. Am J Respir Crit Care Med 172(12):1590–1595.
34. Kim HC, Young T, Matthews CG, Weber SM, Woodward AR, Palta M (1997) Sleep-disordered breathing and neuropsychological deficits. A population-based study. Am J Respir Crit Care Med 156(6):1813–1819.
35. Redline S, Strauss ME, Adams N, et al. (1997) Neuropsychological function in mild sleep-disordered breathing. Sleep 20(2):160–167.
36. Teran-Santos J, Jimenez-Gomez A, Cordero-Guevara J (1999) The association between sleep apnea and the risk of traffic accidents. Cooperative Group Burgos-Santander. N Engl J Med 340(11): 847–851.
37. Young T, Blustein J, Finn L, Palta M (1997) Sleep-disordered breathing and motor vehicle accidents in a population-based sample of employed adults. Sleep 20(8):608–613.
38. Finn L, Young T, Palta M, Fryback DG (1998) Sleep-disordered breathing and self-reported general health status in the Wisconsin Sleep Cohort Study. Sleep 21(7):701–706.
39. Baldwin CM, Griffith KA, Nieto FJ, O'Connor GT, Walsleben JA, Redline S (2001) The association of sleep-disordered breathing and sleep symptoms with quality of life in the Sleep Heart Health Study. Sleep 24(1):96–105.
40. Young T, Hutton R, Finn L, Badr S, Palta M (1996) The gender bias in sleep apnea diagnosis. Are women missed because they have different symptoms? Arch Intern Med 156(21):2445–2451.
41. Tishler PV, Larkin EK, Schluchter MD, Redline S (2003) Incidence of sleep-disordered breathing in an urban adult population: the relative importance of risk factors in the development of sleep-disordered breathing. JAMA 289(17):2230–2237.
42. Faulx MD, Larkin EK, Hoit BD, Aylor JE, Wright AT, Redline S (2004) Sex influences endothelial function in sleep-disordered breathing. Sleep 27(6):1113–1120.

43. Shepertycky MR, Banno K, Kryger MH (2005) Differences between men and women in the clinical presentation of patients diagnosed with obstructive sleep apnea syndrome. Sleep 28(3):309–314.
44. Young T, Peppard PE (2005) Clinical presentation of OSAS: gender does matter. Sleep 28(3):293–295.
45. Patel SR, Palmer LJ, Larkin EK, Jenny NS, White DP, Redline S (2004) Relationship between obstructive sleep apnea and diurnal leptin rhythms. Sleep 27(2):235–239.
46. Hale L, Peppard PE, Young T 2006 Does the demography of sleep contribute to health disparities? in: *Sleep Disorders: Their Impact on Public Health.* 1 ed. (Leger D, Pandi-Perumal SR, eds.) Informa Healthcare, New York.
47. Redline S, Tishler PV, Hans MG, Tosteson TD, Strohl KP, Spry K (1997) Racial differences in sleep-disordered breathing in African-Americans and Caucasians. Am J Respir Crit Care Med 155(1): 186–192.
48. Ancoli-Israel S, Klauber MR, Stepnowsky C, Estline E, Chinn A, Fell R (1995) Sleep-disordered breathing in African-American elderly. Am J Respir Crit Care Med 152(6 Pt 1):1946–1949.
49. Young T, Peppard P, Palta M, et al. (1997) Population-based study of sleep-disordered breathing as a risk factor for hypertension. Arch Intern Med 157(15):1746–1752.
50. Young T, Shahar E, Nieto FJ, et al. (2002) Predictors of sleep-disordered breathing in community-dwelling adults: the Sleep Heart Health Study. Arch Intern Med 162(8):893–900.
51. State-of-Science Conference Statement: National Institute of Health, 2005.
52. Buscemi N, Vandermeer B, Friesen C, et al. (2005) Manifestations and management of chronic insomnia in adults. Evid Rep Technol Assess (Summ) (125):1–10.
53. Chesson AL Jr, Anderson WM, Littner M, et al. (1999) Practice parameters for the nonpharmacologic treatment of chronic insomnia. An American Academy of Sleep Medicine report. Standards of Practice Committee of the American Academy of Sleep Medicine. Sleep 22(8):1128–1133.
54. Morin CM, LeBlanc M, Daley M, Gregoire JP, Merette C (2006) Epidemiology of insomnia: prevalence, self-help treatments, consultations, and determinants of help-seeking behaviors. Sleep Med 7(2):123–130.
55. Phillips B, Mannino D Does Insomnia Kill? Annual Meetings of the Assoicated Professional Sleep Socieites. Denver, 2005.
56. Leger D (2000) Public health and insomnia: economic impact. Sleep 23(Suppl 3):S69–S76.
57. Walsh JK, Engelhardt CL (1999) The direct economic costs of insomnia in the United States for 1995. Sleep 22(Suppl 2):S386–S393.
58. Bixler EO, Vgontzas AN, Lin HM, Vela-Bueno A, Kales A (2002) Insomnia in central Pennsylvania. J Psychosom Res 53(1):589–592.
59. Hajak G (2001) Epidemiology of severe insomnia and its consequences in Germany. Eur Arch Psychiatry Clin Neurosci 251(2):49–56.
60. Ishigooka J, Suzuki M, Isawa S, Muraoka H, Murasaki M, Okawa M (1999) Epidemiological study on sleep habits and insomnia of new outpatients visiting general hospitals in Japan. Psychiatry Clin Neurosci 53(4):515–522.
61. Leger D, Guilleminault C, Dreyfus JP, Delahaye C, Paillard M (2000) Prevalence of insomnia in a survey of 12,778 adults in France. J Sleep Res 9(1):35–42.
62. Leppavuori A, Pohjasvaara T, Vataja R, Kaste M, Erkinjuntti T (2002) Insomnia in ischemic stroke patients. Cerebrovasc Dis 14(2):90–97.
63. Ohayon MM, Partinen M (2002) Insomnia and global sleep dissatisfaction in Finland. J Sleep Res 11(4):339–346.
64. Rocha FL, Guerra HL, Lima-Costa MF (2002) Prevalence of insomnia and associated socio-demographic factors in a Brazilian community: the Bambui study. Sleep Med 3(2):121–126.
65. Rocha FL, Uchoa E, Guerra HL, Firmo JO, Vidigal PG, Lima-Costa MF (2002) Prevalence of sleep complaints and associated factors in community-dwelling older people in Brazil: the Bambui Health and Ageing Study (BHAS). Sleep Med 3(3):231–238.
66. Taylor D, Lichstein K, Durance H (2003) Insomnia as a health risk factor. Behav Sleep Med 1(4):227–242.
67. Terzano MG, Parrino L, Cirignotta F, et al. (2004) Studio Morfeo: insomnia in primary care, a survey conducted on the Italian population. Sleep Med 5(1):67–75.
68. Yeo BK, Perera IS, Kok LP, Tsoi WF (1996) Insomnia in the community. Singapore Med J 37(3):282–284.
69. Broman JE, Lundh LG, Hetta J (1996) Insufficient sleep in the general population. Neurophysiol Clin 26(1):30–39.

70. Dorsey CM, Bootzin RR (1997) Subjective and psychophysiologic insomnia: an examination of sleep tendency and personality. Biol Psychiatry 41(2):209–216.
71. Han SY, Yoon JW, Jo SK, et al. (2002) Insomnia in diabetic hemodialysis patients. Prevalence and risk factors by a multicenter study. Nephron 92(1):127–132.
72. Kappler C, Hohagen F (2003) Psychosocial aspects of insomnia. Results of a study in general practice. Eur Arch Psychiatry Clin Neurosci 253(1):49–52.
73. Lichstein KL, Durrence HH, Bayen UJ, Riedel BW (2001) Primary versus secondary insomnia in older adults: subjective sleep and daytime functioning. Psychol Aging 16(2):264–271.
74. Riedel BW, Durrence HH, Lichstein KL, Taylor DJ, Bush AJ (2004) The relation between smoking and sleep: the influence of smoking level, health, and psychological variables. Behav Sleep Med 2(1):63–78.
75. Ancoli-Israel S, Roth T (1999) Characteristics of insomnia in the United States: results of the 1991 National Sleep Foundation Survey. I. Sleep 22(Suppl 2):S347–S353.
76. Taylor DJ, Lichstein KL, Durrence HH, Reidel BW, Bush AJ (2005) Epidemiology of insomnia, depression, and anxiety. Sleep 28(11):1457–1464.
77. Harvey AG, Greenall E (2003) Catastrophic worry in primary insomnia. J Behav Ther Exp Psychiatry 34(1):11–23.
78. Kawada T, Yosiaki S, Yasuo K, Suzuki S (2003) Population study on the prevalence of insomnia and insomnia-related factors among Japanese women. Sleep Med 4(6):563–567.
79. Pallesen S, Nordhus IH, Kvale G, et al. (2002) Psychological characteristics of elderly insomniacs. Scand J Psychol 43(5):425–432.
80. Kageyama T, Kabuto M, Nitta H, et al. (1997) A population study on risk factors for insomnia among adult Japanese women: a possible effect of road traffic volume. Sleep 20(11):963–971.
81. Kageyama T, Nishikido N, Kobayashi T, Oga J, Kawashima M (2001) Cross-sectional survey on risk factors for insomnia in Japanese female hospital nurses working rapidly rotating shift systems. J Hum Ergol (Tokyo) 30(1–2):149–154.
82. Braga-Neto P, da Silva-Junior FP, Sueli Monte F, de Bruin PF, de Bruin VM (2004) Snoring and excessive daytime sleepiness in Parkinson's disease. J Neurol Sci 217(1):41–45.
83. Hohagen F, Kappler C, Schramm E, Riemann D, Weyerer S, Berger M (1994) Sleep onset insomnia, sleep maintaining insomnia and insomnia with early morning awakening—temporal stability of subtypes in a longitudinal study on general practice attenders. Sleep 17(6):551–554.
84. Ohayon MM, Roth T (2001) What are the contributing factors for insomnia in the general population? J Psychosom Res 51(6):745–755.
85. Winkelman JW, Finn L, Young T (2006) Prevalence and correlates of restless legs syndrome symptoms in the Wisconsin Sleep Cohort. Sleep Med 7:545–552.
86. Van De, Vijver DA, Walley T, Petri H (2004) Epidemiology of restless legs syndrome as diagnosed in UK primary care. Sleep Med 5(5):435–440.
87. Garcia-Borreguero D, Egatz R, Winkelmann J, Berger K (2006) Epidemiology of restless legs syndrome: the current status. Sleep Med Rev 10(3):153–167.
88. Rothdach AJ, Trenkwalder C, Haberstock J, Keil U, Berger K (2000) Prevalence and risk factors of RLS in an elderly population: the MEMO study. Memory and Morbidity in Augsburg Elderly. Neurology 54(5):1064–1068.
89. Hogl B, Kiechl S, Willeit J, et al. (2005) Restless legs syndrome: a community-based study of prevalence, severity, and risk factors. Neurology 64(11):1920–1924.
90. Kutner NG, Bliwise DL (2002) Restless legs complaint in African-American and Caucasian hemodialysis patients. Sleep Med 3(6):497–500.
91. Nomura T, Inoue Y, Miyake M, Yasui K, Nakashima K (2006) Prevalence and clinical characteristics of restless legs syndrome in Japanese patients with Parkinson's disease. Mov Disord 21(3):380–384.
92. Tan EK, Seah A, See SJ, Lim E, Wong MC, Koh KK (2001) Restless legs syndrome in an Asian population: A study in Singapore. Mov Disord 16(3):577–579.

3 Assessment of Insomnia

Edward J. Stepanski, PhD

CONTENTS

INTRODUCTION

Insomnia is the subjective report of difficulty initiating or maintaining sleep, or a report of nonrestorative sleep. This symptom occurs commonly, with about one-third of adults reporting insomnia in a given year *(1–3)*. Most of these cases are transient insomnia and will remit. However, one-third of these patients report insomnia that is chronic or severe *(1)*. Transient insomnia is usually treated by primary care, whereas patients with chronic insomnia may be referred to sleep specialists. The general evaluation strategy described later is designed for cases of chronic insomnia. Strategies to efficiently evaluate a complaint of insomnia with the goal of identifying the contributing factors in a specific case are crucial to treatment planning. Insomnia is a nonspecific symptom that may be exacerbated by a myriad of medical, psychological, and behavioral factors. In cases of chronic insomnia, there are likely to be multiple contributing factors, and identification of these factors is necessary to focus treatment.

INTERVIEW DATA

An initial consultation of 60–90 minutes is needed to carefully explore contributing factors for a patient presenting with a complaint of insomnia. A systematic interview will assess many areas in order to determine what factors are playing a role in causing and maintaining the insomnia (*see* Appendix). A systematic review of the following areas is recommended: medical illness, psychiatric illness, medication effects, behavioral factors, cognitive factors, circadian-rhythm factors, and primary sleep disorders. This process is likely to uncover more than one potential cause of insomnia, and it is also likely that the clinician will not be entirely certain regarding the primary cause of poor sleep after the initial visit. Rather, the goal of this consultation is to uncover all

From: *Current Clinical Practice: Primary Care Sleep Medicine: A Practical Guide*
Edited by: J. F. Pagel and S. R. Pandi-Perumal © Humana Press Inc., Totowa, NJ

possible contributing factors and set up a hierarchy of which factors are the most important to guide treatment.

In many cases, it is not possible at the time of the initial consultation to determine with absolute certainty, which of several potential causes of insomnia is the most important in a given patient. For example, a typical history might find a 62-year-old patient with a 10-year history of insomnia who presents with arthritis, mild depression, an erratic sleep–wake schedule, use of large amounts of coffee, use of sedative-hypnotic medication several nights per week, work-related travel across time zones, increased job-related stress, and the tendency to leave a television on in the bedroom throughout the night. Which of these potential contributing factors is the most important in producing insomnia? The goal of the initial evaluation is to produce a comprehensive view of all possible factors and continue the assessment after treatment is initiated—addressing the most important two or three of these factors.

Medical Factors

A broad range of medical disorders is associated with poor sleep. A study of 3445 patients being treated in a primary care setting with a diagnosis of diabetes, hypertension, congestive heart failure (CHF), postmyocardial infarction, and/or depression found that 50% of this sample had insomnia *(4)*. Odds ratios ranged from 0.8 (diabetes mellitus) to 2.6 (depression) for mild insomnia, and from 0.9 (myocardial infarction) to 8.2 (depression). Medical disorders commonly reported to contribute to insomnia include arthritis, chronic obstructive pulmonary disease, CHF, Parkinson disease, hyperthyroidism, end-stage renal disease, and cancer. Although insomnia, secondary to a primary medical illness, can be considered a diagnostic entity *(5)*, the mechanism causing the insomnia varies across medical disorders. Patients with chronic obstructive pulmonary disease may have increased hypercapnia when lying supine or during sleep, secondary to hypoventilation, and this provides a stimulus to arousal and increased wakefulness *(6)*. CHF can lead to periodic breathing during sleep, and this is disruptive to sleep. End-stage renal disease is associated with both sleep-disordered breathing and restless legs syndrome (RLS)/periodic limb movement disorder (PLMD) *(7)*. Conditions associated with pain are presumed to disturb sleep as a consequence of arousal associated with discomfort.

It is often difficult to be certain if insomnia is secondary to a primary medical disorder. Lichstein *(8)* has suggested guidelines for this, based on the contiguity of the origin and course of the insomnia to the suspected primary disorder. When the insomnia begins in conjunction with the medical disorder and exacerbations of insomnia have occurred in parallel with changes in the medical condition, then the insomnia can be classified "absolutely" as a secondary insomnia. If only the origin or the course of the insomnia is related to the primary disorder then the insomnia is only "partially" secondary. A "specious" relationship exists when the two disorders are comorbid but independent. Determining a relationship between the course of the insomnia and a medical illness is made more difficult when relying on a patient's impression from historical data. A patient may perceive an illusory correlation between sleep and a medical condition or may miss a true correlation that is present. It is often easier for the sleep clinician to find such a relationship when he or she are following a patient during a period of months, particularly with use of daily sleep logs.

Given the uncertainty of determining that a medical or psychiatric disorder is a definite cause of insomnia, a clinician should be cautious in making a diagnosis of secondary insomnia. It is often easier to make the assumption that the insomnia is secondary to a comorbid disorder rather than continuing with further evaluation of insomnia or initiating cognitive–behavioral treatment.

Psychiatric Factors

Mood Disorders

Major depression is almost always associated with disturbed sleep–wake function and is a common cause of insomnia in patients presenting to sleep centers *(9)*. The presence of depression can usually be determined from interview questions that assess mood, appetite and weight changes, crying spells, memory, and social withdrawal. Use of a brief psychometric test, as a screening instrument such as the Beck Depression Inventory *(10)*, may also be helpful in providing an objective measure of depressive symptomatology. Some patients are more candid when completing such a questionnaire than they are when being interviewed and may find it easier to admit to suicidal ideation or other information relevant to a diagnosis of depression on a questionnaire.

Anxiety Disorders

Any anxiety disorder can contribute to insomnia, but post-traumatic stress disorder and panic disorder, in particular, are associated with sleep disturbance *(11,12)*. These disorders are readily identifiable with appropriate interview questions (*see* Appendix). Questions should assess the presence of intrusive thoughts, panic attacks, phobias, compulsive behaviors such as counting or checking rituals, or obsessions. Patients with post-traumatic stress disorder are also noted to have frequent nightmares related to the traumatic event.

Stress/Personality Factors

In addition to identifying specific diagnosable psychiatric disorders as described above, it is also important to characterize the stress level and personality style of the patient at the time of initial consultation. Acute or chronic stress can contribute to insomnia, and issues of job stress, domestic conflict, financial setbacks, or other similar problems may be important factors to consider in treatment.

Personality factors may be more subtle, but are also important in understanding the emotional state of the patient as well as what resources they bring to treatment. For example, when asking what happens during the night when he/she is unable to sleep, some patients will report becoming emotionally upset to the point of tears when unable to sleep. This may not signal a full-blown mood disorder, but may instead reflect poor frustration tolerance and limited coping skills. Some patients will report that they awaken their spouse because this eases their distress during the night, suggesting dependency, anxiety, and limited self-efficacy. The presence of these types of responses to insomnia suggests a bad prognosis for treatment in the sense that the patient has great trouble tolerating even a single night of insomnia. A patient who does not show emotional distress until three or four consecutive nights of poor sleep is more likely to be able to maintain the behavior changes required by cognitive-behavioral therapy, taper hypnotic medication, and better adhere to the overall treatment plan. A patient without sufficient resilience will require much support and psychological work to successfully manage their insomnia without medication.

Table 1
Medications-Associated With Insomnia

Class of drugs	*Examples*
Anticonvulsants	Lamotrigine
Antidepressants	Bupropion
	Phenelzine
	Protriptyline
	Fluoxetine
	Tranylcypromine
	Venlafaxine
β-Blockers	Propanolol
	Pindolol
	Metoprolol
Bronchodilators	Theophylline
Decongestants	Phenylpropanolamine
	Pseudoephedrine
Steroids	Prednisone
Stimulants	Dextroamphetamine
	Methamphetamine
	Methylphenidate
	Modafinil
	Pemoline

Medication Effects

Many medications will affect sleep–wake function. Some may cause unwanted daytime sedation, and others cause insomnia. Medications commonly reported to contribute to insomnia are listed in Table 1. Assessing the impact of medication use on sleep is accomplished by reviewing the contiguity of the sleep disturbance and the initiation of a trial of new medication, or changes in dosages of medications. Because side effects are generally dose-dependent, it is possible that insomnia only begins when a certain medication is increased to a higher dose (e.g., fluoxetine). In some cases, it is possible to taper or discontinue medications suspected of contributing to insomnia, in order to determine positively if that medication is responsible for the insomnia.

Use of hypnotic medication may also contribute to insomnia, but not because of side effects causing changes in central nervous system function, as described above. Instead, hypnotic medication, particularly short-acting compounds are associated with rebound insomnia on the first night of withdrawal *(13)*. Although this effect is increased after multiple consecutive nights of drug administration, it can occur even after a single night of use *(14)*. There are large individual differences in the experience of rebound insomnia, as some patients appear to be much more sensitive to this effect and have a more intense rebound *(14)*. A pattern of rebound insomnia in a patient using hypnotic medication on a PRN (as needed) schedule is the best detected with use of sleep logs. A patient will often not be aware of the rebound, as they assume that poor sleep is a return to their baseline insomnia.

There is another pattern of insomnia related to hypnotic use that will more often occur with intermediate or long-acting compounds. In this situation, a patient is relatively sleep-deprived after several nights of short or poor sleep and is then able to achieve

10 hours of recovery sleep with use of hypnotic medication. On the following night, total sleep time is again reduced, at least in part, because of satiation of sleep drive from excessive sleep the previous night. This situation is, theoretically, the opposite of what is accomplished with sleep restriction therapy, where homeostatic sleep drive is increased in patients with insomnia by systematically decreasing time in bed *(15)*.

Behavioral Factors

This category concerns sleep habits that have been shown to contribute to poor sleep in normal sleepers and are presumed to be relevant in patients with insomnia. These behaviors are referred to as poor sleep hygiene and include the following: excessive use of caffeine or alcohol, spending excessive time in bed, napping, exercising or working close to bedtime, watching television or reading in bed, eating during the night, and sleeping in a noisy bedroom. Identifying these factors is straightforward from interview data but does require that specific questions be asked directly. For example, it is unlikely that a patient will volunteer that they eat upon awakening in the middle of the night unless they are asked. Sleep logs are also very helpful at identifying variation in sleep–wake schedule and napping, and also, in looking for a relation between alcohol or caffeine and insomnia in the context of a specific patient.

Cognitive Factors

Many patients with chronic insomnia have irrational fears about the consequences of insomnia or have unreasonable expectations for the quantity of sleep that causes frustration and anger about their sleep. This situation leads to increased tension and arousal at bedtime that can contribute to insomnia. This aspect of the problem is assessed by asking the patient about their expectations regarding total sleep-time requirements and how poor sleep affects their life. Certain consequences are expected and reasonable such as increased irritability, difficulty concentrating, and fatigue. However, some patients will report that they have not been promoted at work, have not been a good father and/or husband, or have other unreasonable attributions regarding the effects of their insomnia. For some patients, their entire concept of self-worth has been tied to their ability to achieve adequate sleep. Clearly, the experience of getting into bed to relax and sleep is not enhanced if one feels the value of their entire life hangs in the balance, yet this is precisely the situation for certain patients. This causes a ripple effect such that the significance of everyday events is changed; the response to bedtime, as it approaches, awakening and seeing that it is 2 AM, and feeling tired during the day are all experiences that will precipitate worry and increased tension. These common events trigger a cascade of events that do not occur in normal sleepers and did not occur in these patients before the development of their insomnia.

Once a patient decides that "I have a sleep problem that is ruining my life," there are many other changes that follow. When a patient blames insomnia for every failure, there is also the possibility that they receive secondary gain from the insomnia. This further complicates treatment, because there is a high psychological price to be paid if they sleep well they will no longer have an excuse for not achieving their goals. Some patients believe that their physical integrity is being eroded because of lack of sleep. This is especially likely in older patients with medical illness who may even have been told that rest is an essential part of their treatment. They may then spend extra time in bed to get more "rest," but spend time worrying about not acquiring adequate sleep.

Circadian Rhythm Disorders

Delayed sleep-phase syndrome (DSPS) will lead to sleep-onset insomnia, and advanced sleep-phase syndrome is associated with early morning awakenings *(16)*. However, it is DSPS that is encountered most often clinically, especially among adolescents *(17)*. Sleep logs are very helpful in making this diagnosis, and actigraphy can also provide important data about the sleep–wake schedule. The sleep–wake schedule on weekends or days off from work is the key data to be obtained from the clinical interview to establish a diagnosis of DSPS. Patients with DSPS will be able to obtain a normal total sleep time despite their long sleep onset latency. This is in contrast to patients with other causes of insomnia who are usually expected to continue to have short sleep time, even when given the opportunity to sleep through the morning.

Primary Sleep Disorders

Restless Legs Syndrome

RLS can be diagnosed based on clinical symptoms *(16)*. RLS is characterized by an unpleasant sensation in the legs, generally in the calf area that leads to the need to move the legs in order to relieve the sensation. This usually occurs upon lying down in bed at night, but may also occur earlier in the day, especially when the individual is forced to hold their legs still such as during a long car ride or while sitting at a movie theatre. In severe cases, patients report that they must actually arise and walk around the bedroom in order to feel relief. However, the RLS sensations often return once they lay back down in bed.

Although RLS can be diagnosed based on clinical symptoms, polysomnography may be helpful to confirm the diagnosis by documenting a long sleep onset latency with frequent limb movements during this period. Also, polysomnography will document the overall impact of the RLS on total sleep time and sleep quality as well as rule out an additional sleep disorder. Causes of RLS include uremia, iron deficiency anemia (low ferritin), and peripheral neuropathy.

Periodic Limb Movement Disorder

PLMD is marked by repetitive stereotyped movements of the leg muscle during sleep with a rhythmic pattern, typically with movements occurring about 30 seconds apart *(16)*. The movements arise during nonrapid eye movement sleep and usually stop when the patient awakens, such that the patient is not aware of the problem. Therefore, the report of the bed partner is helpful in determining the level of suspicion for this disorder. PLMD often occurs in patients with RLS.

Sleep-Disordered Breathing

Obstructive sleep apnea, central sleep apnea, and sleep-related hypoventilation can all lead to disturbed sleep and a report of insomnia. In the case of obstructive sleep apnea, most patients will present complaining of daytime sleepiness or snoring, rather than insomnia. However, some patients with this disorder report difficulty in maintaining sleep as their primary concern. Interestingly, these patients also often have poor sleep hygiene, giving them an even more insomnia-like presentation. For example, these patients might leave the television on in their bedroom throughout the night and watch intermittently when they awaken. They feel the television is soothing and allows them to return to sleep more readily.

Daytime Sequelae

Assessment of the daytime consequences of insomnia is critical, as daytime impairment generally provides the impetus for patients to seek treatment. Insomnia would not provoke concern for many patients if they were able to sleep just a few hours at night and continue to feel and function normally during the day. To the extent that patients suffer during the day, the insomnia becomes an urgent problem. Patients with insomnia typically experience fatigue during the day, rather than physiological sleepiness *(18)*. They might use the word "sleepy" to describe their daytime state, but further evaluation will reveal that they are not falling asleep unintentionally, but rather, are feeling tired and sluggish. Other common symptoms include cognitive and mood changes. Difficulty concentrating, decreased memory, decreased energy, dysrhythmia, and social withdrawal are common. The extent to which these symptoms interfere with occupational, social, and family roles will determine the significance of the insomnia and how aggressive the treatment should be.

SLEEP LOG DATA

Obtaining 2 weeks of sleep logs before the initial consultation is recommended. This is a good practice for all patients presenting for evaluation of a sleep disorder but is the most crucial for patients with insomnia. This is because of the high night-to-night variability of sleep for these patients, in addition to the tendency to subjectively overestimate the severity of the sleep disturbance. This occurs because patients most often recall the worst nights of sleep, and have the impression that these severe nights are typical. Daily charting of bedtimes and arising times, use of alcohol and caffeine, use of hypnotic medication, fatigue ratings, and napping behavior gives a more precise picture of events than a self-report of habitual behavior given during the consultation. This is not to say that these patients are deliberately misrepresenting their sleep–wake schedules. It is difficult for anyone to reconstruct his or her schedule beyond the most recent week.

ACTIGRAPHY

Increasingly, actigraphy is being used to obtain objective data regarding sleep–wake schedule and total sleep time for patients being evaluated or treated for insomnia. Actigraphy is performed with a wrist monitor that records both the intensity and frequency of movement. These data are then downloaded and analyzed with software designed to score sleep against wakefulness, depending on the movement pattern over time. Patients must use event markers to show bedtime and arising time if sleep parameters such as sleep onset latency and sleep efficiency, are to be derived from these data. Plotting the activity counts across the day provides an estimate of the sleep–wake pattern of the patient (Fig. 1). Although the agreement between actigraphy and electroencephalography measures of sleep show more discrepancies in patients with insomnia, agreement has been shown to be sufficient to provide useful estimates of sleep parameters *(19,20)*.

Actigraphy has the advantage over sleep log data in that it provides objective data regarding the sleep and sleep–wake schedules and, therefore, is not prone to self-report bias. It has an advantage over polysomnography in that it is much less expensive and can be used to monitor sleep for 1 or 2 weeks at a time, as opposed to a single night. This is particularly relevant to evaluate insomnia, as variability in sleep is great in these patients *(21)*.

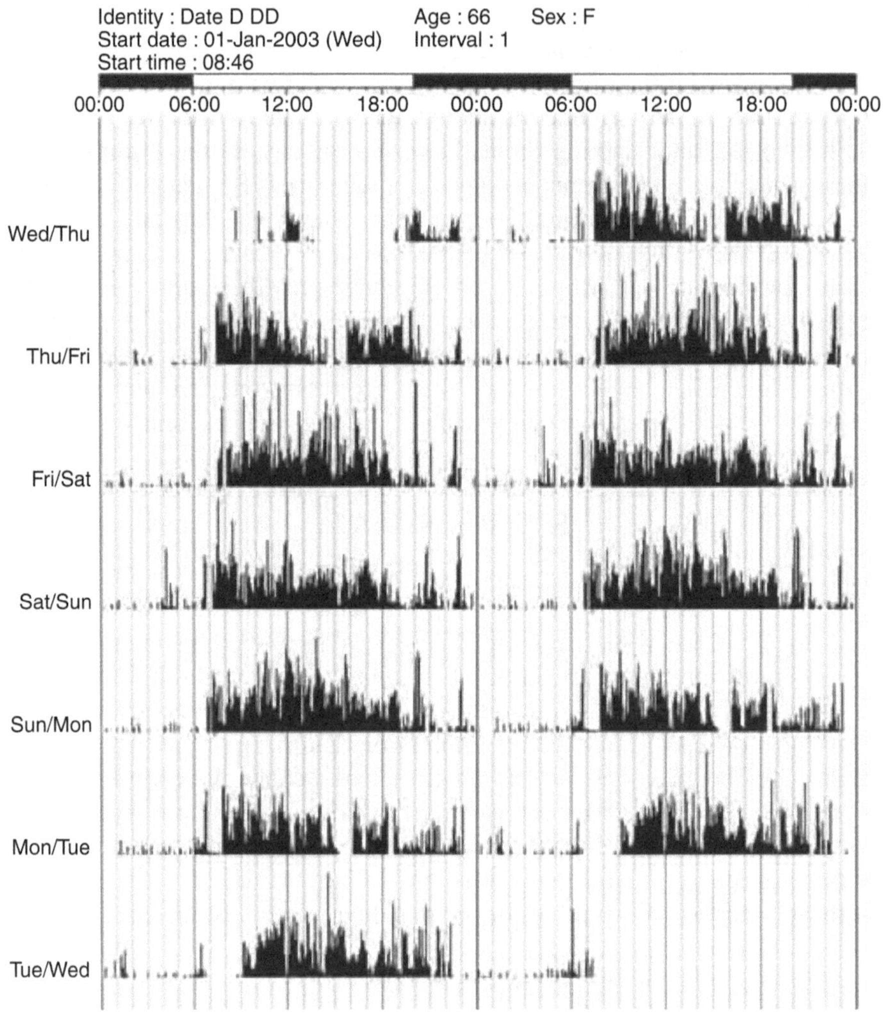

Fig. 1. A printout depicting data downloaded from actigraphy is shown. These data are from a patient complaining of severe insomnia who had not responded to treatment. The pattern of movement shows that the patient is achieving 6–8 hours of total sleep time, which is several more hours of sleep each night than what was reported on an accompanying sleep log.

POLYSOMNOGRAPHY

Although polysomnography is not used as routinely in the evaluation of a complaint of insomnia as in the evaluation of sleepiness, there are circumstances that warrant its use for these patients. First, polysomnography is the only way to definitively diagnose a primary sleep disorder such as PLMD or sleep-disordered breathing. Whereas it is true that sleep-disordered breathing will much more typically present with complaints of daytime sleepiness, some patients with sleep-disordered breathing present with disturbed nocturnal sleep as their primary concern. Second, the only way to diagnose sleep-state misperception is with use of polysomnography. In sleep-state misperception, patients report sleeping little or not at all, despite normal sleep times shown by polysomnography. The diagnosis rests on the discrepancy between subjective reports of sleep and the objective electroencephalogram-defined amount of sleep.

It is not recommended that a polysomnography be obtained for all patients being evaluated for insomnia, but only for those where the suspicion of a primary sleep disorder is increased, based on clinical history. Unfortunately, some sleep specialists routinely perform polysomnography on all patients and only refer the patient for an indepth evaluation for insomnia after a primary sleep disorder is ruled out. A better practice is to first determine the most likely causes of the insomnia and then implement a treatment plan aimed at these factors. If the insomnia is refractory to treatment then this would be an indication for polysomnography to rule out an occult primary sleep disorder or sleep-state misperception. The study results could be interpreted more precisely at this point, because some potential causes of poor sleep would no longer be present.

REFERENCES

1. Melinger G, Balter M, Uhlenhuth E (1985) Insomnia and its treatment. Arch Gen Psych 42:225–232.
2. Foley D, Monjan A, Brown S, et al. (1995) Sleep complaints among elderly persons: an epidemiologic study of three communities. Sleep 18:425–432.
3. Ancoli-Israel S, Roth T (1999) Characteristics of insomnia in the United States: results of the 1991 national sleep foundation survey. I. Sleep 22 (Suppl 2):S347–S353.
4. Katz DA, McHorney CA (1998) Clinical correlates of insomnia in patients with chronic illness. Arch Intern Med 158:1101–1107.
5. American Psychiatric Association. Diagnostic and statistical manual of mental disorders. 4th ed. American Psychiatric Association, Washington, DC, 1994.
6. Sandek K, Andersson T, Bratel T, et al. (1999) Sleep quality, carbon dioxide responsiveness and hypoxaemic patterns in nocturnal hypoxaemia due to chronic obstructive pulmonary disease (COPD) without daytime hypoxaemia. Respir Med 93:79–87.
7. Stepanski E, Faber M, Zorick F, et al (1995) Sleep disorders in patients on continuous ambulatory peritoneal dialysis. J Am Soc Nephrol 6:192–197.
8. Lichstein KL Secondary insomnia. in: *Treatment of late-life insomnia.* (Lichstein KL, Morin CM, eds.) Sage Publications Inc, Thousand Oaks, CA, 2000.
9. Coleman R, Roffwarg H, Kennedy S, et al. (1981) Sleep-wake disorders based on a polysomnographic diagnosis. JAMA 247:997–1003.
10. Beck AT Depression Inventory. Center for Cognitive Therapy, Philadelphia, PA, 1978.
11. Mellman TA, Nolan B, Hebding J (1997) A polysomnographic comparison of veterans with combat-related PTSD, depressed men, and non-ill controls. Sleep 20:46–51.
12. Geraci M, Uhde T (1992) Diurnal rhythms and symptom severity in panic disorder: a preliminary study of 24-hour changes in panic attacks, generalized anxiety, and avoidance behaviour. Br J Psychiatry 161:512–516.
13. Kales A, Scharf M, Kales J (1978) Rebound insomnia: a new clinical syndrome. Science 201: 1039–1040.
14. Merlotti L, Roehrs T, Zorick F, et al. (1991) Rebound insomnia: duration of use and individual differences. J Clin Psychopharmacol 11:368–373.
15. Spielman AJ, Saskin P, Thorpy MJ (1987) Treatment of chronic insomnia by restriction of time in bed. Sleep 10:45–56.
16. American Sleep Disorders Association. The international classification of sleep disorders, revised: diagnostic and coding manual. American Sleep Disorders Association, Rochester, MN, 1997.
17. Carskadon M, Wolfson A, Acebo C, et al. (1998) Adolescent sleep patterns, circadian timing, and sleepiness at a transition to early school days. Sleep 21:871–881.
18. Stepanski E, Zorick F, Roehrs T, et al. (1988) Daytime alertness in patients with chronic insomnia compared with asymptomatic control subjects. Sleep 11:54–60.
19. Ancoli-Israel S, Clopton P, Klauber M, et al. (1997) Use of wrist activity for monitoring sleep/wake in demented nursing-home patients. Sleep 20:24–27.
20. Vallieres A, Morin C (2003) Actigraphy in the assessment of insomnia. Sleep 26:902–906.
21. Wohlgemuth W, Edinger J, Fins A, et al. (1999) How many nights are enough? The short-term stability of sleep parameters in elderly insomniacs and normal sleepers. Psychophysiology 36:233–244.

APPENDIX

Standard Interview Format for the Evaluation of Insomnia

Definition of the problem

1. What time do you go to bed? What time is your final awakening?
2. How long does it take you to fall asleep?
3. Do you awaken during the night? If yes, how many times?
4. How much total sleep time do you get?
5. How much total sleep time do you need to feel rested?
6. How long have you had this sleep pattern?
7. What was your sleep like before you developed this problem?
8. What treatments have you tried for your sleep problem?
9. Did any of these treatments help?

Behavioral insomnia

10. Do you watch TV, read, work, or eat in bed?
11. How do you sleep away from home (e.g., on vacation)?
12. Do you fall asleep more easily on the couch than in bed?
13. Are you easily awakened by noise or light?
14. What do you do while awake at night?
15. Was there a precipitating event when your insomnia first began (e.g., hospitalization or stressful event)?
16. Do you take naps during the day?
17. Do you look at the clock during the night?

Cognitive features

18. Do you feel frustrated or tense when seeing your bed or bedroom?
19. Do you think about your sleep difficulty during the day?
20. Are you afraid of not sleeping? What do you think will happen to you?
21. How does difficulty sleeping affect your life?

Medical

22. Do you have any medical problems? (Review of systems)
23. Do you have any pain at night?
24. What medications do you take? What dosages? How often?

Alcohol/drugs

25. Do you drink alcohol? How much? How often?
26. Do you take any nonprescribed drugs? Diet pills?
27. Have you tried medication for your sleep problem?
28. How much coffee do you drink?

Restless legs/periodic leg movements

29. Have you noticed muscle twitches in your legs at night?
30. Do you ever have painful or itching sensations in your legs that prevent you from sleeping?
31. Has your bed partner ever noticed leg movements while you were sleeping?

(Continued)

Appendix ***(Continued)***

Sleep-disordered breathing

32. Do you snore?
33. Do you ever awaken gasping for breath?
34. Has your bed partner noticed any unusual breathing pattern?
35. Do you have any difficulty breathing through your nose?
36. Have you ever had surgery on your nose or throat?

Psychiatric

37. Have you ever been treated for emotional/psychological problems?
38. Have you felt depressed recently?
39. How is your appetite? Has your weight changed lately? How much?
40. Do you have any phobias? Panic attacks?
41. How is your marriage? Does your spouse understand the problems you have been having with your sleep?
42. Do you have an active sex life? Does this affect your ability to sleep?
43. Do you have a stressful job? Stressful life?

Circadian rhythms

44. Do you find it difficult to get out of bed in the morning?
45. Do you sleep later on weekends (or days off)?
46. What are your working hours?
47. Do you ever change work shifts?

Daytime sequelae/miscellaneous

48. How does poor sleep interfere with your performance the following day?
49. Is your job performance affected?
50. Do you fall asleep at unexpected times during the day?
51. What would you like to see changed about your sleep?
52. How would improved sleep affect your daytime functioning?
53. Do any family members have insomnia, excessive sleepiness, or other sleep disorder?
54. Do you and your bed partner have similar bedtimes?
55. Does your sleep ever improve under certain circumstances?

4 Cognitive–Behavioral Therapy Approaches for Insomnia

Edward J. Stepanski, PhD

CONTENTS

INTRODUCTION

There are many specific treatment approaches for insomnia that fall under the general category of cognitive–behavioral therapy (CBT). Therapies in this area have common elements: patients gain more control on sleep by modifying their sleep–wake schedules, learning relaxation skills, changing sleep-related habits, and/or learning to decrease worry about sleep. These skills can be taught in different ways. The specific CBT approach most likely to be effective in a particular patient presumably depends on the etiology of their insomnia. However, attempts to match patients to particular behavioral therapies have met with limited success. One study did show that patients with increased muscle tension benefited more from electromyograph (EMG) biofeedback, and patients without this tension did better with electroencephalograph (EEG)-based biofeedback *(1)*. However, another study that attempted to match patients to treatment modalities, based on aspects of clinical history, actually found that patients did worse when receiving the predicted "correct" treatment than those receiving the "incorrect"

From: *Current Clinical Practice: Primary Care Sleep Medicine: A Practical Guide*
Edited by: J. F. Pagel and S. R. Pandi-Perumal © Humana Press Inc., Totowa, NJ

treatment *(2)*. The recent trend has been to provide a CBT program that combines different behavioral treatments and cognitive therapy. As all patients are receiving several different treatments, this approach does not require any matching of treatment types to patient's characteristics.

CAUSES OF INSOMNIA

Traditionally, CBT approaches have been recommended only for those patients with primary insomnia *(3)*. The rationale for this rests on the fact that primary insomnia is hypothesized to result from factors that are amenable to cognitive and behavioral treatment approaches. These factors include poor sleep hygiene (SH), somatic arousal, cognitive arousal, and excessive worry regarding the ability to achieve sufficient sleep *(4)*. In contrast, treatment protocols for patients with secondary insomnia recommend targeting the primary medical or psychiatric condition for treatment, with perhaps adjunctive pharmacological treatment of the insomnia. The assumption underlying this plan is that the insomnia will remit with successful resolution of the primary condition. However, it is often the case that a patient with insomnia, apparently because of depression, anxiety, or another primary disorder, continues to report disturbed sleep after the primary condition has remitted *(5)*. These cases suggest that most, if not all, patients who have a chronic case of insomnia ultimately adopt behaviors and cognitions that contribute further to their poor sleep. Spielman and colleagues *(6)* proposed that factors contributing to insomnia be categorized as predisposing, precipitating, or perpetuating. In such a model, it is easy to see how insomnia begins with the introduction of a primary medical or psychiatric disorder (precipitating factor), but then continues because of changes in behavior (perpetuating factors). For example, when an individual is sleeping well, he/she is much less likely to do the following: eat during the night, leave the TV in the bedroom on, stay in bed late into the morning, take an afternoon nap, self-medicate with alcohol at bedtime, spend time during the day worrying about getting sufficient sleep, and so on. These are precisely the types of behaviors that people engage in when sleeping poorly, often as a misguided attempt to improve their sleep or compensate for lack of sleep. For these reasons, CBT may also be efficacious in the treatment of secondary insomnia, as shown by several recent studies *(7,8)*.

SH INSTRUCTIONS

SH rules were first proposed by Hauri *(9)* and included a wide range of recommendations to address presumed behavioral and cognitive contributions to insomnia (Table 1). There are now many versions of SH rules, and they are uniformly recommended in the treatment of insomnia *(3)*. Most lists of SH include recommendations to limit use of caffeine and alcohol, engage in exercise, and to make certain that the sleep environment is sufficiently dark and quiet to be conducive to sleep. Hauri's *(9)* original list also included recommendations to limit time in bed and go to bed only when sleepy. These recommendations overlap with sleep restriction therapy and stimulus control therapy as described later.

Despite the ubiquitous recommendation of SH instructions as a therapy for insomnia, data demonstrating the efficacy of SH as a stand-alone therapy for insomnia are sparse *(10)*. This is not to say that these recommendations are ineffective, but that

Table 1
Original SH Rules

Sleep as much as needed to feel refreshed and healthy during the following day, but not more.
Curtailing time in bed a bit seems to solidify sleep; excessively long times in bed seem related to fragmented and shallow sleep
A regular arousal time in the morning seems to strengthen circadian cycling and finally, lead to regular times of sleep onset
A steady daily amount of exercise probably deepens sleep over the long run, but occasional one-shot exercise does not directly influence sleep during the following night
Occasional loud noises (e.g., aircraft flyovers) disturb sleep even in people who do not awaken because of the noises, and individuals cannot remember them in the morning. Sound attenuating the bedroom might be advisable for people who must sleep close to excessive noise
Although an excessively warm room disturbs sleep, there is no evidence that an excessively cold room solidifies sleep, as has been claimed
Hunger may disturb sleep. A light bedtime snack (especially warm milk or similar drink) seems to help many individuals sleep
An occasional sleeping pill may be of some benefit, but the chronic use of hypnotics is ineffective, at most, and detrimental in some insomniacs
Caffeine in the evening disturbs sleep, even in persons who do not feel it does
Alcohol helps tense people to fall asleep fast, but the ensuing sleep is then fragmented
Rather than trying harder and harder to fall asleep during a poor night, switching on the light and doing something else may help the individual who feels angry, frustrated, or tense about being unable to sleep

Adapted from ref. *9*.

there have not been many studies of SH as an active stand-alone treatment. Current thinking holds that SH instructions are a necessary, but not sufficient, therapy for chronic insomnia *(11)*.

RELAXATION THERAPY

The use of relaxation therapy is based on the theory that hyperarousal causes insomnia, and that if patients learn techniques to reduce arousal, this will lead to improved sleep. The term "relaxation therapy" is a generic term that encompasses many different approaches to accomplish the same general goal. These approaches differ somewhat in terms of how much emphasis is placed on reducing cognitive arousal vs somatic arousal. For example, progressive muscle relaxation is more focused on somatic arousal, whereas guided imagery is more focused on cognitive arousal.

PROGRESSIVE MUSCLE RELAXATION

Progressive muscle relaxation has been used in the treatment of insomnia for many years. These techniques were developed by Edmund Jacobsen in the 1930s, and he applied them to the treatment of insomnia in 1938 *(12)*. In progressive muscle relaxation, the patient is taught to systematically relax each part of the body until the entire body is relaxed *(13)*. The usual procedure for this consists of first tensing up the muscles in that body part, maintaining the tension for a few moments, and then releasing the tension. Many studies of the efficacy of these techniques in the treatment of insomnia have been conducted with good results *(14,15)*.

BIOFEEDBACK

Biofeedback, using both EMG and EEG measures, has been used in the treatment of insomnia *(16)*. Biofeedback teaches relaxation by providing a signal to the patient that reflects the tension level, either based on EMG activity or EEG activity. The theory underlying this treatment approach is that the patient will better learn how to produce relaxation when given immediate feedback regarding increases or decreases in tension, resulting from his/her attempts to control this tension. Use of biofeedback to treat insomnia is not common, probably because of the duration and intensity of this treatment. Patients may require 30–90 individual biofeedback sessions to successfully master relaxation sufficiently to improve sleep.

GUIDED IMAGERY

Guided imagery is a form of meditation and consists of having the patient visualize a specific scene that is associated with a calm and relaxed state. Typically, the patient first engages in a simple relaxation procedure such as deep breathing to become relaxed. Then a specific scene is visualized to deepen the relaxation. Examples of relaxing scenes include lying on a beach, sitting in front of a fire in a cabin in winter, or soaking in a hot bath. Once the patient has practiced this relaxation exercise sufficiently, the relaxation becomes paired with the visual imagery. Then the patient can induce a relaxed state quickly by closing the eyes and focusing on the visual imagery. Theoretically, this approach may be more useful for patients who have cognitive arousal as their primary source of tension, because the imagery provides a distraction from their customary worries and fears.

STIMULUS-CONTROL THERAPY

Stimulus-control therapy (SCT) is a specific type of CBT that is based on the assumption that insomnia is caused by increased tension and arousal that occurs in response to the stimulus of the sleep environment. Spending time in bed, wide awake, strengthens the association between wakefulness and the bedroom, leading to continued insomnia. Therefore, the primary goal is to have the patient in bed only when drowsy or asleep. SCT is aimed at breaking the association between wakefulness and the sleep environment *(17)*. There are six rules for this treatment, as shown in Table 2. Many studies of treatment efficacy have been conducted with SCT *(14,15)*. Research has generally found that SCT is more effective than relaxation training for the treatment of insomnia *(14,15)*. Therefore, this treatment approach is widely used and can be applied to patients with both sleep-onset and sleep-maintenance insomnia.

SLEEP-RESTRICTION THERAPY

Sleep-restriction therapy is a behavioral treatment based on manipulating time in bed according to systematic rules *(18)* (Table 3). Bedtime is delayed and total time in bed is reduced in order to increase homeostatic sleep drive, thereby improving sleep. As sleep improves, patients are allowed to advance their bedtime to increase time in bed, as long as they can continue to fall asleep quickly and sleep most of the night. One drawback to this treatment approach is that patients have been shown to be sleepier during the day during the initial phases of treatment. Additionally, many patients are reluctant to reduce their time in bed, as they perceive that this also reduces their opportunity to obtain adequate sleep time. Adherence to the treatment may be reduced for these reasons.

Table 2
Instructions for Stimulus-Control Therapy

Lie down, intending to go to sleep only when sleepy
Do not use your bed for anything except sleep; that is, do not read, watch television, eat, or worry in bed. Sexual activity is the only exception to this rule. On such occasions, the instructions are to be followed afterward when you intend to go to sleep
If you find yourself unable to fall asleep, get up and go into another room. Stay up as long as you wish, and then return to the bedroom to sleep. Although a person not wanted to watch the clock, he/she is wanted to get out of bed if he/she does not fall asleep immediately. Remember that the goal is to associate his/her bed with falling asleep quickly. If a person is in bed more than about 10 minutes without falling asleep and have not gotten up, he/she is not following this instruction
If a person still cannot fall asleep, repeat rule 3. Do this as often as is necessary throughout the night
Set your alarm, and get up at the same time every morning, irrespective of how much sleep you got during the night. This will help your body acquire a consistent sleep rhythm
Do not nap during the day

Adapted from ref. *17*.

Table 3
Guidelines for Conducting Sleep-Restriction Therapy

Reduce time in bed to the amount of actual total sleep time, as shown by sleep logs, but not less than 4.5 hours
The arising time is fixed, and the bedtime is manipulated, based on the patient's self-reported sleep efficiency. If the sleep efficiency for the previous 5 days is ≥90%, then the patient goes to bed 15 minutes earlier
If the sleep efficiency is more than 85%, then the bedtime is pushed back later to equal the mean total sleep time of the previous 5 days. A decrease in time in bed is not made for at least 10 days from the beginning of treatment, or within 10 days of any other schedule change

Adapted from ref. *18*.

COGNITIVE THERAPY

Cognitive therapy is aimed at addressing the cognitive changes that accompany insomnia and eventually contribute to the problem. Cognitive features of insomnia include irrational fears (e.g., "I will lose my job if I don't get more sleep"), unrealistic expectations (e.g., "I need 8 hours of sleep every night"), and excessive worry regarding sleep (e.g., "I wonder if I will be able to sleep well tonight"). In fact, it could be argued that these cognitive features are the hallmark of insomnia. Many normal sleepers engage in poor SH or have irregular sleep–wake schedules, but insomniacs are singular in their preoccupation, day and night, with their sleep. Common fears about insomnia center around catastrophizing the consequences of daytime impairment associated with poor sleep. Insomniacs fear they will lose their jobs, suffer physical deterioration, or be harmed in yet other ways because of their lack of sleep. These fears place additional pressure on the individual to fall asleep quickly, and this pressure raises tension, and arousal, and further exacerbates insomnia.

Cognitive therapy challenges these beliefs and fears, and provides the individual with other approaches to view their sleep. For example, most individuals with chronic insomnia who report the fear that they will lose their jobs because of fatigue-related impairment, actually compensate and perform adequately despite poor sleep. They have worked many days after a night of little or no sleep without it being noted by coworkers or supervisors. Focussing on this fact can assist them in the avoidance of exaggerating the consequence of poor sleep and modifying their concerns about the effects of poor sleep. Cognitive restructuring is a type of cognitive therapy that modifies dysfunctional cognitive processes. This is accomplished by first systematically identifying cognitive problems. Then, the misattribution, exaggeration, unrealistic expectation, or other inappropriate cognition is challenged and replaced with a more rational interpretation of the situation.

CBT PROGRAMS

Programs that combine several of the treatments described earlier have been designed for patients with insomnia *(19–21)*. These programs are conducted over a period of weeks and may be used to treat patients with insomnia individually or in a group format. Each week, a new treatment is introduced and the treatments from earlier weeks are reviewed. An example of a format for this type of program is described in Table 4. The program described in Table 4 combines SH, SCT, sleep-restriction therapy, relaxation training, and cognitive therapy into an 8-week program. CBT programs have been shown to be as effective as pharmacologic treatment, with better maintenance of benefit at long-term follow-up *(20)*. This treatment requires increased motivation on the part of the patient and also requires more clinician time to implement.

GENERAL TENETS OF PROVIDING CBT

Providing effective CBT, although not complicated, is time-intensive. There are several requirements if these approaches are to be provided in an effective manner. First, the instructions for each treatment must be carefully explained to the patient, along with the rationale for that particular treatment approach. It may not be clear to the patient how changing his/her bedtime or arising time, for instance, could lead to an improvement in sleep. It seems counterproductive to them to use an alarm to arise at a specific time when their primary complaint is that they are not obtaining sufficient sleep time. If the patient does not understand the reason for making the requested changes in behavior, it is less likely that he/she will adhere consistently to that change.

Second, continued reinforcement of the changes is needed. It is unusual for CBT to result in immediate amelioration of insomnia. Instead, it is expected that improvement will be gradual, and changes may be erratic early in treatment. It is common for patients to see progress, only to then have a poor night of sleep for no apparent reason. They may be discouraged at this point, feel that treatment has failed, and return to their previous sleep schedule and habits. The danger of relapse is high in the first couple weeks and is followed by a need for reassurance that transient setbacks are to be expected, along with encouragement to continue with the plan. Regular contact with the clinician during this time is recommended.

For these reasons, simply providing a patient with a handout describing SH, or some other recommended behavior changes, without providing in-depth treatment and ongoing

Table 4
Schedule for a CBT Program for Insomnia

Treatment session 1
Self-monitoring
Program overview
Agenda, sessions 1–8
Overview, self-management approach
Social learning explanation of insomnia
Basic facts about sleep and changes in sleep patterns during the lifetime
Treatment session 2
Self-monitoring
Introduction to behavioral procedures (stimulus control and sleep restriction)
Treatment rationale
Introduction to relaxation procedure
Treatment rationale
Treatment session 3
Self-monitoring
Review of behavioral procedures and rationale
Review of relaxation procedure and rationale
Review of problems found in home practice
Generation of methods to enhance compliance
Review of homework and sleep window
Treatment session 4
Self-monitoring
Review of home practice and problems with behavioral procedures and relaxation procedure
Enhancing compliance
Cognitive therapy
Treatment session 5
Self-monitoring
Review of home practice and problems with behavioral procedures and relaxation procedure
Cognitive therapy
Review of progress and goal attainment
Preview of session 6, SH education
Treatment session 6
Self-monitoring
Review of home practice and problems with behavioral procedures and relaxation procedure
Cognitive therapy
SH education
Treatment session 7
Self-monitoring
Answering questions regarding SH principles
Brief review and integration of all therapy components
Feedback to subject
Review of behavioral procedures
Treatment session 8
Self-monitoring
Brief review and integration of all treatment procedures
Maintaining treatment gains
Relapse prevention
Review of progress and goal attainment

follow-up, is unlikely to be helpful. This approach has been used increasingly in the delivery of SH instructions, where standard written instructions are dispensed to patients with insomnia. The patient is expected to sort through and identify those instructions that apply to each individual's situation, ignore the rules that are less important, and adhere to the recommended changes consistently, despite episodic setbacks. This approach may be beyond the resources of the patient.

Obviously, providing CBT takes a bigger time commitment from the clinician than would be needed to provide pharmacological treatment for insomnia. It also requires a bigger commitment from the patient. The demands on the patient are more than remembering to take a pill at bedtime. In the case of relaxation training, they must practice the relaxation procedures one to two times per day for several weeks before they may be able to use them effectively at bedtime. Sleep restriction therapy requires the patient to reduce time in bed and tolerate increased daytime sleepiness whereas waiting for sleep to improve.

CONCLUSIONS

There are many specific CBT approaches that have been shown effective in the treatment of insomnia, either alone or in combination. The use of CBT in pharmacological treatment is recommended when clinically feasible, despite the need for increased clinician time and patient motivation, because of the superior long-term benefits.

REFERENCES

1. Hauri P, Percy L, Hellekson C, et al. (1982) The treatment of psychophysiologic insomnia with biofeedback: a replication study. Biofeedback Self Regul 7:223–234.
2. Espie C, Brooks D, Lindsay W (1989) An evaluation of tailored psychological treatment of insomnia. J Behav Ther Exp Psychiatry 20:143–153.
3. Buysse D, Reynolds C, Kupfer D, et al. (1997) Effects of diagnosis on treatment recommendations in chronic insomnia: a report from the APA/NIMH DSM-IV field trial. Sleep 20:542–552.
4. Stepanski E Behavioral therapy for insomnia. in: *Principles and Practice of Sleep Medicine*. 3rd ed. (Kryger M, Roth T, Dement W, eds.) WB Saunders, Philadelphia, PA, 2000 pp. 647–656.
5. Zayfert C, DeViva J (2004) Residual insomnia following cognitive behavioral treatment therapy for PTSD. J Trauma Stress 17:69–73.
6. Spielman AJ, Caruso L, Glovinsky P (1987) A behavioral perspective on insomnia. Psychiatric Clin North America 10:541–553.
7. Rybarczyk B, Lopez M, Benson R, et al. (2003) The efficacy of two behavioral treatment programs for comorbid geriatric insomnia. Psychol Aging 48:23–36.
8. Lichstein KL, Wilson NM, Johnson CT (2000) Psychological treatment of secondary insomnia. Psychol Aging 15:232–240.
9. Hauri P *Current Concepts*: *The Sleep Disorders*. The Upjohn Company, Kalamazoo, MI, 1977.
10. Stepanski E, Wyatt J (2003) The efficacy of sleep hygiene in the treatment of insomnia. Sleep Med Rev 7:215–225.
11. Chesson AL, Anderson WM, Littner M, et al. (1999) Practice parameters for the nonpharmacologic treatment of chronic insomnia. Sleep 22:1128–1133.
12. Jacobson E *You Can Sleep Well*. McGraw-Hill Book Company, New York, NY, 1938.
13. Bernstein D, Borkovec T *Progressive Relaxation Training*. Research Press, Champaign, IL, 1973.
14. Morin CM, Culvert JP, Schwartz SM (1994) Nonpharmacological interventions for insomnia: a meta-analysis of treatment efficacy. Am J Psychiatry 151:1172–1180.
15. Murtagh DR, Greenwood KM (1995) Identifying effective psychological treatments for insomnia: a meta-analysis. J Consult Clin Psychol 63:79–89.
16. Hauri P (1981) Treating psychophysiologic insomnia with biofeedback. Arch Gen Psychiatry 38:752–758.

17. Bootzin RR (1972) Stimulus control treatment for insomnia. Proceedings, 80th Annual Convention, APA vol. 395 pp. 395–396.
18. Spielman AJ, Saskin P, Thorpy MJ (1987) Treatment of chronic insomnia by restriction of time in bed. Sleep 10:45–56.
19. Edinger JD, Wohlgemuth WK, Radtke RA, et al. (2001) Cognitive behavioral therapy for treatment of chronic primary insomnia: a randomized controlled trial. JAMA 285:1856–1864.
20. Morin CM, Colecchi C, Stone J, et al. (1999) Behavioral and pharmacological therapies for late-life insomnia: a randomized controlled trial [see comments]. JAMA 281:991–999.
21. Jacobs GD, Pace-Schott EF, Stickgold R, et al. (2004) Cognitive behavior therapy and pharmacotherapy for insomnia: a randomized controlled trial and direct comparison. Arch Intern Med 164:1888–1896.

5 Pharmacological Treatment of Insomnia

James M. Parish, MD, FCCP

CONTENTS

INTRODUCTION

The complaint of trouble sleeping is very common in the practice of sleep medicine, and every physician who wants to be known as a sleep specialist should be knowledgeable about insomnia and have an organized and systematic approach to this problem. It has been estimated that 9% of adults in the United States have a complaint of insomnia, although the prevalance may be as high as 22%. Patients with insomnia view their problem in very emotional terms and for them it is very serious. And when patients see improvement, they are very grateful patients. Additionally, a complaint of insomnia increases morbidity in the elderly, for reasons ranging from falls to coronary events. Utilization of health care resources is higher in patients with severe insomnia. Insomnia should be considered a serious complaint from the patient because of the associated impairment of psychosocial function and quality of life. Insomnia can impair daytime alertness, concentration, memory, and ability to carry out daily tasks.

The patient with insomnia frequently presents a challenge in both the diagnosis and the management. Treatment of chronic or persistent insomnia almost always involves both behavioral therapy and pharmacological therapy and is based on an accurate diagnosis of the underlying cause. Insomnia should be thought of as a symptom, not a disease by itself, in the same sense that fever is a symptom of another disorder, and not a disease or diagnosis on its own. The purpose of the diagnostic evaluation of the patient with insomnia is to identify an underlying etiology that has resulted in the complaint of trouble sleeping. In choosing a drug for the treatment of insomnia, the clinician should

From: *Current Clinical Practice: Primary Care Sleep Medicine: A Practical Guide*
Edited by: J. F. Pagel and S. R. Pandi-Perumal © Humana Press Inc., Totowa, NJ

base that decision in part on an assessment of the underlying basis for the complaint of insomnia and not simply prescribe a hypnotic without a diagnosis in mind.

Primary insomnia is defined as a complaint of difficulty in initiating or maintaining sleep for at least a month, associated with daytime fatigue or impaired performance, and no evidence of another sleep, medical, psychiatric, or substance abuse problem. More often, the complaint of insomnia will be associated with a primary sleep disorder (sleep apnea, restless legs syndrome, circadian rhythm disorders, poor sleep hygiene, or sleep state misperception), a medical disorder (pain, allergies, respiratory disease), a neurological condition (Parkinsonism, dementia, degenerative disorders), or a psychiatric disorder (mood disorders, anxiety disorder, alcoholism). There is a close association between insomnia and depression. Insomnia appears before depression in approx 40% of patients, and patients with insomnia may later develop depression. Patients with primary insomnia are at increased risk of depression 3.5 years after the onset of insomnia.

Drug therapy is clearly useful in patients with transient or short-term insomnia. Short-term insomnia may be related to an adverse life event causing stress, anxiety, or excessive worry. Treating short-term insomnia may prevent long-term psychophysiological insomnia from occurring. It makes sense to use a medication with a half-life appropriate for the complaint. If the patient has initial insomnia, then a medication with a short half-life is appropriate. If the patient has middle insomnia, i.e., 4–5 hours after sleep onset, then a medication with a short half-life does not make sense and a medication with a longer half-life is appropriate. A specific treatment plan should be formulated with an expectation about the duration of treatment, education regarding good sleep habits, and potential side effects and adverse reactions *(1)*.

Very often the complaint of insomnia should be treated regardless of the underlying cause of the insomnia. Long-standing untreated insomnia is associated with sequelae such as daytime fatigue, poor performance, and depression. For example, there is evidence that even when patients are treated optimally for depression, the insomnia complaint that was part of their depression can still exist, and must be treated separately. Patients can be treated for depression with antidepressant medications and even if the depression improves, the complaint of insomnia may not resolve and may in fact get worse. Conversely, patients with both depression and insomnia often experience improvement in general well-being when the symptom of insomnia is addressed separately.

The most effective management of insomnia is a combination of behavioral and pharmacological therapy. In a randomized, controlled clinical trial comparing cognitive therapy, pharmacotherapy, cognitive therapy plus pharmacotherapy, and placebo, the authors found that the combination of cognitive plus pharmacotherapy was superior to any of the other treatment arms *(2)*. A more recent randomized, placebo-controlled study of cognitive–behavioral therapy vs pharmacotherapy found that behavioral cognitive therapy is superior to pharmacotherapy both in the short- and long-term *(3)*. However, there are no studies comparing long-term drug therapy with behavioral or cognitive therapy over a long run.

Nevertheless, certain principles can be applied for the use of drug therapy for the treatment of insomnia. Treatment should be individualized and based on a clinical assessment of causes and related conditions. Pharmacological therapy should be primary for some patients and adjunctive in others. Pharmacological therapy with benzodiazepines, for example, may provide short-term improvement, and behavioral therapy provides long-term improvement. An initial evaluation should identify all contributing medical or psychiatric conditions. Cognitive and behavioral treatment should be initiated in virtually all patients as appropriate. Periodic follow-up should be scheduled to assess efficacy, side effects, and dose escalation.

Even if there is a clear medical problem that is associated with insomnia, it is often important to treat the insomnia separately from the medical condition itself. The point is emphasized in another study of patients with rheumatoid arthritis who had insomnia related to their pain *(4)*. The authors found that was that even when the arthritis was optimally treated, these patients still had insomnia, and the insomnia had to be treated separately for optimal outcome. Therefore, the subjective complaint of insomnia often should be treated pharmacologically, even as the underlying cause of insomnia is being evaluated and treated.

There are times when a drug other than a hypnotic may be the most effective treatment for a complaint of insomnia. Adequate pain medication improves sleep that is disrupted by pain. Steroids or β-agonists may improve sleep that is disrupted by asthma. Dopaminergic agents improve sleep that is disrupted by restless legs syndrome. Proton pump inhibitors improve sleep disrupted by gastroesophageal reflux disease. Angiotensin-converting enzyme inhibitors and diuretics improve sleep disrupted by congestive heart failure. So a comprehensive approach to the diagnosis and treatment of insomnia is important.

Most studies of hypnotics report results on only a short-term basis, usually 4 weeks or less. Therefore, good studies had not been with data about the long-term use of hypnotics in chronic insomnia. In a recent important study, a new hypnotic, eszopiclone was studied for 6 months in adults, the longest study of a hypnotic reported in the literature *(5)*. Eszopiclone is the (S)-isomer of zopiclone, a racemic mixture of (R)- and (S)-isomers that has been used outside the United States. The study was a randomized, double-blinded, placebo-controlled study of 788 subjects with primary insomnia randomly assigned to receive eszopiclone or placebo for 6 months. By the first week of therapy, those in the eszopiclone group showed a significant improvement in virtually all indicators of sleep. Of most significance, there was no evidence of tolerance to the drug. The most common adverse reactions were headache (19.5%) and unpleasant taste (26.1%). There was a slightly higher number of withdrawals because of adverse reactions in the study drug group (12.8 vs 7.1%). Approximately 40% of the participants discontinued treatment in both groups. There are two important findings from this study. First, eszoplicone is effective at treating chronic insomnia. Second, and perhaps more important, long-term pharmacological treatment of chronic insomnia is rational. This study demonstrates that pharmacological approaches to therapy of chronic insomnia can be effective and reasonable.

An important question frequently faced by the sleep specialist regarding the treatment of insomnia is the use of intermittent therapy, rather than nightly therapy, of hypnotics. In many patients insomnia does not occur on a nightly basis, and the time of night at which the sleeplessness occurs may vary as well *(6,7)*. In one large survey, 36% of patients reported insomnia symptoms, and of those, 75% occurred only occasionally. Two-thirds of those with insomnia indicated that middle insomnia was the most common presentation; however, 56% reported initial insomnia and 44% reported awakening too early in the morning as problematic. In patients with chronic insomnia, sleep impairment occurred on average 5.1 nights per week *(7)*. In many patients, insomnia

Table 1
Commonly Used Sedating/Hypnotic Drugs, Onset, Dose, and Half-Life

Drug	*Duration*	*Onset of action (minutes)*	*Hypnotic dose (mg)*	*Mean half-life (hour)*
Zaleplon	Short	15–30	10–20	–
Zolpidem	Short	30	5–10	2.2
Triazolam	Short	15–30	0.125–0.25	2.9
Oxazepam	Intermediate	45–60	15–30	8
Estazolam	Intermediate	15–60	1–2	10–24
Lorazepam	Intermediate	30–60	1–2	14
Temazepam	Intermediate	45–60	15–30	11
Clonazepam	Long	30–60	0.5–1	23
Diazepam	Long	15–30	5–10	43[a]
Flurazepam	Long	30–60	15–30	74[a]
Quazepam	Long	20–45	7.5–15	39[a]

[a]Includes the active metabolites.

occurs intermittently, usually five nights per month, but as often as 16 days per month. The availability of very short-acting hypnotics has even allowed the use of middle-of-the-night drug therapy for patients who experience primarily middle insomnia.

Treatment of insomnia may be accomplished in some patients with intermittent or as-needed use, as insomnia may be intermittent. Intermittent therapy gives patients a more sense of control on their own management of their sleep problem. Flexible use of a hypnotic may prevent progression of intermittent insomnia to a more nightly chronic insomnia. Flexible use may prevent the anxiety and hyperarousal associated with chronic insomnia. Flexible use of hypnotics is not associated with an escalation of dosage. A study by Roehrs and colleagues *(8)* shows that patients do not increase the dose of hypnotics even when given the chance. A long-term, double-blinded, placebo-controlled trial of patients with primary insomnia studied the use of zolpidem three to five nights per week vs placebo three to five nights per week. The zolpidem group showed a 42% reduction in sleep latency, a 52% reduction in the number of awakenings, a 55% decrease in wake-after-sleep-onset time, and a 27% increase in total sleep time. During a 12-week follow-up period of time, the zolpidem group had improved sleep with no evidence of rebound insomnia and no increase in the dose of medication used during the 12 weeks *(9)*.

HYPNOTICS AND SEDATIVES

There are several options in choosing a medication to treat the patient with insomnia (Table 1). There are a variety of medications with capacity to cause sleep and central nervous system (CNS) depression. Alcoholic beverages have been used for centuries to produce sedation and anesthesia. Chloral hydrate and paraldehyde were introduced early in the 20th century. Barbital was introduced in 1903, and phenobarbital was introduced in 1912. The barbiturates were used for sedation, for anesthesia, and as anticonvulsants throughout the last century *(10)*. Their use decreased with the introduction of chlordiazepoxide in 1961, beginning the era of benzodiazepine receptor agonists (BZRAs). Barbiturates have a narrow therapeutic ratio, and patients are known to develop tolerance to them readily. The drugs have a high risk of physical dependence, have many drug interactions, and can result in death when taken as an overdose. Barbiturates cause progressive depression of CNS function in a dose-dependent fashion, initially producing sleep, then unconsciousness, coma, and ultimately respiratory depression and death with progressively higher doses. Notwithstanding, chloral hydrate (Noctec) is still used occasionally and can be an effective hypnotic for a few nights to treat transient insomnia *(11)*. Its drawback is that within a few weeks, its effectiveness can wane, and continued use can lead to physical dependence. Then when the drug is withdrawn, disrupted sleep and intense nightmares often result. Ethchlorvynol (Placidyl) is often associated with dependence and abuse, can be lethal in overdose, and is not often used now *(11)*.

Antidepressants have recently become one of the most frequently used medication classes to treat insomnia and can be successful. According to Walsh and Schweitzer *(12)*, in 1987 four of the five most frequently used medications in the treatment of insomnia (in order, triazolam, flurazepam, temazepam, amitriptyline, and alprazolam) were benzodiazepines *(12)*. In contrast, in 1996, the drug used most frequently was trazadone, an antidepressant with sedating properties. Zolpidem was the second most commonly used drug, followed by temazepam and then amitriptyline, another antidepressant. The authors also reviewed medical records and found that total drug mentions for the treatment of insomnia fell 24.4% during 10 years and hypnotic drug mentions decreased 53.7%, but antidepressant mentions increased by 146%. The use of trazadone for depression decreased significantly, but its use for insomnia increased signficantly *(12)*. The reasons are unclear. There have been few studies on the efficacy and long-term effects of using antidepressants for treating insomnia. A recent meta-analysis of the use of trazadone for sleep *(13)* showed that there were very few data that trazadone improves sleep in patients without a mood disorder. Trazadone does improve sleep in patients who have major depression. Additionally, there are no dose–response data on trazadone and its effect on sleep, and no data on its tolerance regarding sleep. Potential side effects of trazadone include an association with arrhythmias in patients with cardiac disease and priapism. These authors concluded that there are few data supporting the use of trazadone as a hypnotic *(13)*. Another study, however, has found trazadone effective in improving sleep in depressed patients with insomnia who are also treated with selective serotonin uptake inhibitors (SSRIs) *(14)*.

Antihistamines are commonly used as over-the-counter sleep remedies. Despite the popularity of antihistamines for this purpose, there is a paucity of adequate studies on their use, and they have potential for significant adverse reactions. Likewise, antidepressants are commonly used in the treatment of depression, but have less predictable onset and duration of action compared with benzodiazepines.

Benzodiazepine Receptor Agonists

BZRAs are the preferred drugs for the treatment of insomnia in the view of many experts in the field of sleep medicine *(15)*. Benzodiazepines, in contrast to other classes of hypnotic barbiturates, have only a limited capacity to produce coma or respiratory depression or death by themselves. As a result, they have effectively replaced barbiturates as the drugs of choice in the treatment of insomnia. There are more data on the safety of BZRAs in the therapy of insomnia than on the use of antidepressants for the same indication.

The most commonly used agents in the treatment of insomnia now are the BZRAs *(16)*. This term includes the classic benzodiazepines, but also the newer agents, zolpidem and zaleplon, which are chemically unrelated but exert their action through the benzodiapine receptor. The word *benzodiazepine* refers to the common structure of each of these agents, consisting of a benzene ring attached to a seven-membered diazepine ring. The γ-aminobutyric acid-A receptor complex in the brain contains two benzodiazepine receptor subtypes: ω-1 and ω-2. ω-1 Receptors are associated with sedation, whereas ω-2 receptors are associated primarily with anxiety reduction, anticonvulsant activity, memory loss, and motor incoordination. Most benzodiazepines stimulate both the ω-1 and ω-2 receptors; as a result, their sedative effect is often combined with an adverse effect on coordination and memory. It has been observed that patients will perceive an improvement in their sleep from use of a hypnotic without a corresponding objective response in total sleep time. It is interesting to hypothesize that change in perception of sleep duration may be part of the drug's mode of action.

Theoretically, it would be advantageous for a drug to stimulate the ω-1 receptor exclusively. Three drugs have pharmacological profile of selective binding to ω-1 receptors: quazepam, zolpidem, and zaleplon. Quazepam itself is ω-1 selective, but its two long-acting metabolites are not ω-1 selective. Zolpidem is ω-1 selective and has no significant active metabolites. Evidence does suggest that zolpidem may offer a more physiologically normal sleep, produce fewer withdrawal symptoms, and is less likely to induce tolerance. Zaleplon is another nonbenzodiazepine sedative hypnotic with ω-1 receptor selectivity.

Various modifications of these rings, especially attachments to a five-aryl ring, produce the varying pharmacological properties of different drugs in the class. Zolpidem and zaleplon are imidazopyridines. More than 3000 BZRA drugs have been synthesized, at least 120 have been tested clinically, and at least 35 BZRAs are now used in various parts of the world *(17,18)*. All BZRAs possess both sedative and hypnotic properties to some extent, although many were developed primarily for an indication of anxiety. Commonly used drugs in this category for the treatment of insomnia include flurazepam, temazepam, estazolam, quazepam, triazolam, zolpidem, and zaleplon.

The primary pharmacological effects of the BZRAs are sedation, decreased anxiety, muscle relaxation, somnolence, and amnesia. Most BZRAs cause an increase in sleep-related electroencephalography-α activity. The most characteristic effects on sleep architecture of BZRAs are a decreased initial sleep latency, decreased stage 1 sleep, decreased slow-wave sleep, an increase in total sleep time, and an increase in the percentage of stage 2 sleep. Initial rapid eye movement (REM) latency is typically increased and total REM sleep is decreased. REM sleep, however, is not suppressed to the same degree that it is with the barbiturates. Barbiturates suppress REM sleep significantly, and there is often an REM rebound when the barbiturate is discontinued. Slow-wave sleep suppression is also typical of benzodiazepines, usually in a dose-dependent manner. In contrast, zolpidem and zaleplon do not suppress slow-wave sleep.

The most important difference among the various BZRAs is the pharmacokinetics of the drug, i.e., the onset to peak action and the duration of action, which is estimated by the half-life. The different pharmacological profiles of these drugs influence the different properties of the various drugs *(10)*. The onset to action is related to absorption from the GI tract, rapid absorption being related to a quick onset of action and a slower absorption producing a longer onset of action. The half-life is related to the volume of distribution of the drug as well as its metabolism. All benzodiazepines are lipophilic, which results in a wide volume of distribution, including the brain. The drugs are highly protein bound. Many of the metabolites are also pharmacologically active. For example, diazepam is metabolized to desmethyldiazepam, which has a long half-life of 72 hours. Desmethyldiazepam is oxidized to oxazepam, which is also an active drug. If diazepam is taken in repeated doses, the effect on the patient is influenced by concentrations of the combination of diazepam, desmethyldiazepam, and oxazepam. Similarly, flurazepam has a plasma half-life of only 2–3 hours, but its major active metabolite, *N*-desalkylflurazepam has a half-life of 50 hours or more. In contrast, oxazepam, lorazepam, temazepam, triazolam, and midazolam are inactivated by their initial metabolic reaction, and hence, do not have metabolically active metabolites. In treating insomnia and avoiding significant adverse reactions, it is generally more desirable to use the drugs with the most rapid onset of action and the shortest half-life, avoiding the drugs with longer half-lives and active metabolites.

Based on onset and duration of action, BZRAs can be categorized into three categories: short-acting, intermediate-acting, and long-acting drugs. Triazolam, zolpidem, and zaleplon have the most rapid onset of action and the shortest half-lives. These drugs are favored for initial and middle insomnia because they act quickly and are metabolized and inactive by the time the sleep period is completed. Because of its very short half-life of about 1 hour, zaleplon is the only drug that is truly suitable for middle-of-the-night administration. However, in some patients, the drug may not have a long enough duration and they may experience middle- or late-night awakening; in such patients, a drug with a longer duration of action may be more desirable.

Oxazepam, estazolam, temazepam, and lorazepam are examples of drugs that are intermediate in onset and duration of action. The half-life of each varies from 8 to 14 hours. Oxazepam and lorazepam have active metabolites, whereas temazepam and estazolam have no active metabolites. Clonazepam (half-life, 23 hours), quazepam (half-life, 39 hours), diazepam (half-life, 43 hours), flurazepam (half-life, 74 hours), are the longest-acting benzodiazepines and are less desirable as effective treatments for insomnia because of residual daytime effects. However, if daytime anxiety is also present and may be a part of the complaint of insomnia, then it may be desirable to use a long-acting drug to induce nocturnal sleep and reduce daytime anxiety. In addition, certain drugs may have other effects that lead to their use. Clonazepam has been used effectively to treat REM sleep behavior disorder. If started at a low dose and gradually increased, daytime residual sedation is usually minimal.

Zaleplon and zolpidem are nonbenzodiazepines chemically, but are BZRAs in that they bind and activate the benzodiapine receptor *(19–21)*. Zaleplon is a rapid-acting hypnotic that has a shorter duration of action than zolpidem. The sedative properties of zolpidem and zaleplon are more pronounced than the drugs' anxiolytic or muscle relaxant properties. These agents do not alter sleep architecture as much as the benzodiazepines. They do not alter slow-wave sleep or REM sleep as much as the benzodiazepines, and the rebound insomnia following cessation is not as pronounced. They induce little respiratory depression. Zaleplon has not been associated with daytime psychomotor or cognitive impairment *(22)*. In contrast, both triazolam and zolpidem have been associated with mild cognitive impairment *(23)*. Several studies have demonstrated the effectiveness of middle-of-the-night use of zaleplon *(23)*. These properties make zolpidem and zaleplon very effective agents in the treatment of insomnia. However, they are more expensive than benzodiazepines such as temazepam and triazolam.

A new agent, not yet approved by the Food and Drug Administration (FDA) at this time, eszopiclone has a slightly longer half-life (about 4–6 hours) than zolpidem. When this drug is available, there will be a range of nonbenzodiazepine agents with a range of half-lives from ultrashort-acting (zaleplon) to short-acting (zolpidem) to intermediate-acting (eszopiclone).

Adverse Reactions of Benzodiazepines

Benzodiazepines may be associated with residual sedation, also referred to as hangover, characterized by daytime drowsiness, sleepiness, or impairment of daytime cognitive function. Residual sedation is a prolongation of the hypnotic effect of the drug into the daytime. It is derived from the duration of activity of the drug, which is determined by its half-life and the presence of active metabolites. Hence, the short-acting drugs are less likely to cause residual sedation than the intermediate- and long-acting drugs. Zaleplon, the shortest acting of all the hypnotics is associated with the least residual sedation.

Amnesia also occurs with benzodiazepines as an undesirable extension of the desired effect of the drug. Anterograde amnesia occurs for events that occur after the drug is administered. The degree of amnesia is related to the concentration of the drug at the time of the presented information. Therefore, amnesia is most likely to occur at the peak of drug concentration and with higher doses of the drugs. As with other side effects, amnesia is more likely to occur with longer acting drugs because they will still be present during the daytime; in contrast, amnesia of events during the day is less likely to occur with the shorter-acting drugs. Amnesia can also occur with zolpidem or zaleplon if the information is presented during the drug's duration of action.

Virtually, all benzodiazepines result in some rebound insomnia when they are stopped *(24,25)*. Rebound insomnia is the phenomenon whereby sleep time is reduced for several days when a hypnotic drug is stopped, and then returns to the baseline level of sleep. Rebound insomnia may be more significant with shorter-acting drugs and when the drug is used during longer periods of time. Rebound insomnia occurs more often when a higher dose of drug is used. Rebound insomnia occurs with abrupt cessation of 0.5 mg of triazolam after a single night of use, but does not occur with a dose of 0.25 mg *(26)*. Rebound does not seem to occur with zaleplon, even in doses up to 20 mg. However, zolpidem has been associated with rebound after a single night of use in one study *(27)*, but was not associated with rebound in another study *(28)*. A recent randomized, controlled study demonstrated that zolpidem was not superior to temazepam in avoiding rebound insomnia *(29)*. Rebound insomnia can be ameliorated by slowly tapering the dose of drug during several weeks. The longer-acting BZRAs are not associated with rebound because, given their long half-lives, there is a gradual decline in plasma concentration when the drug is stopped. Rebound insomnia differs from a withdrawal syndrome. Withdrawal is associated with not only insomnia, but other symptoms as well, and lasts longer than 2–3 days. The importance of rebound is that it prevents patients from stopping the drug when other behavioral therapy has improved their insomnia. When patients try to stop taking the drug, they experience poor sleep the next night and make the interpretation that they need the drug for sleep. The patients are then unable to stop the drug for a long period of time. If patients are warned about the possibility of rebound and educated about what to expect, then they may be able to tolerate a few nights of bad sleep. Because the longer-acting drugs are less likely to cause rebound insomnia, it may be reasonable to switch a patient from a short-acting drug to a long-acting drug if rebound insomnia is preventing the patient from being able to stop the drug.

There is frequently concern about the addiction potential of BZRAs and their long-term use. This concern has likely resulted in a long-term trend of fewer patients being treated for insomnia with BZRAs in the last decade, and more use of antidepressants as treatment for insomnia *(12)*. However, studies have not supported the concern of long-term addictive use of BZRAs. The self-administration of a hypnotic is determined primarily by the severity of the sleep disruption on the previous night *(15)*; thus, if insomnia is treated effectively, then patients are not likely to increase the dose of the drug. Patients, given the opportunity to self-administer the drug, tend not to increase the dose taken for sleep *(8)*. Most patients using BZRAs for sleep do not self-administer the drug during the day *(30)*. Therefore, in most cases, BZRAs—especially the shorter-acting drugs—should be the treatment of choice for the symptomatic treatment of insomnia. If pharmacological therapy is combined with behavioral therapy for long-term improvement in sleeping, then long-term use of hypnotics should be uncommon.

At the usual doses of BZRAs, respiration is not significantly changed in normal subjects. Higher doses of BZRAs, in contrast, depress alveolar ventilation and may cause mild hypercapnia. This is generally not clinically significant in normal patients without lung disease. However, in patients with chronic obstructive pulmonary disease (COPD), these effects may become important, and high doses of BZRAs should be avoided in patients with chronic lung disease. Lower doses typically are tolerated well in these patients. BZRAs cause severe respiratory depression requiring ventiliatory assistance only when they are combined with other CNS-depressant drugs such as barbiturates or alcohol. BZRAs may worsen obstructive sleep apnea by reducing tone in upper airway muscles or by decreasing carbon dioxide responsiveness. The effect of benzodiazepines is longer apneic events and lower oxyhemoglobin saturations. As a result, alcohol and benzodiazepines are usually considered to be relatively contraindicated in untreated OSA.

Antidepressants in the Treatment of Insomnia

Insomnia and depression share many features clinically, and the symptoms of each may be intertwined *(31)*. Long-standing insomnia is a risk factor for depression, and most studies demonstrate a high prevalence of depressive symptoms in patients with chronic insomnia. Insomnia is a major symptom of depression, occurring in approx 60–70% of patients diagnosed with depression. Conversely, depression is also diagnosed in about 35% of patients with chronic insomnia. There is evidence that insomnia may be a prodrome or a risk factor for depression. Patients with depression have been found to have abnormal sleep architecture. These changes in sleep architecture include reduced stages 3 and 4 sleep, and an increased percentage of REM sleep. Initial REM latency is shortened in patients with endogenous depression, and patients with depression have an increased number of eye movements during REM sleep, described as increased REM density. The shortened REM latency is associated with increased response to antidepressants, but not to psychotherapy.

Given the close linkage between insomnia and depression, it is common to find patients complaining of insomnia who also have symptoms of depression. It follows that antidepressants would play a role in the treatment of certain patients with insomnia.

Four different strategies are available for the treatment of patients with insomnia and mood disorders. A single antidepressant may be used. Alternatively, a combination of two different antidepressants can be used. The third option is a benzodiazepine alone. The fourth major option is a combination of a benzodiazepine and an antidepressant.

Several of the antidepressants have direct sedating properties as well as antidepressant properties. Tertiary tricyclic drugs (amitriptyline, doxepin, trimipramine) are sedating because of the anticholinergic or serotonergic action of the drug. The sedating action is generally immediate in contrast to the antidepressant action of the drug, which may take several weeks to be effective. The sedating action of the drugs also occurs at a lower dose than the antidepressant properties. For example, amitriptyline at dose of 25–50 mg may be effective as a hypnotic, whereas 150–200 mg may be required for its antidepressant effect. Additionally, trazadone, a nontricyclic, non-SSRI antidepressant is frequently used as an effective treatment for insomnia in both depressed and nondepressed patients, again because of its anticholinergic, serotonergic, and/or noradrenergic properties. A dose of 25–150 mg is often effective. Orthostatic hypotension can occur, and rare cases of priapism have been reported. Nefazodone and mirtazapine are useful for treating insomnia. The advantage of using a single drug is avoidance of drug–drug interactions. Potential adverse reactions to tricyclic antidepressants include cardiac arrhythmias, hypotension, and anticholinergic side effects (blurry vision, dry mouth, prostatism). Fortunately, nefazodone and mirtazapine do not share these side effects.

SSRIs are not characterized by direct sedating effects but are also useful for treating insomnia associated with depression. Fluoxetine 20–60 mg, sertraline 50–200 mg, or paroxetine 20–50 mg are effective in improving both the symptoms of depression and the subjective complaint of insomnia. A combination of two antidepressants has been used for treating patients with insomnia and mood disorders. A sedating antidepressant such as a tricylic or nontricyclic drug can be combined with an SSRI or bupropion to achieve maximal improvement in both sleep and depression. Although generally well tolerated, there is a potential for significant sedation, autonomic instability, or the "serotonin syndrome."

The combination of antidepressant therapy and a benzodiazepine has been used when the insomnia complaint is a prominent part of the presentation of depression. The benzodiazepine helps to improve subjective sleep and does not interfere with the antidepressant response. Again shorter acting BZRAs are preferred such as zolpidem, zaleplon, or temazepam. It is uncommon to use a benzodiazepine alone in a patient who has significant depressive symptoms accompanying insomnia. The only exception would be if the patient is being treated actively by a psychiatrist with psychotherapy or electroconvulsive therapy. In this case, a shorter acting drug would be preferable.

SPECIAL CONSIDERATIONS IN THE ELDERLY

Sleep disturbances are common in the elderly, and the use of sedatives is common in this age group *(32)*. Pharmacokinetics are often different in the elderly. There is often reduced hepatic clearance, a longer half-life, and a higher accumulation of the drug. The elderly are more prone to daytime cognitive impairment following the use of BZRAs. The dose of the drugs should be reduced in the elderly, and careful monitoring is warranted. For example flurazepam, with its long half-life and active metabolites with long elimination half-lives, should be used very rarely if at all in the elderly. Daytime cognitive impairment can be significant. Shorter acting BZRAs have a lower profile of daytime impairment in the elderly *(33)*. A multicenter, randomized, placebo-controlled outpatient study examining the effects of zaleplon in 549 patients aged ≥65 years compared zaleplon 5 and 10 mg with zolpidem 5 mg. Zaleplon improved sleep quality in the elderly, had a low incidence of daytime residual effect, and showed little evidence of rebound insomnia *(34)*. Zolpidem did show evidence of rebound insomnia in this study.

Zolpidem, triazolam, and temazepam were compared for efficacy and adverse reactions in 335 elderly hypnotics during a 28-day treatment period. All three drugs improved sleep duration in this study. Zolpidem and temazepam, but not triazolam, improved sleep latency *(35)*. Temazepam was associated with a higher incidence of drowsiness and fatigue compared with placebo and zolpidem. Triazolam was associated with increased nervousness compared with the other two drugs. BZRAs have been associated with tolerance, dependence, and rebound insomnia when therapy is discontinued; data are limited in supporting or refuting these concerns, especially in the elderly. In general, BZRAs with shorter elimination half-lives are more likely to result in rebound insomnia, whereas the prolonged half-life of a drug such as flurazepam provides a pharmacological taper. The available studies indicate that concerns with dependence and rebound are less with zolpidem and zaleplon than with other benzodiazepines *(36)*. This makes the use of these agents even more attractive in treating the insomnia complaint in the elderly population.

Also, there is a high incidence of sleep-disordered breathing, nocturnal myoclonus, depression, and other psychiatric conditions in the elderly, and these underlying causes of insomnia should be sought in the evaluation of insomnia in the elderly. Use of over-the-counter sleep aids such as the antihistamine group can have significant daytime side effects, especially in the elderly. Diphenhydramine is a long-acting agent that can cause daytime sleepiness, cognitive impairment, and anticholinergic side effects. Trazadone has been used as a hypnotic, but its effectiveness and long-term side effects have not been studied in the elderly. Rebound insomnia can occur.

The effectiveness of these drugs as treatments for insomnia can persist for weeks or months, but in all likelihood the drugs can produce some degree of physical dependence, especially with higher doses and more chronic use. Drugs with a short duration of action may cause daytime anxiety and rebound insomnia. Those with a longer duration of action may cause daytime sedation and some degree of motor impairment. Use of benzodiazepines in elderly patients has been associated with an increased incidence of falls and hip fractures and memory impairment *(37)*.

SPECIAL CONSIDERATIONS IN PATIENTS WITH COPD

Concern also exists about the use of hypnotics in patients with COPD. Patients with COPD often complain of poor, disrupted sleep. However, longer-acting benzodiazepines have been associated with increasing hypoxemia during sleep in patients with COPD, and many clinicians have been reluctant to prescribe benzodiazepines to patients with COPD out of fear of worsening the sleep-related hypoxemia. In patients with COPD, flurazepam has been shown to increase the frequency of sleep-disordered breathing events, the frequency and duration of episodes of oxygen desaturation, and the severity of desaturation *(38)*. In contrast, the shorter acting agents, especially zolpidem and zalephlon, have shown no significant adverse effects on breathing and oxygen saturation in patients with mild-to-moderate COPD *(39,40)*. Both of these studies were done in patients with mild-to-moderate COPD, as opposed to severe COPD. Therefore, until further studies are done, long-acting BZRAs should be avoided in patients with COPD, but the shorter-acting drugs, especially zolpidem and zaleplon, appear to be reasonably safe in patients with mild-to-moderate COPD.

ALTERNATIVE TREATMENTS FOR INSOMNIA

Antihistamines provide an over-the-counter alternative to treating insomnia pharmacologically. Diphenhydramine (Nytol, Benadryl, and others) and doxylamine (Unisom and others) are approved by the Food and Drug Administration as "sleep aids." They can cause daytime sedation, impairment of driving skills, dry mouth, and urinary retention. A recent study of rural, elderly, blue-collar individuals showed that over-the-counter diphenhydramine was used by about 8.7% of the population, and resulted in cognitive impairment as measured by the mini-mental status examination *(41)*.

Alcohol typically induces sleep initially but results in fragmented sleep later. Melatonin has received widespread publicity in improving sleep, but controlled trials are lacking and there are questions about the purity of the products on the market. One study showed that in elderly patients with insomnia, both a low dose (0.3 mg) and a higher dose (3 mg) were effective at improving sleep efficiency *(42)*. However, in another recent randomized, double-blinded, crossover study of melatonin at 0.3 mg and 1 mg doses or placebo, no significant improvement in any subjective or objective sleep parameter could be demonstrated *(43)*. Valerian root is an herbal product that may improve sleep. One recent randomized, controlled study showed no signficant subjective improvement in sleep using valerian root *(44)*. However, there were no significant adverse reactions.

LONG-TERM HYPNOTIC PRESCRIPTION

The duration of most studies of hypnotic drugs is rarely longer than 4–5 weeks. Few studies have looked at the issue of use of hypnotics over the long-term. It is not uncommon to see patients who have used a stable dose of a benzodiazepine for many years, and sleep well with it, and have no side effects from it, yet are unable to sleep well without it. No hypnotic is approved for use for more than a few weeks of continuous use. Many patients with persistent insomnia have a chronic, relapsing course. The few studies done show that hypnotics generally maintain efficacy for up to 12 months without significant adverse reactions *(45)*. The continuous long-term use of hypnotics is considered "off-label." However, the long-term use of hypnotics can be reasonably justified if several criteria are met:

1. The insomnia is persistent;
2. Nonpharmacological therapy including behavioral therapy has been prescribed as well;
3. A thorough evaluation for psychiatric disease and medical conditions associated with insomnia has also been performed; and
4. The patient is reevaluated periodically (at least twice a year) to monitor for efficacy, adverse reactions, development of interim medical or psychiatric conditions, and necessity for continued use. It is also advised that the clinician inform the patient that such use of hypnotics is off-label and that continued emphasis be placed on nonpharmacological therapy. The clinician should pay special attention to any escalation of dosage, daytime use, possible adverse reactions, and the development of new medical or psychiatric conditions that should prompt reassessment of the need for long-term hypnotic use.

REFERENCES

1. Sateia MJ, Pigeon WR (2004) Identification and management of insomnia. Med Clin North Am 88:567–596, vii.
2. Morin CM, Colecchi C, Stone J, et al. (1999) Behavioral and pharmacological therapies for late-life insomnia: a randomized controlled trial. JAMA 281:991–999.
3. Jacobs GD, Pace-Schott EF, Stickgold R, et al. (2004) Cognitive behavior therapy and pharmacotherapy for insomnia: a randomized controlled trial and direct comparison. Arch Intern Med 164:1888–1896.
4. Walsh JK, Muehlbach MJ, Lauter SA, et al. (1996) Effects of triazolam on sleep, daytime sleepiness, and morning stiffness in patients with rheumatoid arthritis. J Rheumatol 23:245–252.
5. Krystal AD, Walsh JK, Laska E, et al. (2003) Sustained efficacy of eszopiclone over 6 months of nightly treatment: results of a randomized, double-blind, placebo-controlled study in adults with chronic insomnia. Eur Neuropsychopharmacol 14:793–799.
6. Ancoli-Israel S, Roth T (1999) Characteristics of insomnia in the United States: results of the 1991 National Sleep Foundation Survey. I. Sleep 22:S347–S353.
7. Shochat T, Umphress J, Israel AG, et al. (1999) Insomnia in primary care patients. Sleep 22:S359–S365.
8. Roehrs T, Pedrosi B, Rosenthal L, et al. (1996) Hypnotic self administration and dose escalation. Psychopharmacology 127:150–154.
9. Perlis ML, McCall WV, Krystal AD, et al. (2004) Long-term, non-nightly administration of zolpidem in the treatment of patients with primary insomnia. J Clin Psychiatry 65:1128–1137.
10. Hobbs W, Rall T, Verdoon T. In: *Goodman and Gilman's*: *The Pharmacological Basis of Therapeutics*. 9th ed. (Gilman AG, ed.) McGraw-Hill, New York, NY, 1996, pp. 361–396.
11. Hypnotic drugs. (2000) Med Lett 42:71–72.
12. Walsh JK, Schweitzer PK (1999) Ten-year trends in the pharmacological treatment of insomnia. Sleep 22:371–375.
13. James SP, Mendelson WB (2004) The use of trazodone as a hypnotic: a critical review. J Clin Psychiatry 65:752–755.
14. Kaynak H, Kaynak D, Gozukirmizi E, et al. (2004) The effects of trazodone on sleep in patients treated with stimulant antidepressants. Sleep Med 5:15–20.
15. Roehrs T, Roth T (2003) Hypnotics: an update. Curr Neurol Neurosci Rep 3:181–184.
16. Nicholson A Clinical pharmacology and therapeutics. In: *Principles and Practice of Sleep Medicine*. 2nd ed. (Kryger M, Roth T, Dement W, eds.) WB Saunders, Philadelphia, PA, 1994, pp. 355–363.
17. Consensus conference: drugs and insomnia; the use of medication to promote sleep. (1984) JAMA 251:2410–2414.
18. Greenblatt D (1991) Benzodiazepine hypnotics: sorting the pharmacokinetic facts. J Clin Psychiatry 52(Suppl):4–10.
19. Salva P, Costa J (1995) Clinical pharmacokinetics and pharmacodynamics of zolpidem: clinical implications. Clin Pharmacokinet 29:142–153.
20. Lobo B, Greene W (1997) Zolpidem: distinct from triazolam? Clin Pharmacokinet 29:142–153.
21. Jovanovic U, Dreyfus J (1983) Polygraphic recording in insomniac patients under zopiclone or nitrazepam. Pharmacology 27(Suppl 2):136–145.
22. Walsh JK (2002) Zolpidem "as needed" for the treatment of primary insomnia: a double-blind, placebo-controlled study. Sleep Med Rev 6:S7–S10.
23. Doghramji K (2000) The need for flexibility in dosing of hypnotic agents. Sleep 23:S16–S20.
24. Gillin JC, Spinweber CL, Johnson LC (1989) Rebound insomnia: a critical review. J Clin Psychopharmacol 9:161–172.
25. Roehrs T, Merlotti L, Zorick F, et al. (1992) Rebound insomnia in normals and patients with insomnia after abrupt and tapered discontinuation. Psychopharmacology 108:67–71.
26. Merlotti L, Roehrs T, Zorick F, et al. (1991) Rebound insomnia: duration of use and individual differences. J Clin Psychopharmacol 11:368–373.
27. Elie R, Ruther E, Farr I, et al. (1999) Sleep latency is shortened during 4 weeks of treatment with zaleplon, a novel nonbenzodiazepine hypnotic: Zaleplon Clinical Study Group. J Clin Psychiatry 60:536–544.
28. Schlich D, L'Heritier C, Coquelin JP, et al. (1991) Long-term treatment of insomnia with zolpidem: a multicentre general practitioner study of 107 patients. J Int Med Res 19:271–279.
29. Voshaar RC, van Balkom AJ, Zitman FG (2004) Zolpidem is not superior to temazepam with respect to rebound insomnia: a controlled study. Eur Neuropsychopharmacol 14:301–306.
30. Roehrs T, Bonahoom A, Pedrosi B, et al. (2002) Nighttime versus daytime hypnotic self-administration. Psychopharmacology 161:137–142.

31. Nowell PD, Buysse DJ (2001) Treatment of insomnia in patients with mood disorders. Depress Anxiety 14:7–18.
32. Phillips B, Ancoli-Israel S (2001) Sleep disorders in the elderly. Sleep Med 2:99–114.
33. Grad RM (1995) Benzodiazepines for insomnia in community-dwelling elderly: a review of benefit and risk. J Fam Pract 41:473–481.
34. Ancoli-Israel S, Walsh J, Mangano R, et al. (1999) Zaleplon, a novel nonbenzodiazepine hypnotic, effectively treats insomnia in elderly patients without causing rebound effects. Prim Care Companion J Clin Psychiatry 1(4):114–120.
35. Leppik I, Roth-Schechter G, Gray G (1997) Double-blind, placebo-controlled comparison of zolpidem, triazolan, and temazepam in elderly patients with insomnia. Drug Dev Res 40:230–238.
36. Kummer J, Guendel L, Linden J, et al. (1993) Long-term polysomnographic study of the efficacy and safety of zolpidem in elderly psychiatric in-patients with insomnia. J Int Med Res 21:171–184.
37. Ray WA, Griffin MR, Downey W (1989) Benzodiazepines of long and short elimination half-life and the risk of hip fracture. JAMA 262:3303–3307.
38. Block AJ, Dolly FR, Slayton PC (1984) Does flurazepam ingestion affect breathing and oxygenation during sleep in patients with chronic obstructive lung disease? Am Rev Respir Dis 129:230–233.
39. George CF (2000) Perspectives on the management of insomnia in patients with chronic respiratory disorders. Sleep 23:S31–S35.
40. Steens R (1993) Effects of zolpidem and triazolam on sleep and respiration in mild to moderate chronic obstructive pulmonary disease. Sleep 16:318–326.
41. Basu R, Dodge H, Stoehr GP, et al. (2003) Sedative-hypnotic use of diphenhydramine in a rural, older adult, community-based cohort: effects on cognition. Am J Geriatr Psychiatry 11:205–213.
42. Zhdanova IV, Wurtman RJ, Regan MM, et al. (2001) Melatonin treatment for age-related insomnia. J Clin Endocrinol Metab 86:4727–4730.
43. Almeida Montes LG, Ontiveros Uribe MP, Cortes Sotres J, et al. (2003) Treatment of primary insomnia with melatonin: a double-blind, placebo-controlled, crossover study. J Psychiatry Neurosci 28:191–196.
44. Coxeter PD, Schluter PJ, Eastwood HL, et al. (2003) Valerian does not appear to reduce symptoms for patients with chronic insomnia in general practice using a series of randomised n-of-1 trials. Complement Ther Med 11:215–222.
45. Maarek L, Cramer P, Attali P, et al. (1992) The safety and efficacy of zolpidem in insomniac patients: a long-term open study in general practice. J Int Med Res 20:162–170.

6 Determinants and Measurements of Daytime Sleepiness

Neil S. Freedman, MD, FCCP

CONTENTS

EPIDEMIOLOGY

Daytime sleepiness is the primary complaint of patients who present to sleep clinics. Although the actual prevalence of clinically relevant sleepiness in America is unknown, it has been estimated that significant sleep loss exists in up to one-third or more of normal adults *(1,2)*. Sleepiness has an important impact on general health and functional status, influencing how individuals perceive their energy and fatigue levels *(3)*. Sleep deprivation and sleepiness in general have been associated with poor job performance, anxiety, difficulties in personal relations, and an increased risk for fatal and nonfatal automobile accidents. daytime sleepiness resulting from chronic partial or total sleep deprivation has been demonstrated to result in neurocognitive deficits and alterations in mood, and more recently to cause alterations in physiological and endocrine functions *(4–26)*. Sleep deprivation has also been directly or indirectly linked to several recent catastrophes including the Exxon Valdez oil spill, space shuttle Challenger explosion, and the Three Mile Island near-meltdown.

The 2000 Sleep Foundation Gallup survey *(27)* of 1154 American adults demonstrated that sleep problems and specifically daytime sleepiness are quite common in this country. The study found that

1. 62% of Americans report trouble falling asleep or staying asleep;
2. 33% get more than 6.5 hours sleep per night;
3. 20% report that daytime sleepiness interferes with their daily activities;
4. 8% frequently fall asleep at work; and
5. 19% frequently make errors at work because of sleepiness.

From: *Current Clinical Practice: Primary Care Sleep Medicine: A Practical Guide*
Edited by: J. F. Pagel and S. R. Pandi-Perumal © Humana Press Inc., Totowa, NJ

Interestingly, although the study demonstrated that sleep problems are prevalent, 61% of the respondents had not been asked by a doctor (in their entire lifetime) about how well they slept. These findings validate and confirm results from different studies performed in other industrialized countries *(28,29)*.

Who's at Risk?

Although all individuals suffer from partial sleep loss from time-to-time, there are several groups in which daytime sleepiness is more likely to occur on an ongoing basis. The four groups that appear to be at the highest risk include:

1. Young adults (<25 years old);
2. Older adults (>65 years old);
3. Shift workers; and
4. Individuals with sleep disorders that result in poor sleep quantity or quality. Up to one-third of young adults may be excessively sleepy as evidenced by pathologically reduced sleep latencies on the multiple sleep latency test (MSLT) *(30)*.

This is thought to be secondary to chronic partial sleep deprivation as a result of insufficient sleep time. In a random sample of community-dwelling elderly, 24% suffered from sleep apnea and 45% had periodic limb movements *(31,32)*. Also, older individuals are more likely to suffer from sleep-disruptive medical problems or take medications that may result in daytime sleepiness. Obstructive sleep apnea with hypersomnia is as common as asthma, affecting 2 and 4% of middle-aged women and men, respectively *(33)*. Finally, approx 3.5% of America's workforce work the night shift *(1)*. Night-shift workers experience daytime sleepiness as a result of reduced sleep times as well as circadian influences on the sleep–wake cycle. Permanent night-shift workers average 5.8–6.4 hours of sleep per day, whereas rotating shift workers sleep even less (mean, 5.5 hours per day) when working in the night shift *(34)*.

This chapter will first review the subjective and objective methods used to define and determine daytime sleepiness. The second part of the chapter will review the factors that determine sleepiness as well as those factors that affect an individual's ability to initiate or maintain sleep.

QUANTIFYING SLEEPINESS: MEASURES OF DAYTIME SLEEPINESS

In general, individual subjective reports of sleepiness are imprecise compared with observer reports or tests of sleepiness *(35)*. Several objective and formal subjective measures of sleepiness have been devised to quantify the degree of an individual's sleepiness. This section will review the four most commonly used or referenced instruments for measuring sleepiness. These include the following:

1. The MSLT;
2. The maintenance of wakefulness test (MWT);
3. The Stanford sleepiness scale (SSS); and
4. The Epworth sleepiness scale (ESS).

Pupillometry and the Oxford sleep resistance (OSLER) test will also be briefly reviewed, as these latter two tests may offer more simplified objective measures for assessing daytime sleepiness in the future than the current and more commonly used MSLT and MWT.

Multiple Sleep Latency Test

The MSLT is the most commonly used and experimentally validated objective test of daytime sleepiness *(36–39)*. It is currently the standard for objectively quantifying sleepiness. It has been demonstrated to be a sensitive test of daytime sleepiness in different types of sleep deprivation (partial, complete, acute, and chronic), sleep fragmentation, time of day, and medication protocols *(40–44)*. The test is also used to document the presence of sleep-onset rapid eye movement periods (SOREMPs), which are critical to establishing a diagnosis of narcolepsy *(45)*.

The American Academy of Sleep Medicine (AASM) has recently proposed updated practice parameters for the clinical use of the MSLT *(36)*. The MSLT is indicated as part of the evaluation of patients with suspected narcolepsy and may be useful in the evaluation of patients with suspected idiopathic hypersomnia. It is not routinely indicated for the initial evaluation of patients with obstructive sleep apnea, periodic limb movements, insomnia, circadian-related sleep disorders, or sleepiness resulting from other medical disorders.

The MSLT should be performed on the day following a night time polysomnography to provide objective documentation of the preceding night's sleep *(36,37)*. The overnight polysomnography should be performed during the individual's usual normal sleep period. Four to five 20-minute naps are monitored throughout the day at 2-hour intervals in a sleep-inducing environment. The first nap typically begins 1.5–3 hours after the end of the nocturnal sleep bout. The sleep latency of each nap is calculated as the time elapsed between lights-out and the first 30-second epoch scored as sleep. Rapid eye movement (REM) latency is defined as the time from the beginning of the first epoch scored as sleep to the first epoch of REM sleep *(36,37)*. The five-nap test is currently recommended when the diagnosis of narcolepsy is clinically suspected. The shorter four-nap test is not reliable for the diagnosis of narcolepsy unless at least two SOREMPs have occurred. Also, the diagnosis of narcolepsy may be questioned if the total sleep time on the previous night's polysomnography is less than 6 hours *(36)*.

The individual sleep latencies across all naps are averaged and a mean sleep latency value is calculated. The premise underlying the test is straightforward. Simply, the sleepier the subject is, the faster he will fall asleep. Normal individuals usually demonstrate a mean sleep latency of more than 10 minutes. Pooled data from normal subjects demonstrate that the mean sleep latency is 10.4 ± 4.3 minutes and 11.6 ± 5.2 minutes using the four- and five-nap protocols, respectively *(36)*. Pathological daytime sleepiness has been defined as a mean sleep latency of less than 5 minutes *(46)*. This level of sleepiness has been associated with impaired neurocognitive performance in sleep-deprived normal control subjects. Also, most patients with narcolepsy will fall into this range (mean sleep latency, 3.1 ± 2.9 minutes) *(36)*. Before the latest review of the MSLT, there had been mention of a gray zone for individuals with mean sleep latency values that ranged between 5 and 10 minutes. Given the wide range of mean sleep latency values for normal individuals, the gray zone concept appears to be less valid. From a clinical standpoint, the patient's subjective symptoms and occupation must be taken into account when making a determination of whether the objective findings are clinically significant. Because there is such a wide range of mean sleep latency values in normal subjects, the MSLT should not be used as the sole criterion for determining the presence or severity of excessive daytime sleepiness.

Strict adherence to study protocol must be followed to insure valid and reliable results *(39,47)*. A subject's baseline sleep/wake schedule should be taken into account as sleep latency and the propensity to go into REM sleep will vary depending on the phase of the subject's circadian clock *(43,48,49)*. Medications such as stimulants, depressants, and antidepressants should be strictly avoided as these compounds may influence the ability to fall asleep. Also, the antidepressants as a group are known to suppress REM sleep, which may be important when assessing an individual for the diagnosis of narcolepsy. Depending on a particular patient's motivation (i.e., disability from or ability to continue in a specific occupation), spot drug screening may be required to ensure valid results.

The major disadvantages of the MSLT are that it is time consuming (6.5–8.5 hours), labor intensive, and expensive to perform an adequate test. The test-retest reliability of the standard four- to five-nap session MSLT during a 4- to 14-month time interval is excellent with a correlation coefficient of 0.97 *(38)*. Unfortunately, reducing the MSLT protocol to three or even two naps is not an acceptable alternative. When the MSLT is reduced to three- or two-nap sessions, the correlation coefficient for the mean sleep latency is drastically reduced to 0.85 or 0.65, respectively *(38)*.

A study by Golish et al. *(50)* identified several selected patient groups in which a three-nap MSLT protocol may be used to accurately predict the mean sleep latency as well as SOREMPs. They retrospectively reviewed 588 consecutive MSLTs performed on 522 patients during a 3-year period. Their results demonstrated that the mean sleep latency can be predicted to be normal with 100% accuracy if (1) each of the first three naps has a normal sleep latency, or (2) the patient does not fall asleep in any two of the first three naps. The mean sleep latency can be predicted to be low (<5 minutes) or abnormal (<10 minutes) with 100% accuracy if each of the first three naps has a low or abnormal sleep latency, respectively, along with SOREMPs in any two of these naps. Based on these findings, 23% of the MSLTs could be reduced to three-nap sessions without negatively affecting the validity of the results. Although the four-nap MSLT continues to be the standard, these results may be the most applicable in clinical practice when the MSLT protocol is truncated because of patient and/or technical reasons.

Maintenance of Wakefulness Test

As opposed to the MSLT, which measures sleep tendency, the MWT objectively measures a subject's ability to stay awake. The tendency to fall asleep and the ability to stay awake represent two distinct physiological processes *(51)*. This is evidenced by the fact that the two tests may demonstrate conflicting results when given to the same subject on the same day *(51)*. This difference in results may in part be secondary to the directions given before each test and the posture maintained during each test *(52,53)*. In the MSLT, subjects are instructed to try to fall asleep. Before the MWT, subjects are instructed to try to stay awake. (*See* "Physiological Arousal" for more on the effect of the arousal system on sleep.)

As it has for the MSLT, the AASM has recently proposed new practice parameters for the clinical use of the MWT *(36)*. The MWT is a validated objective measure of the ability of a subject to remain awake for a defined period of time. Unlike the standardized MSLT, the MWT has several different protocols and rules for determining sleep latency *(54)*. The recent AASM practice parameters recommend the use of the four-trial MWT 40-minute protocol in a clinical setting. Four 40-minute sessions are spaced 2 hours apart and should be initiated 1.5–3 hours after the individual's usual wake time. The sleep latency of each trial is determined when the first epoch of any stage of sleep occurs. The trial is terminated after 40 minutes if no sleep occurs or after unequivocal sleep onset (three continuous epochs of stage 1 sleep or one epoch of any other stage of sleep) has occurred. The subject is immediately awakened after sleep onset has been determined to avoid longer sleep periods that could potentially reduce the homeostatic drive for sleep in subsequent trials. Unlike the MSLT, earlier polysmonography is not required as there are no published guidelines to support or refute its use for MWT interpretation.

Limited normative data exist for the mean sleep latency values of the MWT, in large part because of its lack of standardization. Using the four-trial 40-minute protocol, the mean sleep latency control values for the MWT have been suggested to be 30.4 ± 11.2 minutes *(36)*. Using this pooled data, 97.5% of normal subjects should have a mean sleep latency of ≥8 minutes. Staying awake for 40 minutes on all four trials provides the strongest objective data available supporting an individual's ability to stay awake.

Data regarding the utility of the MSLT or MWT to determine an individual's ability to perform safely are limited. Although it has been suggested that the MWT may be a more clinically relevant test to use when assessing the sleepy individual's fitness to drive or work, the predictive value of the mean sleep latency on either test for assessing accident risk in real-world situations is not established. With this in mind, an MWT sleep latency of less than 15 minutes is considered dangerous for driving an automobile in patients with sleep apnea *(55)*. The Federal Aviation Administration uses the MWT to determine whether noncommercial pilots can be licensed after they have been diagnosed with sleep apnea *(56)*. It is recommended that the sleep clinician not solely rely on the mean sleep latency as an indicator of risk for transportation-, work-, or home-related accidents *(36)*.

OSLER Test

The OSLER test is a relatively recently described simplified version of the MWT *(57)*. Subjects are asked to lie in a semirecumbent position in a quiet and darkened room without windows for a maximum testing time of 40 minutes per session. A total of four sessions are conducted at 2-hour intervals. Instead of determining the onset of sleep by electroencephalography criteria, the presence of sleep is assessed behaviorally. Subjects sit in front of a screen that flashes a light regularly at 3-seconds intervals. The subjects are instructed to touch a button every time they see the light flash. The test is terminated after seven consecutive flashes (21 seconds) without a response. The 21-seconds threshold was chosen because it corresponds to the minimal sleep duration generally used to score one epoch of sleep when using standard sleep scoring rules *(58)*. Priest et al. *(59)* demonstrated that the OSLER test had a sensitivity and specificity of 85 and 94%, respectively, for detecting sleep of ≥3 seconds in duration. A mean sleep latency is calculated in a fashion similar to that of the MWT.

Compared with the other objective tests (MSLT and MWT) that are currently used to quantify sleepiness, the OSLER test offers the advantages of simplicity, lower cost, automatic reading, and lower technical requirements for personnel *(59)*. The OSLER test is currently not widely used and requires further testing in larger samples of subjects and different disease populations to confirm its validity and reliability. Although the test has been used to measure sleep tendency in normal control subjects as well as in sleep-deprived individuals and patients with sleep apnea, the studies' sample sizes were small *(59)*.

Stanford Sleepiness Scale

Among the subjective measures of sleepiness, the SSS is the best validated *(60)*. The respondents choose one of seven statements that best describe their current state of sleepiness. The list of statements include:

1. Feeling active and vital, alert, wide awake;
2. Functioning at a high level but not at peak, able to concentrate;
3. Relaxed, awake, not at full alertness, responsive;
4. A little foggy, not at peak, let down;
5. Fogginess, beginning to lose interest in remaining awake, slowed down;
6. Sleepiness, prefer to be lying down, fighting sleep, woozy; or
7. Almost in reverie, sleep onset soon, lost struggle to remain awake.

The advantages of the SSS are that it can be administered multiple times throughout the day and night, it correlates with standard measures of performance, and it reflects the effect of sleep loss. Its major disadvantage is its inability to differentiate sleep-deprived normal subjects from those individuals with sleep disorders. There also appears to be some discordance between choices 1 and 2 and gross behavioral indicators of sleep such as closed eyes *(61)*.

Epworth Sleepiness Scale

The ESS was first published in 1991 and was designed to measure subjective sleep propensity as it occurs in ordinary life situations *(62)*. It is currently the most used subjective test of daytime sleepiness in clinical practice. The questionnaire describes eight situations as follows:

1. Sitting and reading;
2. Watching television;
3. Sitting inactive in a public place;
4. As a passenger in a car riding for an hour without a break;
5. Lying down to rest in the afternoon when circumstances permit;
6. Sitting and talking with someone;
7. Sitting quietly after lunch without alcohol; and
8. In a car, while stopped for a few minutes in traffic.

The participant scores each situation as to its degree of sleep propensity on a scale of 0–3: 0 = would never doze; 1 = slight chance of dozing; 2 = moderate chance of dozing; and 3 = high chance of dozing. A score can range from 0 through 24, with higher scores correlating to increasing degrees of sleepiness.

In general, a score of ≥10 is consistent with excessive daytime sleepiness. This cutoff between normal and abnormal subjective sleepiness is derived from the original study's control group data that demonstrated a mean ESS score of 5.9 ± 2.2 *(62)*. Individual ESS scores of ≥16 are typically seen only in individuals with narcolepsy, idiopathic hypersomnia, or moderate/severe obstructive sleep apnea (respiratory disturbance index, >15). Primary snorers demonstrated ESS scores that were not significantly different from those of control subjects. In patients with periodic limb movement disorder, there is also no significant correlation between the periodic limb movement index and ESS scores. This suggests that daytime sleepiness in patients with periodic limb movement disorder is more likely related to the degree of periodic limb movements causing arousals and not simply to the frequency of the periodic limb movements *(62)*.

It should be emphasized that there is significant controversy regarding the validity of the ESS *(63)*. Although in its original descriptions *(62,64)* the ESS demonstrated a strong correlation (–0.514; $p < 0.01$) with results of the mean sleep latency test, subsequent studies have demonstrated that the ESS has little or no correlation to mean sleep latency values on the MSLT *(65–67)*. Johns *(64)* demonstrated that the sleep propensity as measured by the MSLT was significantly related to only three of the eight items (sitting, inactive in a public place; sitting quietly after lunch; and in a car stopped for a few minutes in traffic) on the ESS. Using these three items from the ESS, the correlation between the MSLT and ESS was significant, with a bivariate correlation coefficient of 0.64. Further research has also demonstrated only a weak correlation with considerable discordant results between the MWT and the ESS in patients with sleep apnea and narcolepsy *(68,69)*. The reasons for the lack of strong association between the ESS and sleep latency on the MSLT and MWT are unclear, but it is likely that these tests measure different but complementary aspects of sleepiness.

One of the main reasons for this discrepancy between the ESS and objective measures of sleepiness is that until recently, there were no large-scale, population-based studies assessing the relationship between the ESS and the results of the MSLT. Punjabi and colleagues *(70)* recently used a population-based sample from the Wisconsin Sleep Cohort Study to better assess this question. They demonstrated that individuals with intermediate (6–11) and high (≥12) ESS scores had a 30 and 69% increased risk for sleep onset, respectively, during the four naps of the MSLT. They concluded that the ESS was moderately associated with objective sleep tendency. These findings help to confirm the validity of the ESS as a measure of sleep propensity.

Assuming that the ESS actually measures sleep propensity, the advantages of the ESS are that it is a validated, reliable tool for assessing subjective sleepiness and that it is able to distinguish normal patients from patients with sleep disorders *(61,62)*. Its disadvantages are that it cannot be used on multiple occasions throughout the day, it is not a good measure of short-term acute sleep loss, and its relationship to more objective measures of sleepiness such as the MSLT is inconclusive *(71,72)*.

Pupillometry

The scientific premise behind pupillometry is that pupil size and stability are inversely related to the degree of subjective sleepiness. Normal pupil size is determined by the interaction between the parasympathetic and sympathetic nervous systems' input to the muscles of the iris, the sphincter, and dilator, respectively. In a state of arousal there is increased sympathetic tone, resulting in mydriasis. Conversely, in a state of drowsiness, there is a predominance of parasympathetic tone, resulting in miosis *(73)*. Sleep-deprived individuals will demonstrate the inability to maintain their pupil size as evidenced by frequent pupillary oscillations during the testing period. A well-rested, alert subject is able to maintain a stable pupil size without oscillation in total darkness for 15 minutes *(74)*. To derive reliable results, patients need to be free of any medications that may affect the parasympathetic or sympathetic pathways.

A recent study demonstrated a strong relationship between ongoing sleep deprivation in normal subjects and typical changes in frequency profiles of spontaneous pupillary oscillations and the tendency toward instability of pupil size *(75)*. With ongoing sleep deprivation, slow pupillary oscillations and SSS scores significantly increased, whereas pupil diameter decreased significantly. Currently, pupillometry is not a widely used clinical measurement of sleepiness, predominantly because the equipment is not readily available. Further research is necessary to determine the role of pupillometry in the assessment of daytime sleepiness in clinical practice.

What's the Best Test for Clinical Practice?

Of the subjective methods, the ESS is more useful than the SSS in clinical practice for assessing daytime sleepiness, as the ESS relates to everyday situations. The SSS is limited in clinical practice, as it allows the clinician to assess the patient's degree of subjective sleepiness at only one point in time. As noted above, there is much debate on the relationship of the ESS to the objective tests used to assess daytime sleepiness. Recent data strengthen the case for the ESS being a valid tool that actually measures objective sleep propensity *(70)*.

The utility of the MSLT and MWT to assess a sleepy individual's ability to work or drive remains unclear, as objective data proving their validity for this purpose are limited. The MSLT does not simulate the environment for operating a motor vehicle and thus has uncertain predictability for driving risk *(76)*. The only study utilizing the MSLT to assess the risk of automobile crashes with sleep disorders did not demonstrate a significant relationship between sleep latency and reported accidents *(77)*. Neither the MSLT nor MWT should be used alone as a method to determine an individual's ability to perform in real-world situations. A combination of clinical history with objective data from the MWT should be used to help and to guide clinical recommendations. In general, the MSLT should be used only to objectively assess daytime sleepiness when the diagnosis of narcolepsy or idiopathic hypersomnia is being entertained.

Overall, debate remains concerning which of the above-described tests is best to use in clinical practice. The most recent recommendations from the AASM help to guide the clinician from the standpoint of using the MSLT and MWT in clinical practice. Typically, a combination of subjective and objective testing along with the clinical history are necessary to best determine the degree of a given patient's daytime sleepiness. In my practice, the ESS is used as a screening tool to assess the degree of subjective sleepiness in all patients. The MSLT is always proceeded to objectively determine the patient's sleep tendency when the patient's sleep complaints are out of proportion to the findings on the overnight polysomnogram or when the diagnoses of narcolepsy and/or idiopathic hypersomnia are in the differential diagnosis. The MWT is typically reserved to objectively determine a patient's ability to remain awake when questions of occupational safety arise such as in the case of a school bus driver with obstructive sleep apnea who has recently begun CPAP therapy. In this last case, the author typically uses a combination of the MWT results, the downloaded CPAP compliance data, and a negative toxicology screen (to rule out stimulant use) to better determine the individual's ability to resume driving safely.

DETERMINANTS OF DAYTIME SLEEPINESS

Not all daytime sleepiness is a result of inadequate amounts of total sleep time. The human sleep–wake cycle is regulated by two primary processes, process S and process C *(78)*. Process S is the homeostatic drive to sleep. This drive increases during wakefulness and decreases during sleep. If a sufficient amount of sleep is not achieved, either through decreased total sleep time (sleep quantity) or sleep fragmentation (sleep quality), the homeostatic drive for sleep increases and results in daytime sleepiness. The amount of slow-wave sleep achieved is primarily linked to process S and the duration of previous wakefulness *(79)*. Process C is the circadian drive for sleep, which acts independently of sleeping and waking. This drive increases sleepiness and alertness during different parts of the subjective day and night. Process C also controls the drive for REM sleep. REM sleep propensity is dependent on the circadian phase and not altered by an increasing homeostatic drive for sleep *(49,79)*.

When encountering the sleepy patient in clinical practice, the differential should be based on the factors that primarily determine sleepiness:

1. *Sleep quantity* and
2. *Sleep quality*, which are related to process S;
3. *Circadian influences*, which are regulated by process C; and
4. *Central nervous system (CNS)-controlled processes*, which are responsible for narcolepsy and CNS (idiopathic) hypersomnia. These primary sleep-inducing processes may act independently of one another or in combination with any or all of the above to produce an additive sleepiness effect.

Sleep Quantity

The number one cause of daytime sleepiness in this and other countries is chronic partial sleep deprivation. The degree of daytime sleepiness is directly proportional to the amount of sleep achieved during the previous night. Total or partial sleep deprivation will result in daytime sleepiness even after only one evening of sleep loss. The total amount of nocturnal sleep that an individual requires to alleviate daytime sleepiness is unknown, and likely varies on an individual basis. The commonly held belief is that most adults require between 7 and 8 hours of sleep per night. This recommendation is based on sleep deprivation studies that demonstrate significant negative changes in neurocognitive function, mood, and subjective and objective sleepiness when sleep times are restricted as little as 1 hour per night *(6,80)*. One well-publicized study using data from the American Cancer Society database found an association between those sleeping either more than 8.5 hours/night or less than 6 hours/night and an increased mortality risk exceeding 15% compared with those sleeping 7–8 hours/night *(81)*. Although these findings are of interest, the validity of these findings has been questioned as the results were not based on a random sample of the population. Other recent studies have also suggested that sleep times of less than 6 and more than 7 hours per night may be associated with higher all-cause mortality in adults *(82,83)*. The possible mechanisms by which short and long sleep times may affect health outcomes are unknown.

It is believed that healthy young adults require between 8 and 8.5 hours of sleep per night *(84)*. A large epidemiological study of young adults has suggested that this group suffers from chronic partial sleep deprivation as their average length of nocturnal sleep achieved on weekdays was only 6.7 hours *(85)*. Conversely, lengthening the nocturnal sleep period beyond 8 hours may result in statistically significant increased alertness and improved reaction times *(86,87)*. Of note, although sleep extension results in statistically significant improvements in performance and decreased slow-wave sleep, some authors debate the clinical significance of these improvements *(88)*, especially in individuals without previous complaints of sleepiness. Studies assessing the effects of late afternoon naps and sleep extension (increasing total sleep time beyond baseline normal levels) have demonstrated significant decreases in the homeostatic drive for sleep *(89–91)*. Daytime naps have also been shown to improve daytime sleepiness after acute sleep deprivation.

The amount of sleepiness that results from sleep restriction not only is dependent on the amount of the nocturnal sleep achieved, but may also be dependent on when that sleep occurs during the evening *(92)*. The preliminary results of a recent study demonstrated that young adults restricted to 4 hours of sleep per night for 7 days in a row were better able to remain awake during the daytime when their 4-hour block of sleep occurred between 2:30 and 6:30 AM vs those who achieved their block of sleep between 11:30 PM and 3:30 AM. The explanation for these results is likely related to the combination of homeostatic and circadian factors influencing sleep. If these results are confirmed by larger studies, these results may have significant implications for instructing patients and the public when to sleep when their busy schedules don't allow them to achieve a full 7.5–8 hours of sleep per night as recommended.

Do all types of sleep deprivation lead to similar results in terms of daytime sleepiness? The effects of selective deprivation of REM sleep on performance, mood, and daytime sleepiness are not well-defined and understood, and therefore the consequences of REM sleep deprivation are described separately. Isolated REM sleep deprivation is rare in clinical medicine, but may be seen in patients with REM-related sleep apnea and in patients on various REM-suppressant medications. REM sleep deprivation in humans under experimental conditions has been shown to result in increased sexual drive, restlessness, and aggression *(93,94)*. Subjects deprived of REM sleep actually display less daytime sleepiness, as assessed by the MSLT, when compared with subjects deprived of equal amounts of non-REM sleep *(94)*. In fact, the REM-deprived individuals do not demonstrate any changes from baseline MSLT values. The mechanism by which REM deprivation exerts its alerting effects is unknown and will require further research.

A question that typically arises is, "Do we ever get used to chronic partial sleep deprivation?" The answer is a resounding no! Data from individuals restricted to 5 hours of sleep per night for seven consecutive nights suggest that cumulative sleep debt has a dynamic and escalating effect in terms of increasing daytime sleepiness and poorer performance on psychomotor vigilance testing, memory problems, and mood evaluations *(6,95)*. A larger study has also demonstrated that sleep restricted to 4 and 6 hours/night for 14 consecutive days results in progressive neurocognitive dysfunction *(4)*. Chronic restriction of sleep to 6 hours or less per night for 2 weeks produced cognitive performance deficits equivalent to up to two nights of total sleep deprivation *(4)*. The subjects in these studies were largely unaware of the increasing and cumulative cognitive deficits over time. These studies confirm that an asymptomatic steady-state sleepiness does *not* appear to be achieved in response to sleep restriction, as elevated sleepiness and performance deficits are demonstrated throughout the sleep restriction period. It should be noted, though that while steady-state sleepiness is not achieved in response to sleep restriction, neurobehavioral deficits from sleep loss vary significantly between individuals and appear to be stable within individuals. These individual differences in the response to sleep deprivation are not explained by variations in sleep history *(96)*.

Sleep Quality

The degree of daytime sleepiness is also regulated by sleep continuity. The sleep continuity theory states that consolidation of sleep is as important as total sleep time.

In general, the degree of daytime sleepiness is directly proportional to the degree of sleep fragmentation *(97)*. Neurocognitive performance deficits are common in individuals experiencing sleep fragmentation *(5,97,98)*. Studies of nocturnal sleep fragmentation demonstrate that daytime sleepiness increases and neurocognitive performance decreases even after one night of sleep fragmentation *(5,97,98)*. The number of stage shifts from other sleep stages to stage 1 sleep or wake, as well as the percentage of stage 1 sleep, correlates with excessive daytime sleepiness in various patient groups *(99)*. It appears that the total number of sleep-fragmenting events is as important as their distribution during the night. Similar numbers of sleep-fragmenting events result in similar deficits in daytime function whether the events are evenly spaced or clustered *(100)*.

In clinical practice, sleep fragmentation may result from primary sleep disorders including obstructive sleep apnea and periodic limb movement syndrome. Several medical disorders are associated with sleep fragmentation including COPD and congestive heart failure (secondary to Cheyne-stokes respirations in stages 1 and 2 sleep) *(101)*. Chronic pain syndromes, including fibromyalgia, are associated with an α–δ sleep pattern that is associated with nonrestorative sleep *(102)*. Frequent awakenings secondary to nocturnal urination are common in older men and in individuals using diuretics. Finally, older age in and of itself is responsible for more frequent awakenings and the diminished ability to consolidate non-REM sleep *(103)*.

Another common question is, "Can we make up for lost or chronically poor sleep?" The good news is that the answer is yes. The amount of sleep needed to recover from a given amount of sleep loss, though, is unclear. The concept of "sleep debt" refers to the need of the body to make up for the hours of sleep lost over time. The size of the sleep debt and the resultant daytime sleepiness are directly proportional to the amount of sleep lost. A sleep debt may develop with one night of partial or total sleep loss or may be accumulated through poor sleep quality secondary to sleep fragmentation. Progressive daytime sleepiness may also result from the accumulation of sleep restriction (as little as 1 hour per night) that occurs during several subsequent nights *(4,6,95)*.

It is unclear if a chronic sleep debt that has accumulated over time needs to be "paid back" on an hour-per-hour basis, or if sleep restoration occurs more quickly than sleep loss accumulation. Several studies (up to 110 hours of sleep deprivation) have suggested that that equal amounts of time are not required to recover from sleep deprivation and that recovery occurs more quickly than the total sleep lost *(104–106)*. Individuals subjected to a consecutive 264 hours of wakefulness required sleep for only 12–15 hours during the initial recovery period *(107)*. Young adults restricted to 5 hours of sleep per night for a week required two full nights of sleep (up to 10 hours per night) to fully recover from performance deficits *(6)*. Horne *(108)* has postulated that only part of the normal night's sleep is essential and that the remaining sleep acts as a buffer. It is possible that sleep restoration may be a logarithmic process, with higher recuperative effects occurring early on in sleep recovery and more minor changes occurring later. Conversely, Dement and Vaughan *(109)* have recently advocated that accumulated sleep debt, whether acutely or chronically accumulated, must be paid back on an hour-for-hour basis. Future studies are needed to answer this question.

Circadian Factors

The circadian system is the internal pacemaker or time clock of the human body. The human sleep–wake cycle, as well as several other neurohormonal cycles, are synchronized to the day–night cycle through the circadian system. The human sleep–wake cycle demonstrates a strong relationship to the deep circadian pacemaker, as it has strong influences on both the timing and duration of sleep in normal individuals *(110)*. There is actually a biphasic pattern of objective sleepiness as demonstrated through multiple sleep latency testing in normal young adults and elderly subjects during a 24-hour period *(44)*. When using core body temperature (CBT) as the surrogate marker for the circadian pacemaker, sleep onset is closely linked to the downslope of the CBT curve *(49,110)*. Two peaks in sleep tendency/troughs in alertness are evident in humans. The major peak in sleep tendency occurs between the hours of 2 and 6 AM and is linked to the nadir and rising limb of the CBT curve. A second, weaker increase in sleep tendency/decrease in alertness occurs during the daytime hours between 2 and 6 PM *(44)*.

Conversely, there is also a biphasic pattern to objective alertness. The two peaks in alertness occur at opposite ends of the clock around 9 AM and 9 PM. This biphasic pattern also correlates with increasing and peak CBT, respectively *(44,111)*. The main troughs in alertness correspond to the aforementioned times of increased sleep tendency.

Because of the biphasic shifts in sleepiness and alertness throughout the 24-hour day, *the major determinant of the duration of sleep is the phase of the endogenous pacemaker rather than the duration of earlier wakefulness (110)*. For these reasons, when normal individuals are placed into environments free of time cues, they demonstrate a shorter sleep duration when a chosen bed time is near the temperature cycle minimum, and a longer sleep length when sleep is initiated near the temperature maximum. As stated above, these patterns persist regardless of the previous length of wakefulness *(110)*.

The differential diagnoses of sleepiness related to circadian disturbances include primary and secondary disorders. Primary circadian disturbances that may result in daytime sleepiness are caused by the patient's internal clock being constantly out of phase, or unsynchronized, with the external environment. These disorders include

1. Delayed sleep phase syndrome;
2. Advanced sleep phase syndrome; and
3. Non-24-hours/irregular sleep–wake syndrome.

Secondary circadian-related sleep disorders occur when

1. The external stimuli that normally entrain the internal clock change abruptly such as in jet lag or rapidly changing shift work or
2. Individuals are required to work at times of the day/night when sleep tendencies are the highest such as in shift workers who work in the night shift routinely. (*See also* Chapter 22, "Shift Work-Related Sleep Disorders.")

Central Factors

Several syndromes that result in daytime hypersomnia are caused by CNS etiologies that have poorly understood mechanisms of disease. The most recognized syndromes in this category include narcolepsy, idiopathic CNS hypersomnia, and Kleine–Levin syndrome. These syndromes will be covered more completely in the chapter concerning narcolepsy and nonapneic hypersomnia. Narcolepsy is the most common neurological cause of excessive daytime sleepiness *(112)*. It is as common as multiple sclerosis, with a prevalence of 0.02–0.09% in the United States *(113)*. The syndrome affects male and female individuals equally. Although the symptoms typically begin during the second decade of life (70–80%), symptoms may occur at any age. Patients typically report poorer quality of life, with disease-related symptoms affecting the personal, social, and professional aspects of their lives *(114,115)*.

PROPOSED MECHANISMS OF DISEASE

Although the underlying mechanisms responsible for narcolepsy still remain unclear, several hypotheses have been put forth. Currently, no structural abnormalities of the brain have been consistently identified in patients with narcolepsy. Genetics likely play a role, with the most likely scenario being that of multiple genes being influenced by environmental factors. A strong association has been demonstrated between two human leukocyte antigen (HLA) haplotypes on human chromosome 6: *HLA-DQB1*0602* and *DQA1*0102* are found in 85–95% of narcoleptics, as compared with 12–38% of the general US population *(116,117)*; the *HLA-DQB1* × *0602* haplotype is more closely associated with cataplexy *(117)*.

Several recent findings have identified a potential biochemical basis for narcolepsy in dogs, mice, and humans *(118–121)*. In the canine model of narcolepsy, a genetic defect in the hypocretin receptor-2 (*Hcrtr2*) gene results in a nonfunctional hypocretin receptor-2 *(119)*. Several human studies have demonstrated that hypocretin A levels are low or undetectable in patients with narcolepsy *(121–123)*. These data suggest that hypocretins (orexins) may be the major neurotransmitters responsible for narcolepsy. The approach to the diagnosis and treatment of narcolepsy will be covered in the chapter/lecture covering this disease.

Idiopathic hypersomnia is a poorly understood condition characterized by excessive daytime sleepiness in the absence of other identifiable conditions such as sleep apnea, narcolepsy, sleep deprivation, and/or medication effects *(124,125)*. Unlike narcolepsy, where the total sleep time per 24-hour period is relatively normal, patients with idiopathic hypersomnia may sleep for unlimited amounts of time throughout the day and night. Objective diagnosis is made through night time polysomnography followed by an MSLT. The polysomnogram is relatively unremarkable. The MSLT typically demonstrates objective evidence of pathological hypersomnolence (mean sleep latency of <5 minutes) without SOREMPs. Neuroimaging studies and HLA evaluation are not indicated. Treatment options are similar to those for narcolepsy and involve a combination of stimulants, regular sleep–wake schedules, and avoidance of sleep deprivation.

The Kleine–Levin syndrome is characterized by intermittent bouts of hypersomnia that may last from days to weeks. The periods between bouts of hypersomnia are characterized by normal levels of alertness and sleep–wake function. Although the syndrome has been classically described as a disease of adolescent boys typically occurring in association with hypersexuality and hyperphagia, it may occur at any time of life as well as in both sexes. The mechanisms of disease and the best treatment options have yet to be defined. Although the syndrome typically occurs in its idiopathic form, it has also been described following head trauma. Anecdotal treatment successes have been reported with both stimulants and lithium. Whether these reports represent true treatment effects or just spontaneous resolution of the symptoms is unclear given the syndrome's periodic nature.

ADDITIONAL FACTORS THAT AFFECT THE ABILITY TO INITIATE OR MAINTAIN SLEEP

Physiological Arousal

We've all had nights where despite feeling tired, we have been unable to initiate or maintain sleep throughout the night. This inability to fall or stay asleep may be explained by the fact that an individual's underlying state of arousal may affect one's ability to fall asleep, independent of the primary drives for sleepiness. Several examples in the literature highlight this point. As emphasized in the MSLT portion of this chapter, stringent adherence to proper MSLT protocol and procedure must be followed to ensure accurate MSLT results *(37)*. State changes in physiological arousal may significantly influence the MSLT results. In a study by Bonnet and Arand *(126)*, normal subjects underwent the MSLT after either a 5-minute walk or lying in bed and watching TV for 15 minutes. Despite similar homeostatic and circadian influences for sleep, sleep latencies were significantly increased in the group who walked before the MSLT, with or without sleep-deprived conditions. These data imply that measured sleepiness is a combination of sleep drive and physiological arousal, which may act independently of each other.

A patient's underlying sleep complaint must also be taken into account when interpreting MSLT results. Several studies have demonstrated that patients with primary insomnia have MSLT values that are significantly longer than those of matched normal control subjects *(127–129)*. It has been argued that because insomniacs have difficulties in initiating sleep, longer sleep latencies in this patient population may be an artifact of their underlying condition rather than a true assessment of their degree of daytime sleepiness *(130)*.

Environmental noise and temperature may affect an individual's response to sleep loss. Environmental noise has been demonstrated to be beneficial in terms of reversing measurable sleepiness in several sleep deprivation studies *(131,132)*. The beneficial effects of noise are thought to be secondary to raising the individual's arousal level. Although noise is effective in countering the effects of sleep deprivation, the beneficial effects of environmental noise may be short-lived. Under monotonous driving conditions, sleep-deprived individuals received no benefit from radio noise as a countermeasure to sleepiness *(133)*. In the same study, cold air to the face also demonstrated no lasting benefits.

A recent study demonstrated that daytime exposure to bright light (1000 lx) can reduce the impact of sleep restriction on daytime sleepiness levels and performance as compared with dim light (<5 lx) *(134)*. These effects occurred independent of the mechanisms responsible for suppression of melatonin secretion, as bright light exposure had no effect on salivary melatonin levels. Although the exact mechanisms responsible for the alerting effects of bright daytime light exposure are not totally clear, one proposed explanation is that bright light exposure increases physiological arousal *(134)*.

Finally, an individual's motivation and body posture may influence the ability to initiate sleep. Bonnet and Arand *(53)* evaluated subjects in several different situations, including:

1. Lie down and sleep.
2. Lie down and stay awake.
3. Sit up and sleep.
4. Sit up and stay awake.
5. Sit in a chair in front of a computer and stay awake.

Despite similar homeostatic and circadian influences for sleep, the results for each condition were significantly different. The mean sleep latency for each condition was as follows:

1. Lie down and sleep, 11.1 minutes.
2. Lie down and stay awake, 21.7 minutes.
3. Sit up and sleep, 17.7 minutes.
4. Sit up and stay awake, 29 minutes.
5. Sit in a chair in front of a computer and stay awake, 30.1 minutes. This study highlights the effects of motivation and posture on the ability to maintain alertness. These arousal effects appear to be additive.

These results emphasize that factors other than sleepiness, i.e., level of physiological arousal and sleep–wake state pathophysiology, may influence the ability to initiate and/or maintain sleep. The above data offer one explanation for why MSLT and MWT results may not always correlate. The MSLT in ideal situations only measures sleepiness whereas the MWT measures the combined effects of the sleep and arousal systems *(53)*.

Medications/Drugs

Medications can have beneficial or adverse effects on daytime sleepiness. CNS stimulants are the most widely studied classes of drugs. Amphetamines and cocaine improve neurocognitive performance and reaction time in sleep-deprived individuals *(135,136)*. The effects of caffeine on daytime sleepiness are not as clear-cut. Caffeine clearly enhances performance and alertness over the short-term (first 24 hours of sleep deprivation) *(137)*. It appears that the beneficial effects of caffeine may decline over time. Some studies of sleep deprivation have found that caffeine used during long periods of time may increase daytime sleepiness by impairing subsequent sleep episodes *(138)*. Modafinil, a CNS stimulant frequently used to combat daytime sleepiness in patients with narcolepsy, improves the ability to remain awake in this patient population. It should be noted that most stimulants improve the ability to remain awake without affecting the underlying drive for sleep. As an example, the modafinil data regarding patients with narcolepsy have demonstrated a significant improvement in the ability to remain awake as measured by the MWT without any significant change in the MSLT scores *(139)*.

The effects of ethanol demonstrate a biphasic response after short-term acute sleep deprivation. At low blood ethanol levels, performance on reaction time and driving tests may actually improve. Increased ethanol consumption in sleep-deprived subjects leads to poorer performance compared with control individuals. Increased basal levels of sleepiness secondary to an ongoing cumulative sleep debt enhance ethanol's sedative effects, even at moderate ethanol doses *(140)*. A complete drug history is essential in the evaluation of the sleepy patient as several over-the-counter and prescription medications may lead to increased daytime sleepiness in both sleep-deprived and nonsleep-deprived individuals. Histamine (H_1) receptor blockers such as diphenhydramine are commonly used in cold and allergy preparations and are known to increase sleepiness and decrease sleep latency *(141,142)*. Antihypertensives such as β-blockers and clonidine may increase subjective daytime sleepiness *(143)*. Several antidepressants (tricyclics), antipsychotics (neuroleptics), and antianxiety medications (benzodiazepines) may cause daytime sleepiness secondary to a long half-life, anticholinergic properties, or induction of sleep fragmentation (i.e., periodic limb movements secondary to tricyclic antidepressants).

CONCLUSIONS

Daytime sleepiness and the abilities to initiate and/or maintain sleep represent a balance between the primary drives for sleepiness (homeostatic, circadian, central, and so on) and modifying factors that affect the arousal system. Factors that affect the degree of sleepiness may act independently or in concert, with the effects on the drive for sleepiness being additive. Alternatively, factors that affect the arousal system may oppose the ability to initiate or maintain sleep. This effect of the arousal system to inhibit sleep is somewhat self-limited, as increasing drives for sleepiness will eventually overcome the ability of the arousal system to maintain wakefulness.

Approach to the Sleepy Patient

Because the etiologies of a given patient's sleepiness can be multifactorial, the approach to treating a patient should take into account all possible factors (homeostatic, circadian, central, and medication/drug). Remember that although inadequate total sleep time is the most common cause of daytime sleepiness, it is not the only etiology. The following is a list of general recommendations to follow when faced with the sleepy patient:

1. Take a complete sleep and medical history including symptoms related to sleep apnea and periodic limb movements. Perform polysomnography, when indicated, and treat objective findings that may be causing sleep fragmentation. Remember that certain chronic medical conditions such as congestive heart failure, renal disease, and Parkinson's disease may cause daytime sleepiness, as they are associated with conditions that lead to sleep fragmentation. Document other factors that may lead to poor sleep quality or quantity such as multiple nocturnal awakenings to urinate related to benign prostatic hypertrophy or evening diuretic dosing.
2. Be aware of the fact that not all patients with sleep disorders will complain of daytime sleepiness as their primary symptom. Symptoms such as lack of energy, tiredness, and fatigue may be the sleep-disordered patient's primary complaint *(144)*.
3. Take a complete medication and social drug use history. Attempt to discontinue any medications/drugs that may lead to daytime sleepiness.
4. From an occupational standpoint, make sure night-shift workers are aware of the circadian influences on sleepiness and awareness.
5. Prescribe a regular sleep–wake schedule for all patients. Even in nonsleep-deprived individuals, regularization of sleep–wake schedules is associated with reduced reported sleepiness and improved sleep efficiency *(145)*.
6. If inadequate nocturnal sleep time is determined to be the etiology of the patient's sleepiness, prescribe increased sleep time.
7. When a given patient's schedule does not allow for increasing the amount of nocturnal sleep time, consider instituting naps as a therapeutic maneuver. For those patients who work the night shift, prophylactic naps before a period of sleep loss help to maintain alertness and performance during the period of sleep loss *(30,146,147)*. In general, longer naps provide more benefit in terms of performance and alertness. For the majority of individuals with daytime occupations, consider instituting short naps (15–60 minutes) into the workday. When prescribing naps during the work period, be aware that sleep inertia may cause difficulty awakening from longer naps. This typically abates spontaneously with in a few minutes.
8. Finally, keep in mind that drivers typically are aware of the signs of sleepiness before falling asleep at the wheel *(148,149)*. Instruct all individuals to be aware of the signs of sleepiness while driving so they can pull over and rest before it is too late.

REFERENCES

1. Bonnet M, Arand D (1995) We are chronically sleep deprived. Sleep 18:908–911.
2. Partinen M (1994) Epidemiology of sleep disorders. In: *Principles and Practice of Sleep Medicine.* (Kryger M, Roth T, Dement W, eds.) WB Saunders, Philadelphia, PA, pp. 437–452.
3. Briones B, Adams N, Strauss M, et al. (1996) Relationship between sleepiness and health. Sleep 19:583–588.
4. VanDongen H, Maislin G, Mullington J, et al. (2003) The cumulative cost of additional wakefulness: dose-response effects on neurobehavioral functions and sleep physiology from chronic sleep restriction and total sleep deprivation. Sleep 26:117–126.
5. Bonnet M (1985) Effect of sleep disruption on sleep, performance and mood. Sleep 8:11–19.
6. Dinges D, Pack F, Williams K, et al. (1997) Cumulative sleepiness, mood disturbance, and psychomotor vigilance performance decrements during a week of sleep restricted to 4-5 h per night. Sleep 20:267–277.
7. Reynolds C, Kupfer D, Hoch C, et al. (1986) Sleep deprivation in healthy elderly men and women: effects on mood and on sleep during recovery. Sleep 9:492–501.
8. Pilcher J, Huffcut A (1996) Effects of sleep deprivation on performance: a meta-analysis. Sleep 19:318–326.
9. Pflug B, Tolle R (1971) Disturbances of the 24-h rhythm in endogenous depression and the treatment of endogenous depression by sleep deprivation. Int Pharmacopsychiatry 6:187–196.
10. Post R, Kotin J, Goodwin F (1976) Effects of sleep deprivation on mood and amine metabolism in depressed patients. Arch Gen Psychiatry 33:627–632.
11. Van den Burg W, van den Hoofdakker R (1975) Total sleep deprivation on endogenous depression. Arch Gen Psychiatry 32:1121–1125.
12. Rechtschaffen A, Bergmann BM, Everson CA, et al. (1989) Sleep deprivation in the rat: X. Integration and discussion of the findings. Sleep 12:68–87.
13. Rechtschaffen A, Gilliland MA, Bergmann BM, et al. (1983) Physiological correlates of prolonged sleep deprivation in rats. Science 221:182–184.
14. Ax A, Luby E (1961) Autonomic responses to sleep deprivation. Arch Gen Psychiatry 4:55–59.
15. Fiorica V, Higgins E, Iampietro P (1968) Physiologic responses of men during sleep deprivation. J Appl Physiol 24:167–176.
16. Horne J (1978) A review of the biological effects of total sleep deprivation in man. Biol Psychol 7:55–102.
17. Johnson L (1969) Physiological and psychological changes following total sleep deprivation. In: *Sleep Physiology and Pathology.* (Kales A, ed.) Lippincott, Philadelphia, PA, pp. 206–220.
18. Kant G, Genser S, Thorne D (1984) Effects of 72 h of sleep deprivation on urinary cortisol and indices of metabolism. Sleep 7:142–146.
19. Kollar E, Pasnau R, Rubin RT, et al. (1969) Psychological, psychophysiological, and biochemical correlates of prolonged sleep deprivation. Am J Psychiatry 126:488–497.
20. Naitoh P, Kelly T, Englund C (1990) Health effects of sleep deprivation. Occup Med 5:209–237.
21. Spiegel K, Leproult R, Van Cauter E (1999) Impact of sleep debt on metabolic and endocrine function. Lancet 23:1435–1439.
22. Horne J, Pettit A (1984) Sleep deprivation and physiological response to exercise under steady-state conditions in untrained subjects. Sleep 7:168–179.
23. Palmblad J, Petrini B, Wasserman J, Akerstedt T (1979) Lymphocyte and granulocyte reactions during sleep deprivation. Psychosom Med 41:273–278.
24. Dinges D, Douglas S, Zaugg L, et al. (1994) Leukocytosis and natural killer cell function parallel neurobehavioral fatigue induced by 64 h of sleep deprivation. J Clin Invest 93:1930–1939.
25. Shouse M (1994) Epileptic seizure manifestations during sleep. In: *Principles and Practice of Sleep Medicine.* (Kryger M, Roth T, Dement W, eds.) WB Saunders, Philadelphia, PA, pp. 801–814.
26. Series F, Roy N, Marc I (1994) Effects of sleep deprivation and sleep fragmentation on upper airway collapsibility in normal subjects. Am J Respir Crit Care Med 150:481–485.
27. 2000 Omnibus Sleep in America Poll. National Sleep Foundation, Washington, DC, 2000.
28. Hublin C, Kaprio J, Partinen M, et al. (1996) Daytime sleepiness in an adult Finnish population. J Intern Med 239:417–423.
29. Liu X, Uchiyama M, Kim K, et al. (2000) Sleep loss and daytime sleepiness in the general population of Japan. Psychiatry Res 93:1–11.
30. Bonnet M (1991) The effect of varying prophylactic naps on performance, alertness, and mood throughout a 52 h continuous operation. Sleep 14:307–315.

31. Ancoli-Israel S, Kripke D, Klauber M, et al. (1991) Sleep-disordered breathing in community dwelling elderly. Sleep 14:486–495.
32. Ancoli-Israel S, Kripke D, Klauber M, et al. (1991) Periodic limb movements in community dwelling elderly. Sleep 14:496–500.
33. Young T, Palta M, Dempsey J, et al. (1993) Occurrence of sleep disordered breathing among middle-aged adults. N Engl J Med 328:1230–1235.
34. Walsh J, Tepas D, Moss P (1981) The twenty four hour workday: proceedings of a symposium on variations of work sleep schedules. Department of Health and Human Services (NIOSH),Washington, DC.
35. Kribbs N, Getsy J, Dinges D (1993) Investigation and management of daytime sleepiness in sleep apnea. In: *Sleeping and Breathing*. (Saunders N, Sullivan C, eds.) Marcel Dekker, New York, NY, pp. 575–604.
36. Littner MR, Kushida C, Wise M, et al. (2005) Practice parameters for clinical use of the multiple sleep latency test and the maintenance of wakefulness test. Sleep 28(1):113–121.
37. Carskadon M, Dement W, Mitler M, et al. (1986) Guidelines for the multiple sleep latency test (MSLT): a standard measure of sleepiness. Sleep 9:519–524.
38. Zwyghuizen-Doorenbos A, Roehrs T, Schaefer M, et al. (1988) Test-retest reliability of the MSLT. Sleep 11:562–565.
39. American Sleep Disorders Association (1992) The clinical use of the multiple sleep latency test. Sleep 15:268–276.
40. Lumley M, Roehrs T, Asker D, et al. (1987) Ethanol and caffeine effects on daytime sleepiness/alertness. Sleep 19:306–312.
41. Carskadon M, Dement W (1982) Nocturnal determinants of daytime sleepiness. Sleep 5(Suppl 2): S73–S81.
42. Levine B, Roehrs T, Stepanski E, et al. (1987) Fragmenting sleep diminishes its recuperative value. Sleep 10:590–599.
43. Carskadon M, Dement W (1992) Multiple sleep latency tests during the constant routine. Sleep 15:396–399.
44. Richardson G, Carskadon M, Orav E, et al. (1982) Circadian variation of sleep tendency in elderly and young adult subjects. Sleep 5:S82–S94.
45. Aldrich M, Chervin R, Malow B (1997) Value of the multiple sleep latency test (MSLT) for the diagnosis of narcolepsy. Sleep 20:620–629.
46. Richardson GS, Carskadon MA, Flagg W, et al. (1978) Excessive daytime sleepiness in man: multiple sleep latency measurement in narcoleptic and control subjects. Electroencephalogr Clin Neurophysiol 45:621–627.
47. Carskadon MA, Dement WC, Mitler MM, et al. (1986) Guidelines for the multiple sleep latency test (MSLT): a standard measure of sleepiness. Sleep 9:519–524.
48. Clodore M, Benoit O, Foret J, et al. (1990) The multiple sleep latency test: individual variability and time of day effect in normal young adults. Sleep 13:385–394.
49. Czeisler C, Zimmerman J, Ronda J, et al. (1980) Timing of REM sleep coupled to the circadian rhythm of body temperature in man. Sleep 2:329–346.
50. Golish J, Sarodia B, Blanchard A, et al. (2002) Prediction of the final MSLT result from the results of the first three naps. Sleep Med 3:249–253.
51. Sangal RB, Thomas L, Mitler MM (1992) Disorders of excessive sleepiness: treatment improves ability to stay awake but does not reduce sleepiness. Chest 102:699–703.
52. Hartse K, Roth T, Zorick F (1982) Daytime sleepiness and daytime wakefulness: the effect of instruction. Sleep 5:S107–S118.
53. Bonnet M, Arand D (2001) Arousal components which differentiate the MWT from the MSLT. Sleep 24:441–447.
54. Mitler MM, Gujavarty K, Browman C (1982) Maintenance of wakefulness test: a polysomnogrpahic technique for evaluating treatment efficacy in patients with excessive somnolence. Electroencephalogr Clin Neurophysiol 53:658–661.
55. Poceta J, Timms R, Jeong D, et al. (1992) Maintenance of wakefulness test in obstructive sleep apnea syndrome. Chest 101:893–897.
56. Department of Transportation. Sleep apnea evaluation specifications. Federal Aviation Administration Specification Letter, October 6, 1992.
57. Bennett L, Stradling J, Davies R (1997) A behavioral test to assess daytime sleepiness in obstructive sleep apnoea. J Sleep Res 6:142–145.

58. Rechtschaffen A, Kales A (1968) A manual of standardized terminology: techniques and scoring system for sleep stages of human subjects. Los Angeles, CA, Brain Info. Serv./Brain Res. Int., UCLA (NIH Publ. 2040).
59. Priest B, Brichard C, Aubert G, et al. (2001) Microsleep during a simplified maintenance of wakefulness test. Am J Respir Crit Care Med 163:1619–1625.
60. Hoddes E, Zarcone V, Smythe H, et al. (1973) Quantification of sleepiness: a new approach. Psychophysiology 10:431–436.
61. Mitler M, Miller J (1996) Methods for testing sleepiness. Behav Med 21:171–183.
62. Johns M (1991) A new method of measuring daytime sleepiness: the Epworth Sleepiness Scale. Sleep 14:540–545.
63. Johns M (2000) Sensitivity and specificity of the multiple sleep latency test (MSLT), the maintenance of wakefulness test and the Epworth sleepiness scale: failure of the MSLT as the gold standard. J Sleep Res 9:5–11.
64. Johns M (1994) Sleepiness in different situations measured by the Epworth Sleepiness Scale. Sleep 17:703–710.
65. Benbadis S, Mascha E, Perry M, et al. (1999) Association between the Epworth Sleepiness Scale and the multiple sleep latency test in a clinical population. Ann Intern Med 130:289–292.
66. Chervin R, Aldrich M, Pickett R, et al. (1997) Comparison of the results of the Epworth Sleepiness Scale and the multiple sleep latency test. J Psychosom Res 42:145–155.
67. Chervin R, Aldrich M (1999) The Epworth Sleepiness Scale may not reflect objective measures of sleepiness or sleep apnea. Neurology 52:125–131.
68. Sangal R, Sangal J, Belisle C (1999) Subjective and objective indices of sleepiness (ESS and MWT) are not equally useful in patients with sleep apnea. Clin Electroencephalogr 30:73–75.
69. Sangal R, Mitler M, Sangal J (1999) Subjective sleepiness ratings (Epworth sleepiness scale) do not reflect the same parameter of sleepiness as objective sleepiness (maintenance of wakefulness test) in patients with narcolepsy. Clin Neurophysiol 110:2131–2135.
70. Punjabi N, Bandeen-Roche K, Young T (2003) Predictors of objective sleep tendency in the general population. Sleep 26:678–683.
71. Miletin M, Hanley P (2003) Measurement properties of the Epworth sleepiness scale. Sleep Med 4:195–199.
72. Chervin R (2003) Epworth sleepiness scale? Sleep Med 4:175–176.
73. Yoss R, Moyer N, Hollenhorst R (1970) Pupil size and spontaneous pupillary waves associated with alertness, drowsiness and sleep. Neurology 20:545–554.
74. Lowenstein O, Feinberg R, Lowenfeld I (1963) Pupillary movements during acute and chronic fatigue: a new test for the objective evaluation of tiredness. Invest Ophthalmol 2:138–157.
75. Wilhelm B, Wilhelm H, Ludtke H, et al. (1998) Pupillographic assessment of sleepiness in sleep-deprived healthy subjects. Sleep 21:258–265.
76. Sleep apnea, sleepiness, and driving risk: American Thoracic Society. (1994) Am J Respir Crit Care Med 150:1463–1473.
77. Aldrich M (1989) Automobile accidents in patients with sleep disorders. Sleep 12:487–494.
78. Borbely A (1982) A two process model of sleep regulation. Hum Neurobiol 1:195–204.
79. Dinges D (1986) Differential effects of prior wakefulness and circadian phase on nap sleep. Electroencephalogr Clin Neurophysiol 64:224–227.
80. Rosenthal L, Roehrs T, Rosen A, et al. (1993) Level of sleepiness and total sleep time following various time in bed conditions. Sleep 16:226–232.
81. Kripke D, Garfinkel L, Wingard D, et al. (2002) Mortality associated with sleep duration and insomnia. Arch Gen Psychiatry 59:131–136.
82. Patel S, Ayas N, Malhotra M, et al. (2004) A prospective study of sleep duration and mortality risk in women. Sleep 27:440–444.
83. Tamakoshi A, Ohno Y (2004) Self-reported sleep duration as a predictor of all-cause mortality: results from the JACC study, Japan. Sleep 27:51–54.
84. Wehr T, Moul D, Barbato G, et al. (1993) Conservation of photo-period-responsive mechanisms in humans. Am J Physiol 265:R846–R857.
85. Breslau N, Roth T, Rosenthal L, et al. (1997) Daytime sleepiness: an epidemiological study of young adults. Am J Public Health 87:1649–1653.
86. Roehrs T, Timms V, Zwyghuizen-Doorenbos A, et al. (1989) A two week sleep extension in sleepy normals. Sleep 12:449–457.

87. Carskadon MA, Dement WC (1979) Sleepiness during extension of nocturnal sleep [abstract]. Sleep Res 8:147.
88. Harrison Y, Horne J (1995) Should we be taking more sleep? Sleep 18:901–907.
89. Feinberg I, Fein G, Floyd T (1982) Computer detected patterns of electroencephalographic delta activity during and after extended sleep. Science 215:1131–1133.
90. Feinberg I, March J, Floyd T, et al. (1985) Homeostatic changes during post nap sleep maintain baseline levels of delta EEG. Electroencephalogr Clin Neurophysiol 61:134–137.
91. Karacan I, Williams R, Finley W, et al. (1970) The effects of naps on nocturnal sleep: influence on the need for stage-1, REM and stage-4 sleep. Biol Psychiatry 2:391–399.
92. Guilleminault C, Powell N, Martinez S, et al. (2003) Preliminary observations on the effects of sleep time in a sleep restriction paradigm. Sleep Med 4:177–184.
93. Vogel G (1975) A review of REM sleep deprivation. Arch Gen Psychiatry 32:749–761.
94. Nykamp K, Rosenthal L, Folkerts M, et al. (1998) The effects of REM sleep deprivation on the level of sleepiness/alertness. Sleep 21:609–614.
95. Carskadon MA, Dement WC (1981) Cumulative effects of sleep restriction on daytime sleepiness. Psychophysiology 18:107–113.
96. Van Dongen H, Baynard M, Maislin G, et al. (2004) Systematic interindividual differences in neurobehavioral impairment from sleep loss: evidence of trait-like differential vulnerability. Sleep 27:423–433.
97. Bonnet M (1989) Infrequent periodic sleep disruption: effects on sleep, performance and mood. Physiol Behav 45:1049–1055.
98. Bonnet M (1989) The effect of sleep fragmentation on sleep and performance in younger and older subjects. Neurobiol Aging 10:21–25.
99. Stepanski E, Lamphere J, Badia P (1984) Sleep fragmentation and daytime sleepiness. Sleep 7:18–26.
100. Martin S, Brander P, Deary I, et al. (1999) The effect of clustered versus regular sleep fragmentation on daytime function. J Sleep Res 8:305–311.
101. Fleetham J, West P, Mezon B, et al. (1982) Sleep, arousals, and oxygen desaturation in chronic obstructive pulmonary disease. Am Rev Respir Dis 126:429–433.
102. Saskin P, Moldofsky H, Lue F (1986) Sleep and post traumatic rheumatic pain modulation disorder (fibrositis syndrome). Psychosom Med 48:319–323.
103. Dijk D, Duffy J, Czeisler C (2001) Age-related increase in awakenings: impaired consolidation of nonREM sleep at all circadian phases. Sleep 24:565–577.
104. Lubin A, Hord DJ, Tracy ML, et al. (1976) Effects of exercise, bedrest and napping on performance decrement during 40 hours. Psychophysiology 13:334–339.
105. Webb W, Agnew H (1973) Effects on performance of high and low energy expenditure during sleep deprivation. Percept Mot Skills 37:511–514.
106. Williams H, Lubin A, Goodnow J (1959) Impaired performance with sleep loss. Psychol Monogr 73:1–26.
107. Johnson L, Slye E, Dement W (1965) Electroencephalographic and autonomic activity during and after prolonged sleep deprivation. Psychsom Med 27:415–423.
108. Horne JA (1985) Sleep function, with particular reference to sleep deprivation. Ann Clin Res 17:199–208.
109. Dement W, Vaughan C (1999) *The Promise of Sleep*. Delacorte Press, New York, NY.
110. Czeisler C, Weitzman E, Moore-Ede M (1980) Human sleep: its duration and organization depend on its circadian phase. Science 210:1264–1267.
111. Dijk D, Duffy J, Czeisler C (1992) Circadian and sleep/wake dependent aspects of subjective alertness and cognitive performance. J Sleep Res 1:112–117.
112. Thorpy M (2001) Current concepts in the etiology, diagnosis and treatment of narcolepsy. Sleep Med 2:5–17.
113. National Institutes of Health. National Heart, Lung, and Blood Institute *Narcolepsy*. Bethesda, MD, 1996.
114. Goswami M (1998) The influence of clinical symptoms on quality of life in patients with narcolepsy. Neurology 50:S31–S36.
115. Broughton W, Broughton J (1994) Psychosocial impact of narcolepsy. Sleep 17:S45–S49.
116. Kadotani H, Faraco J, Mignot E (1998) Genetic studies in the sleep disorder narcolepsy. Genome Res 8:427–434.
117. Mignot E, Hayduk R, Black J, et al. (1997) HLA DQB1*0602 is associated with cataplexy in 509 narcoleptic patients. Sleep 20:1012–1020.
118. Takahashi J (1999) Narcolepsy genes wake up the sleep field. Science 285:2076–2077.

119. Lin L, Faraco J, Li R, et al. (1999) The sleep disorder canine narcolepsy is caused by a mutation in the hypocretin (orexin) receptor 2 gene. Cell 42:365–376.
120. Chemelli R, Willei J, Sinton C, et al. (1999) Narcolepsy in orexin knockout mice: molecular genetics of sleep regulation. Cell 98:437–451.
121. Nishino S, RIpley B, Overeem S, et al. (2000) Hypocretin (orexin) deficiency in human narcolepsy. Lancet 355:39–40.
122. Mignot E, Chen W, Black J (2003) On the value of measuring CSF hypocretin-1 in diagnosing narcolepsy. Sleep 26:646–649.
123. Mignot E, Lammers G, Ripley B, et al. (2002) The role of cerebrospinal fluid hypocretin measurement in the diagnosis of narcolepsy and other hypersomnias. Arch Neurol 59:1553–1562.
124. Bassetti C, Aldrich M (1997) Idiopathic hypersomnia: a series of 42 patients. Brain 120:1423–1435.
125. Billiard M (1996) Idiopathic hypersomnia. Neurol Clin 14:573–582.
126. Bonnet M, Arand D (1998) Sleepiness as measured by the MSLT varies as a function of preceding activity. Sleep 21:477–483.
127. Bonnet M, Arand D (1995) 24-Hour metabolic rate in insomniacs and matched normal sleepers. Sleep 18:581–588.
128. Stepanski E, Zorick F, Roehrs T, et al. (1988) Daytime alertness in patients with chronic insomnia compared with asymptomatic control subjects. Sleep 11:54–60.
129. Schneider-Helmert D (1987) Twenty-four-hour sleep-wake function and personality patterns in chronic insomniacs and healthy controls. Sleep 10:452–462.
130. Stepanski E, Zorick F, Roehrs T, et al. (2000) Effects of sleep deprivation on daytime sleepiness in primary insomnia. Sleep 23:215–219.
131. Gunter T, van der Zance R, Wiethoff M, et al. (1987) Visual selective attention during meaningful noise and after sleep deprivation. Electroencephalogr Clin Neurophysiol 40(Suppl):99–107.
132. Hartley L, Shirley E (1977) Sleep-loss, noise and decisions. Ergonomics 20:481–489.
133. Reyner L, Horne J (1998) Evaluation of "in-car" countermeasures to sleepiness: cold air and radio. Sleep 21:46–50.
134. Phipps-Nelson J, Redman J, Dijk D, et al. (2003) Daytime exposure to bright light, as compared to dim light, decreases sleepiness and improves psychomotor vigilance performance. Sleep 26:695–700.
135. Hartmann E, Orzack M, Branconnier R (1977) Sleep deprivation deficits and their reversal by d- and l-amphetamine. Psychopharmacology 53:185–189.
136. Fischman M, Schuster C (1980) Cocaine effects in sleep-deprived humans. Psychopharmacology 72:1–8.
137. Dinges D, Doran S, Mullington J, et al. (2000) Neurobehavioral effects of 66 h of sustained low-dose caffeine during 88 h of total sleep deprivation [abstract]. Sleep 23:A20.
138. Wyatt J, Dijk D, Ritz-De Cecco A, et al. (2000) Low-dose, repeated caffeine administration as a countermeasure to neurobehavioral deficits during a forced desynchrony protocol [abstract]. Sleep 23:A45.
139. Mitler M, Harsh J, Hirshkowitz M, et al. (2000) Long-term efficacy and safety of modafinil (Provigil) for the treatment of excessive daytime sleepiness associated with narcolepsy. Sleep Med 1:231–243.
140. Zwyghuizen-Doorenbos A, Roehrs T, Lamphere J, et al. (1988) Increased daytime sleepiness enhances ethanol's sedative effects. Neuropsychopharmacology 1:279–286.
141. Nicholson A (1983) Antihistamines and sedation. Lancet 2:211–212.
142. Weiler J, Bloomfield J, Woodworth G, et al. (2000) Effects of fexofenadine, diphenhydramine, and alcohol on driving performance: a randomized, placebo-controlled trial in the Iowa driving simulator. Ann Intern Med 132:354–363.
143. Paykel E, Fleminger R, Watson J (1982) Psychiatric side effects of antihypertensive drugs other than reserpine. J Clin Psychopharmacol 2:14–39.
144. Chervin R (2000) Sleepiness, fatigue, tiredness, and lack of energy in obstructive sleep apnea. Chest 118:372–379.
145. Manber R, Bootzin R, Acebo C, et al. (1996) The effects of regularizing sleep-wake schedules on daytime sleepiness. Sleep 19:432–441.
146. Bonnet M, Gomez S, Wirth O, et al. (1995) The use of caffeine versus prophylactic naps in sustained performance. Sleep 18:97–104.
147. Bonnet M, Arand D (1994) Impact of naps and caffeine on extended nocturnal performance. Physiol Behav 56:103–109.
148. Horne J, Reyner L (1995) Driver sleepiness. J Sleep Res 4:23–29.
149. Horne J, Reyner L (1999) Vehicle accidents related to sleep: a review. Occup Environ Med 56:289–294.

7 Central Sleep Apnea

Implications for the Failing Heart

Virend K. Somers, MD, PhD

Contents

INTRODUCTION

Central sleep apnea (CSA), which refers to a periodic breathing pattern occurring during sleep has been increasingly recognized as a potentially important pathophysiological characteristic, and perhaps mechanism, in the pathogenesis of heart failure. CSA may also occur in premature infants and healthy individuals, particularly those at high altitudes, and may also manifest in response to certain medications as well as after structural damage to the central nervous system.

It is clear that heart failure is a systemic disease and that neuroendocrine adaptations that accompany heart failure may in fact contribute to symptoms and to disease pathophysiology. Strategies that seek to attenuate the neuroendocrine manifestations of heart failure include blocking the renin–angiotensin systems, the aldosterone system, and the sympathetic nervous system *(1–3)*. All of these approaches have yielded considerable benefit in terms of functional status as well as hard cardiovascular end points. Nevertheless, despite multiple available options for treating heart failure, the rapid increase in heart failure prevalence and the high associated mortality has placed great importance on identification of prognostic markers and alternative treatment strategies. Recognition of the potential importance of CSA in heart failure has been highly enhanced by speculative mortality benefits that may be conferred by treatment of CSA.

This review will examine the mechanisms by which CSA may occur in patients with heart failure, the prevalence of CSA in the heart failure population, the cardiovascular consequences of central apnea and its potential implications for mortality, and the effects of treatment of central apnea on outcomes in heart failure patients.

From: *Current Clinical Practice: Primary Care Sleep Medicine: A Practical Guide*
Edited by: J. F. Pagel and S. R. Pandi-Perumal © Humana Press Inc., Totowa, NJ

MECHANISMS ELICITING CSA IN HEART FAILURE

The genesis of central apnea in the heart failure patient population is complex and not well understood. Several hypotheses have been proposed including that periodic breathing is a self-sustaining oscillation that occurs secondary to the loss of stability in the closed-loop chemical control of ventilation *(4,5)*. This instability may be secondary to an enhanced-loop gain (hyperventilation), delayed circulation time between lungs and chemoreceptors, and abnormalities in chemoreflex sensitivity. During nonrapid-eye-movement sleep, hyperventilation from whatever cause may lower PCO_2 below the apnea threshold, thus inducing apnea. Consequent hypoxia elicits chemoreflex activation and subsequent hyperventilation. In the presence of instability in this control loop, periodic breathing may be initiated, with oscillations of PCO_2 more than and less than the apnea threshold.

A potential important contributor to the periodic breathing pattern may be an enhanced sensitivity to CO_2, which has been demonstrated in heart failure patients with central apnea as compared with those without central apnea *(6)*. A unifying hypothesis attempting to reconcile the clinical controversies regarding the pathogenesis of central apnea in heart failure has been proposed using a model theory *(7)*. Factors implicated in facilitating ventilatory instability in heart failure that were cited included low-cardiac output, low ventilation, small lung volumes, a high alveolar-atmospheric CO_2 difference, and a long lag to chemoreflex response. The major contributors appear to be the enhanced hypercapnic chemoreflex gain and a prolonged lag to ventilatory response.

It is likely that other factors, including pulmonary congestion with decreased lung compliance and increased intracardiac filling pressures may be involved *(8–11)*. The likelihood of CSA is increased in patients with higher pulmonary capillary wedge pressures, and afterload reduction with consequent decrease in cardiac filling pressures has been shown to acutely attenuate CSA.

Prevalence of CSA in Congestive Heart Failure

A clear understanding of the true prevalence of central apnea in heart failure has been very limited by selection biases in population samples from the different studies. For example, prevalence data based on referrals to the sleep laboratory would reflect a biased population, namely those who would be selected as probably having sleep apnea. Furthermore, diagnostic criteria for central apnea may differ between studies. Also important is that changes in heart failure severity may affect the severity of central apnea at any given time. Because heart failure is such a dynamic and often unstable disease condition, the prevalence of central apnea may vary according to the nature of the disease. In understanding the relative likelihood of obstructive or CSA in heart failure, it is also important to recognize that central apnea tends to be present in the more lean heart failure patient. How increased obesity in the heart failure population may be affecting the prevalence and type of apnea is not known. Whether recent innovations in treatment of heart failure may affect CSA prevalence also remains unclear. For example, because the autonomic nervous system contributes so importantly to chemoreflex control, do β-blockers have any discernible effect on the prevalence of central apnea in the heart failure population?

Recognizing these limitations, it nevertheless appears that up to 50% of patients in a heart failure patient population may have significant CSA *(12,13)*. The prevalence in unselected patients with diastolic heart failure remains unclear. Also important is that in studies of patients with left ventricular (LV) dysfunction, before the development of overt heart failure, there appears to be a significant likelihood of CSA, as high as 50% *(14)*. Whether the CSA in the LV dysfunction population potentiates the subsequent development of overt heart failure is not known.

Implications of CSA in Heart Failure

A number of studies have implicated CSA as a marker of poorer prognosis in heart failure patients *(15–17)*. In a clinically stable population with moderate-to-severe heart failure, an apnea/hypopnea index 30 or more is accompanied by very high 2-year cardiac mortality, independent of other known risk factors including ejection fraction, peak VO_2, and noninvasive indices of elevated filling pressure. More recent data have also suggested that the presence of a periodic breathing pattern during exercise may also independently predict cardiac mortality in chronic heart failure patients awaiting cardiac transplantation *(18)*. Whereas central apnea may be a consequence of heart failure, it has hence also been proposed that the repetitive apneas and arousals during sleep may themselves contribute to the cardiovascular pathophysiological process, as described next.

Heart failure patients with CSA appear to have higher levels of sympathetic activation, as evidenced by plasma and urine norepinephrines *(19)*. This may be in large part linked to chemoreflex activation, because even though resting sympathetic traffic is high in patients with heart failure, sympathetic activation increases even further during apneic episodes *(20)*. These increases in sympathetic drive during apnea elicit cyclical changes in blood pressure, which—although relatively modest compared with the pressor response to obstructive apnea—may be problematic in the context of the failing heart.

Other autonomic problems that may occur with central apnea include bradyarrhythmias *(21–23)*. Bradyarrhythmias facilitated by the diving reflex—as described in Chapter 9 (Evidence and Mechanisms Linking Obstructive Sleep Apnea to Cardiovascular Disease)—may be less easily tolerated by the failing heart. Whether bradyarrhythmias are potentiated in the heart failure patient population is not known. The relevance of any bradyarrhythmias during apnea in the heart failure population in terms of mortality is also not known. An increased likelihood of daytime ventricular arrhythmias has been noted in heart failure patients and LV dysfunction patients with CSA vs those without CSA. Whereas obstructive apnea has been linked to multiple neuroendocrine changes such as higher levels of endothelin and systemic inflammation, the effects of central apnea on atrial natriuretic peptide, brain natriuretic peptide, and vasoactive substances remain to be determined.

Whether the arrhythmias and/or neuroendocrine activation may be implicated in the heightened mortality present in heart failure patients with CSA remains unclear. Namely, the pathophysiological characteristics of heart failure patients with CSA may be part of the underlying heart failure pathophysiology, with CSA as an epiphenomenon. Alternatively, CSA occurring during heart failure may activate pathological mechanisms that contribute to progression of heart failure and to increased mortality. These questions remain unanswered and are addressed later.

Treatment of CSA in Congestive Heart Failure

It is generally accepted that improved heart failure management reduces central apnea severity. This may in part relate to decreases in pulmonary congestion, improved circulation times, blunted neurohumoral activation, and decreased cardiac filling pressures.

Other strategies that have been tried to include administration of low levels of oxygen during sleep *(24–26)*. Theophylline, a phosphodiesterase inhibitor has been shown to significantly attenuate CSA in heart failure *(27)*. However, given the potential adverse cardiovascular effects of phosphodiesterase inhibitors in heart failure, any long-term benefit of this strategy in the heart failure patient population remains unproven. Other strategies that seek to modulate ventilatory control, particularly by acting on carbon dioxide levels, include acetazolamide. Again, long-term benefits are not known.

Continuous positive airway pressure and refinements on this approach such as the use of adaptive ventilation (Servo Ventilator; Siemens-Elma AB; Sweden) and bilateral pressure ventilation (BiPAP ventilation system; Respironics Inc; Murrysville, PA) have also been proposed as treatment strategies in heart failure patients *(28–30)*. Heart failure patients are often less tolerant of mechanical approaches to breathing control. Nevertheless, several studies have suggested that these approaches may significantly decrease the severity of central apnea. Indeed, one long-term study noted that more than 5 years, heart failure patients with CSA randomly assigned to receive continuous positive airway pressure treatment had an improved transplant-free survival compared with those randomly assigned to receive no treatment *(31)*. However, when analyzed on an intention-to-treat basis, these results fell short of showing significant benefit. A large randomized study addressing this overall question, the CANPAP (Canadian Positive Airway Pressure) trial *(32)* was prematurely discontinued and outcome results from the study are pending.

Recent evidence has suggested that cardiac pacing may confer some benefit in sleep apnea. In one of the earliest studies in this area, in a population without heart failure, it was shown that atrial overdrive pacing significantly attenuated both obstructive and CSA *(33)*. The mechanisms for any such benefit are not easily understood. More mechanistically appealing is the potential benefit of biventricular pacing or cardiac resynchronization therapy in attenuating central apnea. This therapeutic approach has been shown to significantly decrease mortality in heart failure patient populations with ejection fractions less than 30%. Given the high cost of cardiac resynchronization therapy and the high and rising prevalence of heart failure, the cost effectiveness of placing biventricular pacemakers for heart failure in eligible patients has been widely debated. Consequently, there is great importance in identifying more specifically those heart failure patients who are most likely to benefit from cardiac resynchronization therapy. Recent data suggest that in patients with a low ejection fraction of around 24% and left bundle branch block, cardiac resynchronization therapy significantly lowered the severity of CSA and highly improved sleep quality *(34)*. The mechanisms of this benefit are not known, but may relate to changes in intracardiac filling pressures. An intriguing possibility is that it may be that those heart failure patients who also have CSA who are most likely to benefit from cardiac resynchronization therapy. However, at this time, any such assertion remains speculative.

CONCLUSIONS

It is clear that CSA is an important problem in heart failure. Whether the abnormal breathing pattern is a cause or consequence of cardiac dysfunction remains unclear. Another factor needing consideration is that disrupted sleep in response to severe central apnea in heart failure may contribute in part to the daytime fatigue and other problems that are manifested in the heart failure patient population. How CSA and its implications relate to the presence of periodic breathing patterns, without apnea, during resting, wakefulness, and exercise also needs to be addressed. Limited available options for effectively treating central apnea in heart failure as well as the multiple comorbidities that accompany heart failure have made it difficult to identify any compelling etiological link between central apnea and heart failure outcome. Most important is that it is not known whether treatment of the central apnea has beneficial or detrimental effects on heart failure outcomes. The advent of cardiac resynchronization therapy in the treatment of selected heart failure patients provides some early promise in improving both the understanding of and the treatment options for patients with heart failure and CSA.

REFERENCES

1. Hunt SA, Baker DW, Chin MH, et al. (2001) ACC/AHA Guidelines for the Evaluation and Management of Chronic Heart Failure in the Adult: Executive Summary A Report of the American College of Cardiology/American Heart Association Task Force on Practice Guidelines (Committee to Revise the 1995 Guidelines for the Evaluation and Management of Heart Failure); Developed in Collaboration With the International Society for Heart and Lung Transplantation; Endorsed by the Heart Failure Society of America. Circulation 104:2996–3007.
2. Effects of enalapril on mortality in severe congestive heart failure: results of the Cooperative North Scandinavian Enalapril Survival Study (CONSENSUS); The CONSENSUS Trial Study Group. (1987) N Engl J Med 316:1429–1435.
3. Effect of metoprolol CR/XL in chronic heart failure: Metoprolol CR/XL Randomised Intervention Trial in Congestive Heart Failure (MERIT-HF). (1999) Lancet 353:2001–2007.
4. Khoo MCK, Kronauer RE, Strohl KH, et al. (1982) Factors inducing periodic breathing in humans: a general model. J Appl Physiol 53:644–659.
5. Pinna GD, Maestri R, Mortara A, et al. (2000) Periodic breathing in heart failure patients: testing the hypothesis of instability of the chemoreflex loop. J Appl Physiol 89:2147–2157.
6. Javaheri S (1999) A mechanism of central sleep apnea in patients with heart failure. N Engl J Med 341:949–954.
7. Francis DP, Willson K, Davies CL, et al. (2000) Quantitative general theory for periodic breathing in chronic heart failure and its clinical implications. Circulation 102:2214–2221.
8. Solin P, Bergin P, Richardson M, et al. (1999) Influence of pulmonary capillary wedge pressure on central apnea in heart failure. Circulation 99:1574–1579.
9. Lanfranchi PA, Somers VK (2003) Sleep-disorderd breathing in heart failure: characteristics and implications. Respir Physiol Neurobiol 136:153–165.
10. Giannuzzi P, Imparato A, Temporelli PL, et al. (1994) Doppler-derived mitral deceleration time of early filling as a strong predictor of pulmonary capillary wedge pressure in postinfarction patients with left ventricular systolic dysfunction. J Am Coll Cardiol 23:1630–1637.
11. Dark DS, Pingleton SK, Kerby GR, et al. (1987) Breathing pattern abnormalities and arterial oxygen desaturation during sleep in the congestive heart failure syndrome: improvement following medical therapy. Chest 91:833–836.
12. Javaheri S, Parker TJ, Liming JD, et al. (1998) Sleep apnea in 81 ambulatory male patients with stable heart failure: types and their prevalences, consequences, and presentations. Circulation 97: 2154–2159.
13. Sin DD, Fitzgerald F, Parker JD, et al. (1999) Risk factors for central and obstructive sleep apnea in 450 men and women with congestive heart failure. Am J Respir Crit Care Med 160:1101–1106.
14. Lanfranchi PA, Somers VK, Braghiroli A, et al. (2003) Central sleep apnea in left ventricular dysfunction, prevalence and implications for arrhythmic risk. Circulation 107:727–732.
15. Hanly PJ, Zuberi-Khokhar NS (1996) Increased mortality associated with Cheyne-Stokes respiration in patients with congestive heart failure. Am J Respir Crit Care Med 153:272–276.
16. Lanfranchi PA, Braghiroli A, Bosimini E, et al. (1999) Prognostic value of nocturnal Cheyne-Stokes respiration in chronic heart failure. Circulation 99:1435–1440.
17. Findley LJ, Zwillich CW, Ancoli-Israel S, et al. (1985) Cheyne-Stokes breathing during sleep in patients with left ventricular heart failure. South Med J 78:11–15.

18. Leite JJ, Mansur AJ, de Freitas H, et al. (2003) Periodic breathing during incremental exercise predicts mortality in patients with chronic heart failure evaluated for cardiac transplantation. J Am Coll Cardiol 41:2175–2188.
19. Naughton MT, Benard DC, Liu PP, et al. (1995) Effects of nasal CPAP on sympathetic activity in patients with heart failure and central sleep apnea. Am J Respir Crit Care Med 152:473–479.
20. van de Borne P, Oren R, Abouassaly C, et al. (1998) Effect of Cheyne-Stokes respiration on muscle sympathetic nerve activity in severe congestive heart failure. Am J Cardiol 81:432–436.
21. Guilleminault C, Connolly SJ, Winkle RA (1983) Cardiac arrhythmia and conduction disturbances during sleep in 400 patients with sleep apnea syndrome. Am J Cardiol 52:490–494.
22. Grimm W, Hoffmann J, Menz V (1996) Electrophysiologic evaluation of sinus function and atrioventricular conduction in patients with prolonged ventricular asystole during obstructive sleep apnea. Am J Cardiol 77:1310–1314.
23. Daly MD, Angell-James JE, Elsner R (1979) Role of carotid-body chemoreceptors and their reflex interactions in bradycardia and cardiac arrest. Lancet 1(8119):764–767.
24. Hanly PJ, Millar TW, Steljes DG, et al. (1989) The effect of oxygen on respiration and sleep in patients with congestive heart failure. Ann Intern Med 111:777–782.
25. Staniforth AD, Kinnear WJ, Starling R, et al. (1998) Effect of oxygen on sleep quality, cognitive function and sympathetic activity in patients with chronic heart failure and Cheyne-Stokes respiration. Eur Heart J 19:922–928.
26. Javaheri S, Ahmed M, Parker TJ, et al. (1999) Effects of nasal O_2 on sleep-related disordered breathing in ambulatory patients with stable heart failure. Sleep 22:1101–1106.
27. Javaheri S, Parker TJ, Wexler L, et al. (1996) Effect of theophylline on sleep-disordered breathing in heart failure. N Engl J Med 335:562–567.
28. Issa FG, Sullivan CE (1986) Reversal of central sleep apnea using nasal CPAP. Chest 90:165–171.
29. Naughton MT, Liu PP, Benard DC, et al. (1995) Treatment of congestive heart failure and Cheyne-Stokes respiration during sleep by continuous positive airway pressure. Am J Respir Crit Care Med 151:92–97.
30. Teschler H, Döhring J, Wang YM, et al. (2001) Adaptive pressure support servo-ventilation: a novel treatment for Cheyne-Stokes respiration in heart failure. Am J Respir Crit Care Med 164:614–619.
31. Sin DD, Logan AG, Fitzgerald FS, et al. (2000) Effects of continuous positive airway pressure on cardiovascular outcomes in heart failure patients with and without Cheyne-Stokes respiration. Circulation 102:61–66.
32. Bradley TD, Logan AG, Floras JS (2001) Rationale and design of the Canadian Continuous Positive Airway Pressure Trial for Congestive Heart Failure patients with Central Sleep Apnea—CANPAP. Can J Cardiol 17:677–684.
33. Garrigue S, Bordier P, Jais P, et al. (2002) Benefit of atrial pacing in sleep apnea syndrome. N Engl J Med 346:404–412.
34. Sinha A, Skobel EC, Breithardt O, et al. (2004) Cardiac resynchronization therapy improves central sleep apnea and Cheyne-Stokes respiration in patients with chronic heart failure. J Am Coll Cardiol 44:68–71.

8 Obstructive Sleep Apnea

Clinical Presentation

Charles W. Atwood, Jr., MD, FCCP

CONTENTS

INTRODUCTION

Obstructive sleep apnea (OSA) is associated with a decreased quality of life *(1)* and increased morbidity, particularly an increased risk for driving accidents because of falling asleep or inattention *(2)* and cardiovascular disease *(3)*. However, before sleep apnea can be diagnosed, it must be considered as a possible diagnosis. Clinical presentation and recognition is crucial in considering OSA as an explanation for a group of symptoms and clinical findings. How do patients present when they have OSA? Whom do they go to for evaluation? Are there differences between genders and races? These questions will be addressed in this chapter.

OBSTRUCTIVE SLEEP APNEA

OSA is condition of abnormal pharyngeal narrowing and closure during sleep. During sleep, some degree of pharyngeal narrowing is normal in healthy humans. Thus, OSA is a disorder of degrees and thresholds. OSA is dependent on how frequently narrowing occurs, how severe it is, and for how long it occurs. Although the optimal way to define sleep apnea is not known, the most common metric of defining sleep apnea is the apnea-hypopnea index (AHI). This measure takes into account the number of apneas and hypopneas recorded per hour of sleep. The denominator in this

From: *Current Clinical Practice: Primary Care Sleep Medicine: A Practical Guide*
Edited by: J. F. Pagel and S. R. Pandi-Perumal © Humana Press Inc., Totowa, NJ

metric is the total sleep time, because the total sleep time is known from the polysomnogram. A similar metric is the respiratory disturbance index (RDI). The RDI differ from the AHI in two ways. One is that, in addition to measuring apneas and hypopneas, the RDI may also measure other respiratory abnormal findings such as inspiratory flow limited events. Another difference is that the denominator used may be the total recording time, instead of the total sleep time. This metric is most commonly used in portable sleep studies in which sleep *per se* is not measured, but rather is estimated from the total recording period. This may lead to a slight tendency for portable monitors to underestimate sleep-disordered breathing, because the total recording time is always less than the total sleep time.

EPIDEMIOLOGY

Realizing how common the disease is in the general population is the first step in understanding its clinical presentation. OSA syndrome is a very common condition that affects approx 5% of Western populations *(4,5)*. This value is probably somewhat of an underestimate, as most prevalence studies in the United States tended to underrepresent minorities, some of which are strongly suspected of having a higher prevalence. Some minority groups such as African-Americans, probably have a higher prevalence than whites, but only one large study has examined these potential ethnic differences in disease prevalence *(6)*. Men have a higher prevalence than women. In the Wisconsin Sleep Cohort study, the difference was about twofold *(4)*. Similar findings were noted in a similar prevalence trial from the Pennsylvania State University study *(7,8)*.

CLINICAL PRESENTATION

The way in which patients present with OSA depends on several factors, including age, gender, race, and comorbidities. However, several symptoms are common to most clinical presentations. These include loud and frequently socially embarrassing or disruptive snoring, nocturnal choking, and gasping episodes that awaken the patient from sleep, and excessive daytime sleepiness (EDS).

Snoring

Snoring is common. Habitual snoring affects up to 50% of men and up to 30% of women in the general population *(9)*. The noise results in disturbed sleep for the bed partner and other household members. This may lead to bed partners sleeping apart, marital discord, and higher risk for divorce *(10)*. When sleep clinic populations are studied, the symptom of snoring is roughly equal between men and women *(11)*. If community populations are studied, then men have a higher prevalence of snoring, compared with women. Snoring is the most common symptom of OSA, and it is the symptom that brings patients to clinical attention more than any other. However, it is not a particularly good predictor of sleep apnea, because it is so common in the general population *(12)*. Snoring is also an important symptom to use in long-term management of OSA, because its recurrence after OSA treatment may signal a need to re-evaluate the therapy.

Nocturnal Choking/Gasping

This is a somewhat difficult symptom to understand. Bed partners will often report that the patient has periods of witnessed breathing cessation that ends with an episode of choking, gasping, or sputtering followed by resumption of normal breathing. Patients themselves will experience such an episode that culminates in an awakening long enough for them to be aware of it. Choking/gasping episodes, because of sleep apnea, need to be differentiated from other causes of startled awakenings such as paroxysmal nocturnal dyspnea with congestive heart failure, nocturnal panic disorder, acute dyspnea from bronchospasm associated with asthma, or chronic obstructive pulmonary disease (COPD). Occasionally, patients with gastroesophageal reflux will complain of nocturnal fullness or choking sensation in their pharynx. Distinguishing between these different conditions can usually be done by taking a careful history of the events and by knowing the patient's other medical or psychiatric problems.

Excessive Daytime Sleepiness

EDS is also a common symptom in OSA. As with snoring, EDS, though common, does not reliably differentiate a normal state from disease state, because sleepiness is a common symptom in the general population. Sleepiness in OSA is thought to be caused by sleep fragmentation. This is probably only partially true. As the understanding of brain mechanisms of sleepiness improves, it is very likely that a more complete understanding of EDS will emerge. As a symptom, sleepiness may be confused with fatigue or lethargy. This is particularly difficult to sort out. Many sleep medicine physicians resort to standardized questionnaires and formal inquiry about EDS. The most commonly used instrument is the Epworth sleepiness scale *(13)*. Others include the Stanford sleepiness scale and the Karolinska scale and are generally reserved for research applications. The Epworth scale is popular, because it is short (eight questions) and has good face validity and psychometric properties (test/retest and correlation with other instruments of sleep sleepiness) *(14)*.

However, it is clearly not the same as an objective measure of sleep such as the multiple sleep latency test (MSLT). Benbadis and colleagues *(15)* compared the subjective Epworth scale with the objective MSLT in 102 clinic patients with a variety of sleep disorders. The overall degree of correlation between the two tests was 0.17 (using Pearson's *r*-test). Benbadis and colleagues concluded that there was no significant correlation between the two tests. Interestingly, in a community-based sample of subjects who underwent MSLT and Epworth, a better correlation was found *(16)*. Physiologically and psychologically, these two tests appear to measure somewhat related, but largely nonoverlapping aspects of sleepiness. Nonetheless, the Epworth scale is widely used and is useful in clinical practice, as is the MSLT. A number of validated fatigue self-report instruments have been developed such as the fatigue impact scale *(17)*.

Excessive sleepiness is a hallmark symptom of OSA, but it is also common in other disorders. At present, there have been no instruments that can distinguish subtypes of sleepiness across different disorders (if subtypes even exist). Some clinicians (personal conversations) feel that the sleepiness of narcolepsy is worse (more intense) than the sleepiness associated with OSA, but these differences are not easily quantifiable. In clinical practice, measurement of sleepiness is important. However, for routine management of OSA, subjective testing is adequate. A recent position paper from the American Academy of Sleep Medicine did not endorse routine use of the MSLT in OSA *(18)*.

OTHER COMMON PRESENTING SYMPTOMS OR SIGNS

Patients with OSA present with other symptoms besides the aforementioned cardinal symptoms.

Morning Headache

The exact frequency of this symptom is not known, nor is the mechanism. The headaches tend to be frontal and dull. They gradually dissipate during the ensuing period of wakefulness. Sleep apnea-related headaches tend to improve with treatment.

Restless Sleep

Patients with OSA may complain of this symptom or their bed partner may mention it. Patients with OSA tend to move around frequently in bed. Most of the time they are unaware of it while it occurs, but they may note that bed linens and bed partners are no longer in or on the bed when they awaken the next morning.

Obesity

Many, but not all, obese individuals have OSA. In an unpublished study of approx 506 morbidly obese men (24% of population) and women (76% of population), the author found that 56% of these patients had OSA, as defined by an AHI of 15 or more. This is a slightly higher prevalence of OSA in morbid obesity, body mass index of more than 35 kg/m^2, compared with other reports of the frequency of OSA in obesity, which have reported values in the 45–50% range *(19,20)*. In severe obesity, OSA may be present irrespective of symptoms and should be considered as part of a routine assessment of their health status.

Nocturia

Frequent urination at night is a bothersome symptom. Its prevalence is estimated to be approx 48% in a severe population of patients with sleep apnea in a typical sleep disorders clinic population *(21)*. In a recent study by Hajduk and colleagues *(22)*, 60% of women with OSA and 41% of men were affected. Treatment of OSA with continuous positive airway pressure decreased nocturia in a study published in Japan *(23)*.

Dry Mouth or Pharynx

This is a common symptom that is probably because of mouth breathing. In some cases, it may be a prominent cause for seeking attention for OSA, but more commonly, it is one of several reported symptoms referable to upper airway problems.

GENDER DIFFERENCES IN PRESENTATION OF OSA

Several excellent reviews of some gender differences in OSA have been published in the past 5 years *(24–27)*. These papers summarize the existing literature on this subject. Several highlights from these and some original research on this subject and reviews are presented.

1. Young and colleagues *(28)* present original research from the Wisconsin sleep cohort study about gender differences. In this study, women with an AHI of 15 or higher had more depressive symptoms, morning headache, and anxiety than men. No significant differences were found between men and women for the common sleep apnea symptoms of snoring, choking/gasping episodes, and daytime sleepiness. This is reassuring; it indicates that OSA is probably not a fundamentally different disorder across genders but that there are some moderate differences in particular aspects of presentation.
2. Another finding from Young and colleagues *(28)* is that women are more likely to be symptomatic from OSA at lower level of AHI than men. Women with an AHI of 2–5 were as symptomatic as women with an AHI of 5–15 and significantly more symptomatic than

women with an AHI of 0–2, whereas men with an AHI of 2–5 were indistinguishable from men with an AHI of 0–2.

3. Pregnancy is a vulnerable time for the development of OSA. Sleep problems in general are ubiquitous during pregnancy. The vast majority of women endure sleep problems during pregnancy rather than seek treatment for them *(24)*.
4. In an intriguing study from Canada, women were significantly more likely to present with insomnia symptoms with OSA rather than with EDS. Sherpertycky and colleagues *(27)* found that 17% of women in their population of 130 retrospectively and randomly selected female subjects with OSA had insomnia, compared with 5% of 130 randomly selected men from their database. This results in an odds ratio of 4.20, with 95% confidence intervals more than 1. In this study, men and women were otherwise similar in terms of percentage of patients with snoring, EDS, and witnessed apneas by bed partners. The reason for this difference is not known, but it is possible that it relates to the tendency of female patients with OSA to develop depressive symptoms.

RACIAL AND ETHNIC DIFFERENCES IN OSA PRESENTATION

Limited data exist on ethnic differences in presentation of OSA whereas relatively more data exist on racial differences in OSA severity and response to treatment *(11,29)*. Scharf and colleagues *(29)* studied African-American and white sleep apnea referrals to their sleep disorders program in Baltimore, MD. They found that there were no differences in symptoms at presentation between African-Americans and whites. At presentation, African-Americans were younger (by 5 years), were significantly heavier (body mass index of 39.7 ± 10.7 vs 33.4 ± 9.2 kg/m^2), and had lower incomes. Fortunately, treatment efficacy and adherence were no different between races.

PRESENTATION TO NONSLEEP MEDICINE SPECIALISTS

Patients present to doctors with symptoms and complaints and not diagnoses. This is true of sleep apnea as much as any other disorder. Patients with sleep apnea may present to their general or primary care physician with a variety of complaints that may lead that physician to consider sleep apnea. According to one study *(30)* about the behavior of physicians in diagnosing OSA, conducted in a staff model HMO, primary care physicians in the United States are reasonably good at identifying sleep apnea in very obese patients with classic symptoms of snoring, choking, and gasping episodes. However, in this study, the primary care physicians referred fewer than 1% of their patient panel for sleep evaluations, suggesting that they were missing many cases of sleep apnea that did not meet the "extremely obvious" level of recognition. Improved recognition of sleep apnea by primary care physicians is a crucial step in more awareness by the public in general.

Patients may present to other specialists with sleep complaints. The specialist physician may or may not recognize the presenting symptoms as being related to a sleep disorder. For example, a patient with cardiomyopathy and daytime fatigue may or may not be referred for sleep apnea evaluation, depending on if the cardiologist recognizes that cardiomyopathy patients are at high risk for OSA (and other forms of sleep-disordered breathing). An urologist may evaluate an obese young male for nocturia and recognize that OSA may be a significant contributor to this problem and that OSA therapy may result in decreased symptoms. Neurologists may refer patients for headache evaluations to determine if the recurrent headaches are because of OSA. Many nonsleep specialists have seen sleep apnea and remained unaware of it.

CONCLUSIONS

OSA is a common disorder that is easy to recognize if the common presentations are kept in mind. Unfortunately, the majority of patients with OSA continue to go unevaluated and, therefore, untreated. Less-than-optimal clinical recognition by physicians is one cause. Patient awareness is growing. Physician awareness is growing, as well. The current generation of trainees is in an era of more sleep-disorder awareness, compared with the generation before them. This should help with recognition, evaluation, and ultimately, treatment.

REFERENCES

1. Jenkinson C, Davies R, Mullins R, et al. (1999) Comparison of therapeutic and subtherapeutic nasal continuous positive airway pressure for obstructive sleep apnoea: a randomized prospective parallel trial. Lancet 353:2100–2105.
2. George C (2004) Sleep. 5: Driving and automobile crashes in patients with the apnoea/hypopnoea syndrome. Thorax 59:804–807.
3. Peker Y, Hedner J, Norum J, et al. (2002) Increased incidence of cardiovascular disease in middle-aged men with obstructive sleep apnea: a 7-year follow-up. Am J Respir Crit Care Med 166:159–165.
4. Young T, Palta M, Dempsey J, et al. (1993) The occurrence of sleep-disordered breathing among middle-aged adults. N Engl J Med 328:1230–1235.
5. Young T, Peppard PE, Gottlieb DJ (2002) Epidemiology of obstructive sleep apnea: a population health perspective. Am J Respir Crit Care Med 165:1217–1239.
6. Tishler PV, Larkin EK, Schluchter MD, et al. (2003) Incidence of sleep-disordered breathing in an urban adult population: the relative importance of risk factors in the development of sleep-disordered breathing. JAMA 289:2230–2237.
7. Bixler EO, Vgontzas AN, Lin H-M, et al. (2001) Prevalence of sleep-disordered breathing in women. effects of gender. Am J Respir Crit Care Med 163:608–613.
8. Bixler EO, Vgontzad AN, Ten Have T, et al. (1998) Effects of age on sleep apnea in men. I: prevalence and severity. Am J Respir Crit Care Med 157:144–148.
9. Ohayon M, Guilleminault C, Priest R, et al. (1997) Snoring and breathing pauses during sleep: telephone interview survey of a United Kingdom population sample. BMJ 314:860–863.
10. Grunstein R, Senlof K, Hedner J, et al. (1995) Impact of self-reported sleep-breathing disturbances on psychosocial performance in the Swedish obese subjects (SOS) study. Sleep 18:635–643.
11. Redline S, Kump K, Tishler PV, et al. (1994) Gender differences in sleep-disordered breathing in a community-based sample. Am J Respir Crit Care Med 149:722–726.
12. Viner S, Szalai J, Hoffstein V (1991) Are history and physical examination a good screening test for sleep apnea? Ann Intern Med 115:356–359.
13. Johns M (1991) A new method for measuring daytime sleepiness: the Epworth Sleepiness Scale. Sleep 14:540–545.
14. Johns M (1992) Reliability and factor analysis of the Epworth Sleepiness Scale. Sleep 15:376–381.
15. Benbadis S, Mascha E, Perry M, et al. (1999) Association between the Epworth Sleepiness Scale and the Multiple Sleep Latency Test in a clinical population. Ann Intern Med 130:289–292.
16. Punjabi N, Bandeen-Roche K, Young T (2003) Predictors of objective sleep tendency in the general population. Sleep 26:678–683.
17. Fisk J, Ritvo P, Ross L, et al. (1994) Measuring the functional impact of fatigue: initial validation of the fatigue impact scale. Clin Infect Dis 18:S79–S83.
18. Littner M, Kushida C, Wise M, et al. (2005) Practice parameters for clinical use of the Multiple Sleep Latency Test and the Maintenance of Wakefulness Test. Sleep 28:113–121.
19. van Kralingen K, de Kanter W, de Groot G, et al. (1998) Assessment of sleep complaints and sleep-disordered breathing in a consecutive series of obese patients. Respiration 66:312–316.
20. Laaban J-P, Cassuto D, Orvoen-Frija E, et al. (1998) Cardiorespiratory consequences of sleep apnoea syndrome in patients with massive obesity. Eur Respir J 11:20–27.
21. Hajduk I, Jasani R, Strollo P, et al. (2001) Nocturia in sleep disordered breathing. Sleep Med 1:263–267.
22. Hajduk I, Strollo P, Jasani R, et al. (2002) Prevalence and predictors of nocturia in obstructive sleep apnea-hypopnea syndrome (osahs): a retrospective study. Sleep 26:61–64.

23. Akashiba T, Otsuka K, Yoshizawa T, et al. (1991) Effects of nasal continuous positive airway pressure (NCPAP) on nocturnal renal function in obstructive sleep apnea syndrome (OSAS). Jpn J Thor Dis 29:573–577.
24. Collop N, Adkins D, Phillips B (2004) Gender differences in sleep and sleep-disordered breathing. Clin Chest Med 25:257–268.
25. Kapsimalis F, Kryger M (2002) Gender and obstructive sleep apnea syndrome, part 1: clinical features. Sleep 25:409–416.
26. Schlosshan D, Elliot M (2005) Sleep 3: Clinical presentation and diagnosis of the obstructive sleep apnoea hypopnoea syndrome. Thorax 59:347–352.
27. Sherpertycky M, Banno K, Kryger M (2005) Differences between men and women in the clinical presentation of patients diagnosed with obstructive sleep apnea syndrome. Sleep 28:309–314.
28. Young T, Hutton R, Finn L, et al. (1996) The gender bias in sleep apnea diagnosis: are women missed because they have different symptoms. Arch Intern Med 156:2445–2451.
29. Scharf S, Seiden L, DeMore J, et al. (2004) Racial differences in clinical presentation of patients with sleep-disordered breathing. Sleep Breath 8:173–183.
30. Kramer N, Cook T, Carlisle C, et al. (1999) The role of the primary care physician in recognizing obstructive sleep apnea. Arch Intern Med 159:965–968.

9 Obstructive Sleep Apnea/Hypopnea Syndrome

Epidemiology and Pathogenesis

Brian A. Boehlecke, MD, MSPH, FCCP

CONTENTS

INTRODUCTION

The obstructive sleep apnea/hypopnea syndrome (OSAHS) includes a constellation of symptoms, most prominently excessive daytime somnolence and unrefreshing sleep, associated with sleep-disordered breathing (SDB). The periodic respiratory events constituting SDB may be complete cessation of airflow (apneas), reductions in airflow of various degree (hypopneas), increased respiratory "effort" events with no increase in airflow (flow limitation events), or a combination of these events occurring at various times during the sleep period. Unrefreshing sleep and excessive daytime somnolence are thought to be because of disruption of the normal sleep architecture from recurrent brief arousals associated with the respiratory events, usually resulting in reduced "deep" (slow wave) and rapid eye movement sleep. Oxyhemoglobin desaturation, often severe, usually accompanies the respiratory events and may be a major factor in the cardiovascular morbidity associated with OSAHS. However, this satisfyingly simple and logical construct for OSHAS is likely an oversimplification. The lack of universally accepted criteria for defining a specific disease entity and the lack of certainty about the causal relationship of the various types of respiratory events and associated arousals/desaturations with symptoms and the pathophysiological consequences, limit the understanding of the prevalence, risk factors, and natural history of clinically important SDB.

From: *Current Clinical Practice: Primary Care Sleep Medicine: A Practical Guide*
Edited by: J. F. Pagel and S. R. Pandi-Perumal © Humana Press Inc., Totowa, NJ

In 1998, Young and Finn *(1)* pointed out several important epidemiological aspects of SDB still needing further study. They cited inadequate information on the causal role of SDB in the development or exacerbation of adverse health outcomes, the effect of aging on SDB, and the impact of risk-factor reduction and treatment on the natural history of SDB. Much has been learned as this paper and a previous review by this author *(2)*, both from additional studies of population-based samples providing a better understanding of the syndrome in the general population, compared with that in patients presenting to sleep disorders clinics and clinical/laboratory studies in humans and animals. However, many questions remain about its epidemiology and pathogenesis.

Proper understanding of the natural history and the effects of intervention on this syndrome are important because of its potential impact on health outcomes and the consequent costs to the health-care system. Sleep apnea patients used approximately twice as many health-care services defined by physician claims and overnight stays in the hospital in the 10 years before their initial diagnostic evaluation for OSAHS, compared with controls *(3)*. What is not clear at the present time is how much the difference is directly attributable to the SDB and how much is associated to conditions having their own adverse health consequences, which would not necessarily be completely ameliorated by interventions targeting only the SDB component *(4)*. With these caveats in mind, current information on the epidemiology and pathogenesis is presented as follows.

PREVALENCE

Estimates of prevalence depend on the criteria used to define the syndrome, especially those pertaining to the definition of a "scorable" respiratory event on polysomnography. In 2001, the Clinical Practice Review Committee of the American Academy of Sleep Medicine published criteria for "scorable" hypopneas, which require at least a 30% reduction in airflow with an associated 4% or higher desaturation *(5)*. Applying these criteria would eliminate hypopneas associated with a microarousal, but less than a 4% desaturation from contributing to the apnea/hypopnea index (AHI) and, thus, would reduce the apparent severity of SDB for individuals in previously reported studies using less stringent criteria. Nevertheless, an important estimate of the prevalence of SDB in a nonclinic population was published by Young and colleagues in 1993 *(6)*. They studied a random sample of 602 Wisconsin state employees aged 30–60 years from a group of 3513 respondents to a survey questionnaire. Based on results of overnight polysomnography, they estimated the prevalence of an apnea/hypopnea rate of five or more per hour (considered to be abnormal) to be 9% in women and 24% in men. They noted men to be 2–3.7 times as likely as women to have SDB, depending on age group. The prevalence appeared to increase with age. Prevalence of SDB associated with self-reported hypersomnolence was estimated to be present in 2% of women and 4% of men. They noted that male gender and obesity were risk factors in SDB, and age was also related, but not after the midadult years of 40–49. This paper raised awareness of the possibility that there were numerous, undiagnosed persons suffering from SDB in the general community.

Subsequent studies in the United States and from around the world have confirmed that a large number of undiagnosed cases of SDB are likely to be present in the community. An investigation in a small town in the Netherlands *(7)* studied a sample of symptomatic questionnaire respondents with in-home overnight airflow measurements by thermistry, followed by an overnight polysomnogram for those with signs of SDB on the home study. From the results, they estimated a prevalence of "clinically significant" sleep apnea syndrome in men more than the age of 35 years in their community of at least 0.45%. Their estimate for the prevalence of SDB with excessive somnolence for a population comparable with that studied by Young was only 0.9%. However, only 4 of 25 patients they studied with polysomnography had a body mass index (BMI) of 30 or more. Therefore, their study population appeared to have a low prevalence of the significant risk factor of obesity.

A study *(8)* of persons 50–70 years old from a small city in Spain showed a much higher prevalence of SDB, with 15.8% of subjects studied having an AHI of 10 or more. However, only 6.8% of men studied had SDB, plus symptoms of snoring or apneas observed at home. A much younger population was studied by Hui and colleagues *(9)*. They sampled first-year students at the University of Hong Kong, with a mean age of 19.4 years, and performed home polysomnography on a sample that had responded to a questionnaire. They found 75% snored, and 9% snored at least 10% of the night, but only 2.3% had a respiratory disturbance index of five or more. They estimated a minimum prevalence of SDB of 0.1% in this population. Again, this population had a low prevalence of obesity, with a mean BMI of 20.

Kripke and colleagues *(10)* performed home interviews and sleep monitoring for three nights on a sample of 190 men and 165 women, ages 40–64. Their overall estimate of the prevalence of SDB, defined as 4% desaturation events occurring at least 15 times per hour, in the age range of the study by Young and colleagues *(6)* was 20.3% for men and 7.6% for women. However, their estimates for whites were very similar to those of Young and colleagues *(6)*, indicating that the nonwhites in their study had a much higher prevalence. They concluded that race was a significant risk factor for SDB. A community study in Pennsylvania found a prevalence of an AHI of 20 or more in 6.3% of men, age 45–64 years, and 13.3% in those age 64–100 years *(11)*. However, a diagnosis of OSAHS by "Sleep Disorders Clinic Criteria" peaked at 4.7% in the 45- to 64-year-old group and fell to 1.7% in the older group. Note that in the Sleep Heart Health Study, with more than 5000 participants, the severity of self-reported sleepiness using the Epworth Sleepiness Scale (ESS) was not closely associated with the AHI *(12)*. The mean score on ESS was 7.2 in those with an AHI less than 5 and only 9.3 for those with AHI of 30 or more. The scale runs from 0–24, and values more than 10 have been considered indicative of "excessive sleepiness." Thus, a high AHI does not predict self-perceived sleepiness.

Overall, these studies indicate that there are a large number of persons with SDB who do not present for medical attention. However, the prevalence of symptomatic SDB is lower than that based only on the AHI. The natural history of clinically important OSAHS (i.e., that which responds to treatment with reduction in symptoms and/or improved long-term morbidity) may also be different from that based only on currently used objective indices of SDB *(13)*.

RISK FACTORS

Obesity

Obesity has clearly been shown to be a risk factor for SDB, increasing the risk by 10–14-fold over that for the nonobese. However, obesity alone is neither necessary nor sufficient for significant SDB, and other risk factors clearly modify its effect. Several studies have shown neck circumference to be one of the best predictors of the presence of SDB. This has been postulated to be because of the effect of fat accumulation in the neck that causes narrowing of the airway and increases the chances of airway closure during sleep. Ferguson and colleagues *(14)* studied craniofacial features and soft tissue measurements in men with SDB, separated into three groups based on neck circumference. They found retrognathia was more prominent in patients with smaller neck circumference. Soft tissue measures such as tongue length, cross-sectional area, soft palate length, and thickness were positively associated with neck size, i.e., they increased as neck circumference increased. The authors postulated that patients with obstructive sleep apnea fall into three groups:

1. Obese with abnormal, upper airway soft tissue structures;
2. Nonobese with abnormal craniofacial structures; and
3. A group with abnormalities in both upper airway soft tissue structures and craniofacial structures.

However, even nonobese patients with sleep apnea/hypopnea syndrome may have excess neck fat, as shown on magnetic resonance imaging *(15)*. Nonobese patients were found to have no increase in neck circumference, compared with controls, but an increase in total body fat and an increase in fat volume in the anterolateral segments of the neck. Visceral fat may also be a risk factor for sleep apnea, distinct from overall obesity *(16)*. Schotland and colleagues *(17)* demonstrated increased fat in the genioglossus muscle of patients with obstructive sleep apnea, compared with controls. This difference was found to be present even when patients and controls were matched for BMI. They also noted changes consistent with increased edema of the tongue in the patients. One limitation of the study was the small number of subjects (nine apneics and nine controls), with only three apneics and three controls matched for BMI. It is well-recognized clinically that many patients present to medical attention after having had a recent weight gain. Phillips and colleagues *(18)* found that 53 out of 77 patients referred for suspicion of this condition were documented to have obstructive sleep apnea had gained an average of 6.8 kg for the men and 8 kg for the women for the previous year. Whereas the 24 patients found not to have sleep apnea had, on average, lost 0.46 kg during the same time period.

The Wisconsin cohort showed that a 10% increase in weight was associated with a sixfold increase in risk for developing OSAHS during a 4-year follow-up period *(19)*. Interestingly, Bixler and colleagues *(20)* found that 100% of premenopausal women and postmenopausal women taking hormone replacement therapy (HRT) who had an AHI of 15 or more, were obese (BMI 32.3 or more), whereas only 49% of postmenopausal women not taking HRT with this level AHI were obese. Thus, the effect of obesity appears to be moderated by a protective effect of female hormones.

There appears to be an overall increasing risk in a "dose–response" manner, with increasing BMI, neck circumference, and waist–hip ratio, but other factors modify the relationship within individuals. The association with the latter indices indicates the importance of central obesity. Thus, the distribution of fat appears to play a role in the risk of SDB.

Gender

It has been widely recognized that more men than women present to sleep clinics with symptoms of SDB. This has prompted investigation of possible mechanisms for increased risks for SDB in men. One postulate was that premenopausal hormonal status protected women from reductions in ventilation and upper airway narrowing and closure during sleep. Carskadon and colleagues *(21)* showed no effect of clinical menopausal status or measurements of serum hormone levels on women's response to experimental nasal occlusion. They studied polysomnography in women, aged 45–55, with and without artificial occlusion of the nares. They found that nasal occlusion increased the AHI approximately fourfold, and the average arousal index increased from 20 to 35 per hour. The size of the respiratory response to nasal occlusion was predicted by BMI, neck circumference, and cephalometric measurements, but not by menopausal status or hormonal levels. They concluded that weight and facial morphometry were more important than hormonal factors in the risk of development of SDB during midlife in women.

Women have been found to have higher levels of electromyogram activity in the genioglossus muscle during the waking state, than men *(22)*, and an increased electromyogram response to inspiratory loading (not observed in men). This could provide partial protection from airway collapse; however, no difference in pharyngeal resistance was found between the normal women and men in this study. The critical closing pressure of the pharynx in men with sleep apnea was increased above that for women. That is, the men's upper airways were more collapsible *(23)*. However, the critical closing pressure was not correlated with neck circumference or BMI, two known strong predictors of SDB in both sexes. The authors concluded that several factors may play a role in the predisposition to pharyngeal collapse and thus, may lead to differences between men and women in risk of SDB. One of these factors may be deposition of fat in the neck *(24)*.

Normal men matched with normal women for BMI, ESS scores, and age had a more percentage of fat in the neck than the body as a whole (22 vs 17%), whereas the reverse was true for women (29 vs 33%). The men had two regions with larger absolute volume of fat: (1) anterior inside the mandible and (2) posterior at the level of the palate. Forty-six percent of the total neck fat was at the palatal level in men vs 33% in women. Thus, the extra fat loading in these segments of the neck in men might contribute to airway narrowing, especially when supine and asleep.

In a commentary on this study, Schwab *(25)* noted several potential reasons why men and women may differ in the risks for sleep apnea. However, he also noted that the more recent epidemiological studies cited above tend to show a male to female ratio of 2:1, rather than the 8:1 male predominance previously reported in studies of symptomatic patients presenting to medical attention. Thus, sleep apnea is also relatively common in women. Its prevalence may still be underestimated in women, if there is a difference in the predelection for reporting symptoms, as many epidemiological studies oversample persons reporting symptoms consistent with sleep apnea. Interestingly, Young and Finn *(1)* found women patients with an AHI of more than five had significantly lower survival rates than their male counterparts, despite similar apnea/hypopnea indices.

A recent study found that nocturnal sudden death may be increased in patients with OSAHS, suggesting the possibility of early "drop-out" of women with unsuspected SDB *(26)*. In the population studies, postmenopausal women clearly had higher prevalence of OSAH. In the Wisconsin cohort, postmenopausal women had a threefold increase not accounted for by BMI, age, or other risk factors *(27)*. In the Pennsylvania study *(20)*, postmenopausal women not using HRT had a fourfold increased risk, whereas, in the Sleep Heart Health Study, postmenopausal women using HRT had half the risk of nonusers *(28)*. In a recent, 3-month, randomized, controlled, crossover trial of estrogen therapy, a small but significant reduction in apnea frequency occurred with therapy, but there was no change in number of episodes of partial airway obstruction or oxyhemoglobin desaturations *(29)*. The study was limited by the relatively short time-course and the use of a static-charge-sensitive bed method for estimating respiratory events. Thus, the true difference in relative risk for SDB between the sexes is not clear, but it is likely influenced by menopausal status. It is not clear whether the consequences of the condition once developed are different in the two sexes.

Ethnicity

Community studies have often found an increased prevalence of SDB in nonwhite individuals. For example, Kripke and colleagues *(10)* estimated population prevalences of SDB of 4.9% in whites and 16.3% in nonwhites. Ancoli-Israel and colleagues *(29)* studied a random sample of persons more than 65 years of age from the community with home, overnight monitoring. The overall prevalence of SDB, defined as a respiratory disturbance index of more than 15 per hour was approximately the same in whites (30%) as in African Americans (32%), but more African Americans had severe SDB with a respiratory disturbance index of more than 30 (17 vs 8%). Logistic regression showed that African American race as well as male gender, older age, and an increased BMI were independent risk factors for a respiratory disturbance index of more than 30. The odds ratio for African Americans for severe SDB was 2.55, compared with whites, even after adjustment for BMI, sex, and age. A case–control study that also included family members of patients with obstructive sleep apnea showed that African Americans with SDB tended to be younger than their white counterparts *(31)*. For subjects less than 25 years old, the African Americans had significantly higher respiratory disturbance indices than their white counterparts, even after adjustment for obesity, sex, familial clustering, and proband sampling. Interestingly, cephalometric measurements on a subsample, mostly from persons who had a relative with sleep apnea, showed whites to have more association of both bony and soft tissue risk factors, whereas the African Americans had an association only with soft tissue risk factors. The authors concluded that young African Americans may be at increased risk for sleep apnea, but the cause for this excess risk was not clear. Cephalometric measurements also showed differences between whites and Asians with obstructive sleep apnea *(32)*. The Asians had a larger posterior air space, but narrower cranial base angle. Obesity was not as significant a risk factor in the Asians, only 4% of whom had a BMI of more than 35 vs 22% of the whites. Respiratory disturbance index was similar in the two groups (56.6 and 55.6, respectively). Overall, these studies suggest differences among ethnic groups in the distribution of risk factors and possibly underlying genetic differences in susceptibility to SDB.

CRANIOFACIAL MORPHOLOGY

Both soft tissue and bony may play a role in the risk for OSAHS. Children with enlarged tonsils and adenoids are known to be at risk for SDB and may be at risk for abnormal growth patterns of the lower face and jaw, leading to increased risk as adults *(33,34)*. Patients with OSAHS tend to have smaller upper airways lumens, because of a variety of structural features, including reduction in the length of the mandible, retroposition of the hyoid bone and maxilla, increased tongue volume, elongated soft palate, and increased parapharyngeal fat pads *(35)*. Many of these features are likely to be inherited and play a role in the familial aggregation of OSAHS. A recent study found that both Asians and Caucasians with OSAHS had a more crowded posterior oropharynx (judged by Mallampati score) and steeper thryomental plane (line through soft tissue mentum and thryroid prominence) than the controls *(36)*. The Asians tended to have more severe airway narrowing by these measures and more severe OSA after accounting for BMI and neck circumference. Brachycephaly, a head form associated with reduced anterior–posterior cranial dimensions, appears to be associated with a risk for an AHI of 15 or more in whites but not in African Americans *(37)*. Thus, craniofacial abnormality may be an important risk factor for SDB, but its importance may vary among different ethnic groups.

Nasal Obstruction

As described earlier *(21)*, experimental nasal obstruction appeared to increase both the AHI and the frequency of arousals on overnight polysomnogram in women aged 45–55. This suggested that nasal obstruction could play a role in worsening naturally occurring sleep apnea. Young and colleagues *(37)* found that symptoms of chronic rhinitis were significantly associated with habitual snoring, chronic excessive daytime somnolence, and complaints of nonrestorative sleep—even after adjustment for age, sex, and BMI. Adjusted odds ratios ranged from 2 to 2.4 for these symptoms. These investigators also measured nasal patency with rhinometry and found a trend toward an association of increasing frequency of snoring with decreased nasal airflow, but there was no linear relationship between decreased nasal flow and the AHI. There was a significant association of apnea/hypopnea indices of more than 15 and nasal congestion secondary to reported allergies. The authors concluded that allergic rhinitis may be a risk factor for SDB, but there was no clear relationship between nasal obstruction and the severity of SDB. Kushida and colleagues *(38)* reviewed this topic and felt that the literature supported at least a minor influence on the pathogenesis of upper airway collapse and OSA from nasal obstruction. Mirza and Lanza *(39)* provided a discussion of multiple mechanisms by which nasal obstruction could lead to SDB, including obstructive sleep apnea. These include the increased negative upper airway pressure produced by inspiratory efforts against a partially occluded nasal airway, turbulence, nasal reflexes, and snoring causing damage to the upper airway soft tissues. This latter mechanism will be discussed under pathophysiology.

In a study of children with obstructive sleep apnea *(41)*, 68% were found to have a family history of allergies, compared with only 28% of those without sleep apnea. Redline and colleagues *(42)* looked at risk factors for SDB in children and adolescents as part of a epidemiological genetic study. Participants were family members of an index case with SDB. An AHI of 10 or more was found to be associated with obesity, as expected, but was also found to be associated with African-American race, sinus problems, symptoms of wheezing, cough, and physician-diagnosed asthma. After adjustment for obesity and African-American race, there was still a significant association of SDB with respiratory illnesses. There was a fourfold risk associated with physician-diagnosed asthma and a fivefold risk associated with a history of sinus problems. There was no association of asthma and sinus problems in these data, nor was there an association of obesity with sinus problems or asthma. There was no association of passive smoke exposure with this risk.

Thus, allergies and upper respiratory problems appear to be related to the risk of obstructive sleep apnea in children. Of note is that an association of increased risk of SDB with race persisted after an adjustment for obesity, asthma, sinus problems, and wheezing was performed. African-American race was independently associated with an approximate threefold increase in the rate of SDB. In contrast to the findings relating to exposure to smoke in children, adult smokers in the Wisconsin cohort had a threefold increased risk of OSAHS, compared with never and former smokers *(43)*. These studies suggest that nasal obstruction, especially that associated with allergies, may be a significant exacerbating factor for SDB. It does not account for the increased risk in African Americans.

FAMILIAL/GENETIC FACTORS

The following is a summarization and interpretation for nongeneticists, by a nongeneticist, of the excellent recent discussion by Redline *(44)*. There is no standardized phenotypic definition of OSAHS, so AHI has been used as a marker to define the phenotype in most genetic studies. Significant familial clustering of the AHI and/or symptoms consistent with OSAHS has been observed in studies from many countries. The prevalence of OSAHS in first-degree relatives of OSA index cases has been reported to be 22–84%. The odds ratio of OSA of family members carrying this diagnosis has been reported to be from 2 to 46. Segregation analysis models suggest recessive Mendelian inheritance of AHI in whites, which accounts for 21–27% of the variance of the trait. In African Americans, this analysis suggests a codominant gene, accounting for 35% of total variance of AHI trait. The findings were strengthened in African Americans when adjusted for BMI, suggesting that risk factors independent of those affecting BMI are heritable in African Americans.

Given the findings discussed in this and preceding sections, it appears that multiple genes affecting obesity, body fat distribution, craniofacial morphology, and other factors not discussed here (e.g., ventilatory control and sleep cycles/architecture) play an important role in the risk for OSAHS.

Age

Both snoring and measured respiratory disturbance indices have tended to increase with age up to middle age, but show no increase or decrease in prevalence thereafter. As part of the Tucson Epidemiologic Study of Obstructive Airway Disease, respondents answered questions on symptoms, including habitual snoring *(45)*. Risk factors for developing habitual snoring over a span of 5.8 years between surveys included male gender and (for women only) obesity and respiratory symptoms. For men of increasing age, especially more than the age of 65, habitual snoring was associated with remission of habitual snoring. In a community study of 441 volunteers weighted toward those being overweight and reporting symptoms of snoring or sleep problems, Olsen and colleagues *(4)* found the prevalence of respiratory disturbance index higher than 15 tended to increase in age groups, starting with age 35–39, up to the 50–54 age group, and then was relatively constant up to age 64. In this study a high prevalence was found in the 65–69 age group, but again, the sample was biased toward those who were overweight and symptomatic.

Bixler and colleagues *(11)* performed overnight polysomnography on 741 men from a telephone survey of 4364, with the study sample weighted toward those reporting risk factors of snoring, excessive daytime somnolence, obesity, and hypertension. They found the overall prevalence of OSAHS defined by an AHI of more than 10 plus clinical symptoms to be 3.3%, with a maximum prevalence in the 45- to 64-year-old group of 4.7%. It was lower in both the younger and older subjects (1.2% in the 20- to 44-year-olds and 1.7% in the 65- to 100-year-olds). The peak prevalence appeared to be in the 50- to 59-year-old range. Interestingly, they found that in using only an AHI criterion to define the condition, there was a monotonic increase in prevalence with age. Central apneas turned out to be much more frequent in the over 65-year-old group and appeared to account for the overall monotonic increase of the apnea index with age. The severity of SDB, as judged by the number of respiratory events and the minimum oxygen saturation, decreased with age when BMI was controlled. Overall, the authors found that obstructive sleep apnea appeared to increase in prevalence, up to approximately the age of 55, and then decrease or remain constant, depending on the diagnostic criteria used. Obstructive sleep apnea appeared to be less severe in the elderly.

In a study of older Japanese-American men *(46)*, excessive daytime sleepiness was more prevalent at older ages, but habitual snoring declined. Excessive sleepiness was associated with a higher prevalence of heart disease, cognitive impairment and dementia, chronic obstructive pulmonary disease (COPD), and diabetes, so that its association with SDB was not clear. Three-year mortality was not associated with these symptoms after adjusting for prevalent heart disease and cognitive impairment. In a prospective study of the course of SDB, Lindberg and colleagues *(47)* performed polysomnograms on 29 subjects who had been studied 10 years previously after reporting symptoms suggestive of SDB on a questionnaire and having had received no treatment in the interim. They found an increase in mean AHI from 2.1 to 6.8, with 8% of subjects having an AHI of more than 10 on the second study vs 1% on the first study. Mean BMI was unchanged from 26 at baseline to 26.3 on follow-up. Using a criterion of at least a 50% change in AHI, 72% of those studied were worse, 7% were improved, and 21% were "stable." There were no specific predictors of a change in AHI of five or more; variables considered included baseline BMI, baseline AHI, change in BMI, baseline physical activity, smoking, and alcohol dependence.

The authors concluded that without treatment, SDB tended to worsen during a 10-year period, independent of age, initial BMI, weight gain, or smoking in middle-aged men who had reported snoring and excessive daytime somnolence during the initial study. Although bias in sampling and/or dropout of persons with the most severe SDB because of its complications may have influenced the findings, these studies suggest that age and other risk factors interact in a complex manner to affect the prevalence and severity of SDB.

ENDOCRINE ABNORMALITIES

A study by Isono and colleagues *(48)* of patients with acromegaly showed their pharyngeal airway to be highly collapsible. The authors felt that anatomic abnormalities, especially at the base of the tongue, also appear to play a significant role in SDB in this condition. Androgen therapy may precipitate obstructive sleep apnea in men and short-term administration of high-dose testosterone was shown to worsen sleep and increase SDB events in older men *(49)*. However, testosterone levels are often depressed in men with established OSAHS, and its role in the development of OSAHS is unknown.

Hypothyroidism has been suspected as a potential cause for sleep apnea because of abnormalities in the upper airway and perhaps of ventilatory drive. Skodt and colleagues *(50)* found that 2.4% of patients with obstructive sleep apnea have previously undiagnosed hypothyroidism. They found that treatment with thyroxine therapy alone resulted in resolution of SDB symptoms and nocturnal hypoxia when thyroid deficiency had been resolved. However, Mickelson and colleagues *(51)* screened 834 patients referred to their office for evaluation of snoring or obstructive sleep apnea. Only 10 of these patients, or 1.2%, were discovered to have previously undiagnosed clinical hypothyroidism. Four of the 10 patients with newly diagnosed hypothyroidism had obstructive sleep apnea. They were treated with thyroid hormone replacement and underwent repeat polysomnography once they had achieved a euthyroid state. There was no significant difference between their pre- and post-treatment respiratory disturbance index. The authors concluded that the prevalence of hypothyroidism in patients referred for the evaluation of snoring and SDB is no more than that in the general population. Because thyroid HRT did not result in resolution of sleep apnea in the few patients with both conditions, no evidence of an association was demonstrated. Several studies have demonstrated an association between OSAHS and insulin resistance *(52,53)*. However, this is a topic unto itself and will not be addressed further here.

PATHOGENESIS

Two excellent reviews of this topic have been published recently *(54,55)*. In humans, the upper airway is not a rigid structure, so its patency depends on the balance of forces acting on the walls (trans-mural pressure) and the resistance of the walls to collapse (wall elastance, i.e., the inverse of compliance). During inspiration, the negative intraluminal pressure tends to collapse the airway and the activity of upper airway dilating muscles (e.g., the genioglossus) phasically increases to counteract this collapsing force and maintain patency. Other upper airway muscles (e.g., tensor palatine) have a more constant tonic activity and maintain a level of wall stiffness to resist collapse. Inspiratory phasic muscle activity is normally maintained during sleep after a transitory drop during the wake–sleep transition. However, tonic muscle activity appears to fall as sleep deepens. This causes a decrease in airway luminal cross-section and an increase in upper airway resistance to airflow. During wakefulness, upper airway muscles respond to a burst of negative pressure with a reflex-like increase in activity. If a more forceful inspiratory effort is made in response to a stimulus (e.g., an increased $PaCO_2$ or decreased PaO_2), producing a more negative intraluminal pressure, a compensatory increase in dilating force occurs. This response is reduced during sleep with the loss of the "wakefulness stimulus."

At a given inspiratory flow rate, intraluminal pressure will be more negative if the airway cross-sectional area is reduced. Patients with OSAHS usually have some degree of anatomic narrowing of the upper airway, as discussed earlier. Upper airway lumen cross-sectional area also decreases somewhat during sleep because of the loss of "tracheal tug," because lung volume falls on assuming the recumbent position. The fall in lung volume is accentuated in obese persons, including those with OSAHS, further compromising the airway. In addition, persons with OSAHS have increased activity of both phasic and tonic upper airway muscles while awake, compared with those without this condition, possibly as a compensatory mechanism to maintain patency of their anatomically compromised airway. However, with the onset of sleep, this augmented activity is lost and the already-small upper airway is subject to collapse and closure. In some patients with OSAHS, an unstable respiratory control system appears to promote cycling of respiratory effort. This produces varying levels of upper airway intraluminal-negative pressure and the inadequate compensatory increase in phasic dilator muscle activity predisposes the airway to collapse. Brief microarousals following apneas cause an increase in respiratory effort and accentuate the changes in ventilation. This results in fluctuations in the level of PaO_2 and $PaCO_2$ feedback to neural respiratory control centers augmenting and perpetuating respiratory cycling.

Even lesser degrees of anatomic upper airway narrowing or collapse may lead to progressive changes in the upper airway musculature, predisposing to further worsening airway narrowing and collapse. A hypothesis has been put forth that vibratory damage to upper airway soft tissues may worsen or induce the obstructive sleep apnea syndrome *(56)*. Friberg and colleagues *(57)* studied biopsy data of the upper airway of control subjects, snorers, and patients with obstructive sleep apnea. Data were taken from other muscles (e.g., anterior tibialis) as control sites. All patients had abnormalities on the upper airway biopsy, and 71% had morphometric signs such as fascicular atrophy and grouped atrophy consistent with neurogenic lesions. Only 20% of controls had slight changes of these types. The tibialis muscle biopsy data were normal in 20 of the 21 patients, indicating that no generalized muscle or neurological abnormality was present. The degree of abnormality in the upper airway biopsy data was correlated with the percentage of time spent in periodic breathing on an overnight monitoring study. The fiber-type distribution was not different between controls and patients, but the fiber-size spectrum was abnormal in 75% of the patients with increased numbers of hypertrophied or atrophied fibers. There was no correlation between the degree of morphological abnormality or spectral abnormality with age, but the BMI was correlated with the degree of morphometric abnormality. The authors concluded that trauma from snoring may contribute to neurogenic lesions of the upper airway, leading to increased collapsibility and increased risk for SDB. However, whether such trauma is a primary causal phenomenon or merely a secondary change because of SDB, caused by other risk factors, cannot be determined from this study. Such a mechanism could partially account for the association of allergic nasal obstruction with snoring and SDB.

Upper airway patency is determined by the interaction of a number of structural and functional factors. Patients with OSAHS appear to have varying degrees of anatomic narrowing, combined with reduced neuromuscular dilatory compensatory mechanisms during sleep. Ventilatory controller instability may contribute to a propensity for periodic breathing and partial or complete airway closure in some patients.

CONCLUSIONS

SDB is an important public health problem with significant health consequences for affected individuals. It is highly prevalent, but the exact prevalence depends on the definition used and the populations surveyed. There are likely differences in prevalence between sexes and races, but the exact causes are unclear. The natural history of the condition is still unclear, especially in relationship to aging. It is likely that selective participation or dropout from the population of those most affected have affected the observed relationships of SDB in studies to date. The pathogenesis is multifactorial in most affected persons, with obesity and various craniofacial anatomic abnormalities being major factors. Other potential risk factors such as chronic allergic rhinitis and hypothyroidism are less well-documented.

REFERENCES

1. Young T, Finn L (1998) Epidemiological insights into the public health burden of sleep disordered breathing: sex differences in survival among sleep clinic patients. Thorax 53(Suppl 3):S16–S19.
2. Boehlecke B (2000) A Epidemiology and Pathogenesis of sleep disordered breathing. Curr Opin Pulm Med 6:471–478.
3. Ronald J, Delaive K, Roos L, et al. (1999) Health care utilization in the 10 years prior to diagnosis in obstructive sleep apnea syndrome patients. Sleep 22:225–229.
4. Olson L, King M, Hensley M, et al. (1995) A community study of snoring and sleep disordered breathing. Am J Respir Crit Care Med 152:717–720.
5. Meoli AL, Casey KR, Clark RW, et al. (2001) Hypopnea in sleep-disordered breathing in adults. Sleep 24:469–470.
6. Young T, Palta M, Dempsey J, et al. (1993) The occurrence of sleep-disordered breathing among middle-aged adults. N Engl J Med 328:1230–1235.
7. Neven A, Middlekoop H, Kemp Kamphuisen H, et al. (1998) The prevalence of clinically significant sleep apneoa syndrome in the Neverlands. Thorax 53:638–642.
8. Zamarron C, Gude F, Otero Y, et al. (1999) Prevalence of sleep-disordered breathing and sleep apena in 50- to 70-year-old individuals. Respiration 66:317–322.
9. Hui D, Chan J, Ho A, et al. (1999) Prevalence of snoring and sleep-disordered breathing in a student population. Chest 116:1530–1536.
10. Kripke DF, Ancoli-Israel S, Kaluber MR, et al. (1997) Prevalence of sleep-disordered breathing in ages 40-64 years: a population-based survey. Sleep 20:65–76.
11. Bixler EO, Vgontzas AN, Ten Have T, et al. (1998) Effects of age on sleep apnea in med: I. prevalence and severity. Am J Respir Crit Care Med 157:144–148.
12. Gottbib D, Whitney C, Bonekat W, et al. (1999) Relation of sleepiness to respiratory disturbance index: The Sleep Heart Health Study. Am J Respir Crit Care Med 159:502–507.
13. Stradling J, Davies R (2004) Sleep: obstructive sleep apnoea/hypopnea syndrome: definitions, epidemiology, and natural history. Thorax 59:73–78.
14. Ferguson K, Ono T, Lowe A, et al. (1995) The relationship obesity and craniofacial structure in obstructive sleep apnea. Chest 108:375–381.
15. Mortimore IL, Marshal I, Wraith PK, et al. (1998) Neck and total body fat deposition in nonobese and obese patients with sleep apnea compared with that in control subjects. Am J Respir Crit Care Med 157:280–283.
16. Shinoha E, Kihara S, Yamashita S, et al. (1997) Visceral fat accumulation as an important risk factor for obstructive sleep apnea syndrome in obese subjects. J Int Med 241:11–18.
17. Schotland HM, Inso EK, Schwab RJ (1999) Quantitative magnetic resonance imaging demonstrates alterations of the lingual musculature in obstructive sleep apnea. Sleep 22:605–613.
18. Phillips B, Hisel T, Kato M, et al. (1999) Recent weight gain in patients with newly diagnosed obstructive sleep apnea. J Hypertension 17:1297–1300.
19. Peppard PE, Young T, Palta M, et al. (2000) Longitudinal study of moderate weight change and sleep disordered breathing. JAMA 284:3015–3021.
20. Bixler EO, Vgontaz AN, Lin HM, et al. (2001) Prevalence of sleep-disordered breathing in women: effects of gender. Am J Respir Crit Care Med 163:608–613.
21. Carskadon M, Bearpark H, Sharkey K, et al. (1997) Effects of menopause and nasal occlusion on breathing during sleep. Am J Respir Crit Care Med 155:205–210.
22. Popovic R, White D (1995) Influence of gender on waking genioglossal electromyogram and upper airway resistance. Am J Respir Crit Care Med 152:725–731.
23. Sforza E, Petiau C, Weiss T, et al. (1999) Pharyngeal critical pressure in patients with obstructive sleep apnea syndrome. Am J Respir Crit Care Med 159:149–157.
24. Whittle A, Marshall I, Mortimore I, et al. (1999) Neck soft tissue and fat distribution: comparison between normal men and women by magnetic resonance imaging. Thorax 54:323–328.
25. Schwab R (1999) Sex differences and sleep apnoea. Thorax 54:284–285.
26. Young T, Finn L (1998) Epidemiological insight into the public health burden of sleep disordered breathing. Thorax 53(Suppl 3):S16–S19.
27. Young T, Finn L, Austin D, et al. (2003) Menopausal status and sleep-disordered breathing in the Wisconsin sleep cohort study. Am J Respir Crit Care Med 167:1181–1185.
28. Shahar E, Redline S, Young T, et al. (2003) Hormone replacement therapy and sleep-disordered breathing. Am J Respir Crit Care Med 167:1186–1192.

29. Ancoli-Israel S, Klauber M, Stepnowsky C, et al. (1995) Sleep-disordered breathing in African-American elderly. Am J Respir Crit Care Med 152:1946–1949.
30. Redline S, Tishler P, Hans M, et al. (1997) Racial differences in sleep-disordered breathing in African-Americans and Caucasians. Am J Respir Crit Care Med 155:186–192.
31. Li K, Powell N, Kushida C, et al. (1999) A comparison of Asian and white patients with obstructive sleep apnea syndrome. Laryngoscope 109:1937–1940.
32. Riley RW, Powell NB, Li KK, et al. (2000) Surgery and obstructive sleep apnea: long-term clinical outcomes. Otolaryngol Head Neck Surg 122:415–421.
33. Arens R, Marcus C (2004) Pathophysiology of upper airway obstruction: a developmental perspective. Sleep 27:997–1019.
34. Fogel R, Malhotra A, White D (2004) Sleep 2: pathophysiology of obstructive sleep apnea/hypapnea syndrome. Thorax 59:159–163.
35. Lau B, Ip M, Teneh E, et al. (2005) Craniofacial profile in Asian and white subjects with obstructive sleep apnea. Thorax 60:504–510.
36. Cakirer B, Hans M, Graham G, et al. (2001) The Relationship between craniofacial morphology and obstructive sleep apnea in whites and in African-Americans. Am J Respir Crit Care Med 163:947–950.
37. Young T, Finn L, Kim H (1997) Nasal obstruction as a risk factor for sleep-disordered breathing. J Allergy Clin Immunol 99:S757–S762.
38. Kushida C, Guilleminault C, Clerk A, et al. (1997) Nasal obstruction and obstructive sleep apnea: a review. Allergy Asthma Proc 18:69–71.
39. Mirza N, Lanza DC (1999) The nasal airway and obstructed breathing during sleep. Otolaryngol Clin North Am 32:243–262.
40. Harvey J, O'Callaghan M, Wales P, et al. (1999) Aetiological factors and development in subjects with obstructive sleep apnoea. J Paediatr Child Health 35:140–144.
41. Redline S, Tishler P, Schluchter M, et al. (1999) Risk factors for sleep-disordered breathing in children. Am J Respir Crit Care Med 159:1527–1532.
42. Redlinc S (2005) Genetics of obstructive sleep apnea. In: *Principles and Practice of Sleep Medicine*. 4th ed. (Kryger MH, Roth R, Dement W, eds.) Saunders/Elsevier, Philadelphia, PA, pp. 1013–1022.

10 Evidence and Mechanisms Linking Obstructive Sleep Apnea to Cardiovascular Disease

Virend K. Somers, MD, PhD

CONTENTS

INTRODUCTION

Obstructive sleep apnea (OSA) has been recognized as a cause of sleep disruption and daytime somnolence. During the past two decades, emerging evidence has implicated OSA as a comorbidity in a number of cardiovascular disease conditions *(1)*. More recently, the effects of OSA have been linked to the activation of a number of mechanisms that may contribute to the development and progression of cardiovascular disease. Treatment of OSA in patients with existing cardiovascular disease conditions has been associated with improvements in these disease conditions. However, much of the evidence is still circumstantial and etiological evidence for OSA in initiating cardiovascular damage remains debatable. This review will examine the possible mechanisms by which sleep apnea may contribute to cardiovascular dysfunction and disease, those cardiovascular disease conditions that frequently exist as comorbidities with OSA, and the effects of treatment of sleep apnea on these cardiovascular disease conditions.

MECHANISMS BY WHICH OSA MAY ELICIT CARDIAC AND VASCULAR DYSFUNCTION

Sympathetic Activation

The sympathetic nervous system is likely to be a key contributor to any cardiac and vascular dysfunction that may occur secondary to OSA. In otherwise healthy patients

From: *Current Clinical Practice: Primary Care Sleep Medicine: A Practical Guide*
Edited by: J. F. Pagel and S. R. Pandi-Perumal © Humana Press Inc., Totowa, NJ

with sleep apnea, sympathetic nerve traffic—even during normoxic quiet resting daytime wakefulness—is substantially higher than that which is seen in normal control subjects *(2)*. The reason for this high central sympathetic outflow in sleep apneics is not known. Tonic chemoreflex activation may be involved, as administration of 100% oxygen to healthy awake patients significantly reduces not only sympathetic traffic, but also heart rate and blood pressure *(3)*. Awake and otherwise healthy patients with OSA also have disturbances in heart rate and blood pressure control that are reflected in faster heart rates, decreased heart rate variability, and increased blood pressure variability *(4)*. These three characteristics are each linked to an enhanced long-term risk for cardiovascular disease, in particular hypertension *(5)*.

At night, during sleep, episodes of OSA elicit both hypoxemia and CO_2 retention. Hypoxemia and hypercapnia act synergistically at the peripheral and central chemoreceptors. During apnea, when the inhibitory influence of hyperventilation is absent, the sympathetic neural response to hypoxia and hypercapnia is potentiated *(6,7)*. Thus, episodes of OSA result in increases in sympathetic traffic during the apnea, more even than is seen in measurements obtained during wakefulness. This sympathetic vasoconstrictor activity raises blood pressure. Surges in blood pressure are most marked at the end of apnea, when breathing resumes. This may be related to the increase in venous return and hence, cardiac output that occurs during breathing at the end of apnea. The net result of the sympathetic vasoconstriction and increased cardiac output includes surges in blood pressure to very high levels, sometimes as high as 240/120 mmHg *(2)*. These increases in pressure occur repetitively through the night and the stress of maintaining this high blood pressure level occurs simultaneously with the hypoxemic and metabolic stress elicited by apnea. Thus, sympathetic activation, during wakefulness and especially with apneic sleep, may contribute importantly to the long-term development of heart and blood vessel damage in patients with sleep apnea.

Endothelial Dysfunction

There are many reasons for supposing that endothelial dysfunction may be present in patients with sleep apnea. Indeed, some data suggest that the smaller arterioles do not dilate appropriately in response to acetylcholine, suggesting that they have a blunted ability to produce nitric oxide (resistance vessel endothelial dysfunction). These data are nevertheless not consistent across studies *(8–10)*. Whether the large vessel (conduit vessel) endothelial function is also impaired in sleep apnea is also controversial. Some studies have noted decreased conduit vessel endothelial function with improvement after continuous positive airway pressure therapy *(11)*. An important consideration is the early morning reduction of conduit vessel endothelial function evident in healthy normal subjects *(12)*, which may confound studies when conduit vessel dilation is measured in the morning in sleep apneics, but later in the day in control subjects.

Thus, although endothelial dysfunction is an appealing disease mechanism to explain the presence of cardiovascular disease in sleep apnea, evidence for endothelial dysfunction in sleep apneic patients without other diseases that may cause endothelial dysfunction (such as hypertension, diabetes, smoking, and hyperlipidemia) remains inconsistent.

Inflammation

Hypoxemia and sleep deprivation are important causes for increases in C-reactive protein *(13,14)*. Sleep apnea is characterized by both hypoxemia and by sleep deprivation. A number of studies have suggested that patients with OSA have high levels of C-reactive protein *(15)*. The effects of body fat distribution on these findings are not yet known. Other evidence suggesting a systemic inflammatory state in patients with sleep apnea include findings of heightened levels of serum amyloid A, increased cytokines, increased adhesion molecules, and increased binding of leukocytes from apneic patients to endothelial cells in culture *(16–19)*. The presence of a systemic inflammatory state in sleep apnea may be an important causative mechanism for damage to the endothelium because activated white cells would bind to endothelial cells, thus enhancing permeability to low-density lipoprotein and macrophages.

Oxidative Stress

The repetitive nocturnal hypoxemia and reperfusion that characterizes sleep apnea suggests a likely substrate for the production of reactive oxygen species with consequent damage to cardiovascular tissue. However, the data regarding the presence of increased oxidative stress in sleep apnea are not consistent *(20,21)*.

Production of Vasoactive Substances

The severe hypoxemia in sleep apnea has been implicated as a possible cause for the release of vasoactive substances such as endothelin *(22,23)*. Sleep apnea also may trigger release of atrial natriuretic peptide, which may be implicated in nocturia in sleep apnea patients. However, brain natriuretic peptide, which has been used as an index of the presence and severity of congestive heart failure, does not appear to increase overnight in untreated sleep apneics, whether or not heart failure is present *(24)*.

METABOLIC MECHANISMS

Extensive data have suggested that sleep apnea is accompanied by a state of metabolic dysregulation and that sleep apnea may be an important component of and perhaps contributor to the metabolic syndrome *(25)*. Certainly, patients with sleep apnea have been noted to have increased insulin resistance *(26,27)*. They also may have enhanced leptin resistance so that leptin levels in male sleep apneics are higher than that which would be present in similarly obese men *(28)*. In the year before diagnosis, sleep apneics appear to be more likely to gain weight. Obesity is an established and independent mechanism for the development of cardiovascular disease. Potentiation of any propensity to obesity by OSA would be an important mechanism by which sleep apnea may elicit cardiac and vascular disease.

CHANGES IN INTRATHORACIC PRESSURE

Because of the upper airway obstruction, very significant intrathoracic negative pressures are generated during repetitive Mueller maneuvers in OSA patients *(29)*. Negative pressures of −40 mmHg or more may have significant mechanical effects on cardiac trans-mural pressures. The pressure gradient between the inside and outside of the cardiac chambers would be consequently increased resulting in increased cardiac wall stress. The effects of negative pressure may be especially significant for the thin-walled atria, and may be implicated in any relationship between atrial fibrillation and OSA.

CARDIOVASCULAR DISEASES ASSOCIATED WITH OSA

Hypertension

The Wisconsin Cohort Study has shown that over a 4-year follow-up, OSA (classified as an apnea/hypopnea index of >15) is independently linked with a threefold increase in the likelihood of new hypertension developing, as compared with patients without apneas during sleep *(30)*. Further evidence suggesting an interaction between OSA and hypertension emerges from studies where treatment of OSA has resulted in significant reductions in blood pressure not only at night, but also in the morning *(31,32)*. The evidence implicating OSA in hypertension has prompted the most recent Joint National Committee 7 Guidelines for the management of hypertension to list OSA as first of the identifiable causes of hypertension. Furthermore, emphasis is placed on excluding OSA in patients with resistant hypertension (those taking three or more antihypertensive drugs).

Heart Failure

Although central sleep apnea is the most prominent type of sleep-disordered breathing in heart failure, OSA may be present in 10% or more of heart failure patients. This prevalence may be increasing as the heart failure population becomes more obese. Several studies have suggested that treatment of OSA improves ejection fraction in heart failure patients *(33–35)*. Effects on blood pressure are less clear-cut. Based on sympathetic activation and the other consequences of OSA, it is persuasive that prevention of the obstructive apneas and consequently of hypoxemia would improve cardiac function. However, whether there is any mortality benefit from treatment of OSA in heart failure patients is not known.

Atrial Fibrillation

The hypoxemia, sympathetic activation, increased blood pressures, and abrupt increases in intrathoracic negative pressures provide a reasonable basis for linking OSA to risk for atrial fibrillation. Indeed, patients with OSA are more likely to develop atrial fibrillation postoperatively *(36)*. Based on responses to questionnaires assessing risk for OSA, about 50% of patients coming to cardioversion for atrial fibrillation have a high risk for OSA *(37)*. Of those who are cardioverted successfully, the presence of untreated significant OSA is accompanied by an 80% risk of recurrence of atrial fibrillation over 1 year, about double the risk of recurrence seen in patients whose OSA has been treated *(38)*. However, there are not yet any clear data unequivocally implicating OSA as an independent risk factor for the development of atrial fibrillation.

Cardiac Ischemia

Severe stresses elicited by OSA, including hypoxemia and increased afterload, would also be reasonably expected to increase the likelihood of nocturnal cardiac ischemia in those patients with significant coronary artery disease. ST depression, which is suggestive of cardiac ischemia, is more frequent in patients with coronary artery disease who have more severe OSA, and appears to be related to oxygen desaturation *(39)*. The duration of ST depression in sleep apneics is significantly attenuated by continuous positive airway pressure treatment. Patients with established coronary artery disease and OSA have an increased 5-year mortality compared with those who do not have OSA *(40)*. However, whether OSA independently predicts coronary events and cardiac mortality, and whether treatment of OSA may diminish this risk is not yet known.

Stroke

Evidence linking OSA to stroke is also circumstantial. A history of snoring is accompanied by increased stroke risk *(41–43)*, and sleep apnea is highly prevalent in patients with stroke and is associated with adverse outcomes *(41–43)*. Nevertheless, there are as yet no data clearly implicating OSA as an independent risk factor for the development of stroke.

Arrhythmias

Apart from atrial fibrillation, which has been discussed earlier, sleep apnea has also been linked to premature ventricular contractions and ventricular tachycardia. Because of problems in subject selection and comorbidities, whether OSA in and of itself predisposes to a higher risk of ventricular arrhythmias remains unclear. However, the hypoxemia and apnea associated with OSA is known to elicit bradyarrhythmias by activation of the diving reflex *(44)*. This reflex triggers increased sympathetic activation to peripheral blood vessels except to the brain and to the heart, where the vessels dilate. The other component of the diving reflex is increased cardiac vagal drive resulting in bradycardia, so as to minimize cardiac oxygen consumption during hypoxemic apnea. The consequence of this can be seen in a minority of patients with OSA in whom bradyarrhythmias may manifest as asystole lasting up to 10 seconds or more. These severe bradyarrhythmias can occur in the setting of a completely normal cardiac conduction system, and treatment requires treatment of the apnea; if this treatment is effective, it will result in resolution of the arrhythmia.

CONCLUSIONS

There is clear evidence of the acute activation of multiple cardiovascular disease mechanisms during episodes of OSA. There is also evidence suggesting that even in otherwise healthy patients with OSA, subtle evidence of abnormalities in cardiovascular control may be evident. It is possible that in the long-term, functional abnormalities in patients with OSA, together with the development of structural cardiovascular changes, may predispose to an increased risk for overt cardiovascular disease. However, yet there are no clear data to support this, except in the context of hypertension. Also important is that although effective treatment of OSA attenuates the acute changes described earlier, may improve ejection fraction in heart failure patients, and may lower blood pressure in hypertensive patients, there are no objective, prospective, long-term data showing any improvement in hard cardiovascular end points or cardiovascular mortality with OSA treatment.

REFERENCES

1. Shamsuzzaman ASM, Gersh BJ, Somers VK (2003) Obstructive sleep apnea: implications for cardiac and vascular disease. JAMA 290:1906–1914.
2. Somers VK, Dyken ME, Clary MP, et al. (1995) Sympathetic neural mechanisms in obstructive sleep apnea. J Clin Invest 96:1897–1904.

3. Narkiewicz K, van de Borne PJ, Montano N, et al. (1998) Contribution of tonic chemoreflex activation to sympathetic activity and blood pressure in patients with obstructive sleep apnea. Circulation 97:943–945.
4. Narkiewicz K, Montano N, Cogliati C, et al. (1998) Altered cardiovascular variability in obstructive sleep apnea. Circulation 98:1071–1077.
5. Singh JP, Larson MG, Tsuji H, et al. (1998) Reduced heart rate variability and new-onset hypertension: insights into pathogenesis of hypertension; the Framingham Heart Study. Hypertension 32:293–297.
6. Somers VK, Zavala DC, Mark AL, et al. (1989) Influence of ventilation and hypocapnia on sympathetic nerve responses to hypoxia in normal humans. J Appl Physiol 67:2095–2100.
7. Somers VK, Zavala DC, Mark AL, et al. (1989) Contrasting effects of hypoxia and hypercapnia on ventilation and sympathetic activity in humans. J Appl Physiol 67:2101–2106.
8. Carlson JT, Rangemark C, Hedner JA (1996) Attenuated endothelium-dependent vascular relaxation in patients with sleep apnoea. J Hypertension 14:577–584.
9. Kato M, Roberts-Thomson P, Phillips BG, et al. (2000) Impairment of endothelium-dependent vasodilation of resistance vessels in patients with obstructive sleep apnea. Circulation 102:2607–2610.
10. Kraiczi H, Hedner J, Peker Y, et al. (2000) Increased vasoconstrictor sensitivity in obstructive sleep apnea. J Appl Physiol 89:493–498.
11. Ip MS, Tse H, Tsang KW, et al. (2003) Endothelial function in obstructive sleep apnea and response to treatment. Am J Respir Crit Care Med 169:348–353.
12. Otto ME, Svatikova A, Barretto R, et al. (2004) Early morning attenuation of endothelial function. Circulation 109:2507–2510.
13. Hartmann G, Tschop M, Fischer R, et al. (2000) High altitude increases circulating interleukin-6, interleukin-1 receptor antagonist and C-reactive protein. Cytokine 12:246–262.
14. Meier-Ewert HK, Ridker PM, Rifai N, et al. (2004) Effect of sleep loss on C-reactive protein, an inflammatory marker of cardiovascular risk. J Am Coll Cardiol 43:678–683.
15. Shamsuzzaman AS, Winnicki M, Lanfranchi P, et al. (2002) Elevated C-reactive protein in patients with obstructive sleep apnea. Circulation 105:2462–2464.
16. Chin K, Nakamura T, Shimizu K, et al. (2000) Effects of nasal continous positive airway pressure on soluble cell adhesion molecules in patients with obstructive sleep apnea syndrome. Am J Med 109:562–567.
17. Dyugovskaya L, Lavie P, Lavie L (2002) Increased adhesion molecules expression and production of reactive oxygen species in leukocytes of sleep apnea patients. Am J Respir Crit Care Med 165:934–939.
18. El-Solh AA, Mador MJ, Sikka P, et al. (2002) Adhesion molecules in patients with coronary artery disease and moderate-to-severe obstructive sleep apnea. Chest 121:1541–1547.
19. Svatikova A, Wolk R, Shamsuzzaman AS, et al. (2003) Serum amyloid A in obstructive sleep apnea. Circulation 108:1451–1454.
20. Schulz R, Mahmoudi S, Hattar K, et al. (2000) Enhanced release of superoxide from polymorphonuclear neutrophils in obstructive sleep apnea: impact of continuous positive airway pressure therapy. Am J Respir Crit Care Med 162:566–570.
21. Wali SO, Bahammam AS, Massaeli H, et al. (1998) Susceptibility of LDL to oxidative stress in obstructive sleep apnea. Sleep 21:290–296.
22. Kourembanas S, Marsden PA, McQuillan LP, et al. (1991) Hypoxia induces endothelin gene expression and secretion in cultured human endothelium. J Clin Invest 88:1054–1057.
23. Phillips BG, Narkiewicz K, Pesek CA, et al. (1999) Effects of obstructive sleep apnea on endothelin-1 and blood pressure. J Hypertension 17:61–66.
24. Svatikova A, Shamsuzzaman AS, Wolk R, et al. (2004) Plasma brain natriuretic peptide in obstructive sleep apnea. Am J Cardiol 94:529–532.
25. Coughlin S, Mawdsley L, Mugarza JA, et al. (2004) Obstructive sleep apnoea is independently associated with an increased prevalence of metabolic syndrome. Eur Heart J 25:735–741.
26. Punjabi NM, Sorkin JD, Katzel LI, et al. (2002) Sleep-disordered breathing and insulin resistance in middle-aged and overweight men. Am J Respir Crit Care Med 165:677–682.
27. Ip MS, Lam B, Ng MM, et al. (2002) Obstructive sleep apnea is independently associated with insulin resistance. Am J Respir Crit Care Med 165:670–676.
28. Phillips BG, Kato M, Narkiewicz K, et al. (2000) Increases in leptin levels, sympathetic drive, and weight gain in obstructive sleep apnea. Am J Physiol Heart Circ Physiol 279:H234–H237.

29. Leung RS, Bradley TD (2001) Sleep apnea and cardiovascular disease. Am J Respir Crit Care Med 164:2147–2165.
30. Peppard PE, Young T, Palta M, et al. (2000) Prospective study of the association between sleep-disordered breathing and hypertension. N Engl J Med 342:1378–1384.
31. Pepperell JC, Ramdassingh-Dow S, Crosthwaite N, et al. (2002) Ambulatory blood pressure after therapeutic and subtherapeutic nasal continuous positive airway pressure for obstructive sleep apnoea: a randomised parallel trial. Lancet 359:204–210.
32. Becker HF, Jerrentrup A, Ploch T, et al. (2003) Effect of nasal continous positive airway pressure on blood pressure in patients with obstructive sleep apnea. Circulation 107:68–73.
33. Malone S, Liu PP, Holloway R, et al. (1991) Obstructive sleep apnea in patients with dilated cardiomyopathy: effects of continuous positive airway pressure. Lancet 338:1480–1484.
34. Kaneko Y, Floras JS, Usui K, et al. (2003) Cardiovascular effects of continuous positive airway pressure in patients with heart failure and obstructive sleep apnea. N Engl J Med 348:1233–1241.
35. Mansfield DR, Gollogly NC, Kaye DM, et al. (2004) Controlled trial of continuous positive airway pressure in obstructive sleep apnea and heart failure. Am J Respir Crit Care Med 169:361–366.
36. Mooe T, Gullsby S, Rabben T, et al. (1996) Sleep-disordered breathing: a novel predictor of atrial fibrillation after coronary artery bypass surgery. Coron Artery Dis 7:475–478.
37. Gami AS, Pressman G, Caples SM, et al. (2004) Association of atrial fibrillation and obstructive sleep apnea. Circulation 110:364–367.
38. Kanagala R, Murali N, Friedman P, et al. (2003) Obstructive sleep apnea and the recurrence of atrial fibrillation. Circulation 107:2589–2594.
39. Franklin KA, Nilsson JB, Sahlin C, et al. (1995) Sleep apnoea and nocturnal angina. Lancet 345:1085–1087.
40. Peker Y, Hedner J, Kraiczi H, et al. (2000) Respiratory disturbance index: an independent predictor of mortality in coronary artery disease. Am J Respir Crit Care Med 162:81–86.
41. Palomaki H, Partinen M, Erkinjuntti T, et al. (1992) Snoring, sleep apnea syndrome, and stroke. Neurology 42:75–81.
42. Partinen M (1995) Ischaemic stroke, snoring and obstructive sleep apnoea. J Sleep Res 4:156–159.
43. Dyken ME, Somers VK, Yamada T, et al. (1996) Investigating the relationship between stroke and obstructive sleep apnea. Stroke 27:401–407.
44. Daly MD, Angell-James JE, Elsner R (1979) Role of carotid-body chemoreceptors and their reflex interactions in bradycardia and cardiac arrest. Lancet (1)8119:764–767.

11 Treatment for Obstructive Sleep Apnea

Surgical and Alternative Treatments

James M. Parish, MD, FCCP

Contents

INTRODUCTION

No area in sleep-disorders medicine has been marked by as much controversy as the surgical treatment for obstructive sleep apnea (OSA). The literature has been hampered frequently by poorly defined outcomes or outcomes that varied from study to study. The exact surgical procedures being done often vary, making two papers are difficult to compare as the surgical techniques are different. In recent years, however, the literature of surgical therapy has improved and there are now many papers with sound methodology using well-defined end points. However, no single surgical procedure has ever been found to be entirely satisfactory for the treatment of OSA. As a result, there is continued intensive investigation finding the ideal surgical treatment for OSA.

Most people agree that continuous positive airway pressure (CPAP) is the first-line therapy. CPAP reverses the underlying pathophysiology of OSA by stenting the upper airway open with positive air pressure. CPAP eliminates snoring, obstructive apneas, and hypopneas. It is noninvasive and has no major complications. Its limiting factor is the cumbersome nature of the device and patients' ability to tolerate its use. Many patients are unable to tolerate CPAP and as a result, alternative treatments including oral appliances and surgery have been investigated for these patients. This review will consider conservative treatments such as weight loss and positional therapy, and then will discuss surgical approaches *(1)*.

From: *Current Clinical Practice: Primary Care Sleep Medicine: A Practical Guide*
Edited by: J. F. Pagel and S. R. Pandi-Perumal © Humana Press Inc., Totowa, NJ

CONSERVATIVE TREATMENTS FOR OSA

Weight Reduction

Excess body weight is often associated with OSA. In many studies, approximately two-thirds of patients with OSA are obese as defined by higher than 120% of ideal body weight *(2)*. Obesity is a major risk factor for OSA, especially, if there is significant fat accumulation in the neck. Weight gain has been also associated with increases in the severity of OSA in several studies *(3)*. Also, weight reduction has been shown to reduce the overall apnea/hypopnea index (AHI). However, it is known that many obese patients do not have significant OSA. Therefore, obesity is just one variable that interacts with other variables such as the shape and size of the mandible and maxilla and the overall size and configuration of the posterior pharynx. The mechanism of weight gain causing increased severity of OSA is likely related to the effect of the regional fat deposition in the tissues surrounding the pharynx. The excess adipose tissue reduces the area of the posterior pharyngeal airway, reducing the trans-mural pressure and favoring pharyngeal occlusion during inspiration. Weight loss therefore results in a reduction in upper airway collapsibility *(4)*.

Most efforts at voluntary weight loss, including caloric restriction show a success rate of approx 10% at the end of a year. One study found that only 3% of patients with OSA who had a significant improvement in sleep apnea following weight reduction were able to maintain their weight loss for 3 years *(5)*. However, bariatric surgery results in a significant degree of weight reduction in many patients. Several studies, examining the effects of weight loss associated with bariatric surgery have shown marked reductions in the AHI associated with improvements in the lowest oxygen saturation, sleep architecture, and general quality of life *(6,7)*. Recent improvements in the surgical techniques including the use of the laparoscopic Roux-en-Y procedure have produced successful weight loss with a very low degree of morbidity *(8)*. Morbidity is significantly lower using the laparoscopic approach compared with the open surgical procedure. Bariatric surgery results in more predictable and larger amounts of weight loss compared with voluntary dietary restriction.

Alcohol and Other Respiratory Depressants

Alcohol suppresses the dilator muscles of the upper airway, increases collapsibility, increases inspiratory airway resistance, and predisposes to obstructive apneas. Alcohol increases the frequency of obstructive apneas during sleep in both normals and patients who have known OSA. A similar reduction in upper airway dilator muscle activity and increase in severity of OSA occurs with benzodiazepines, narcotics, and barbiturates. These same substances also suppress the arousal response to hypoxia and hypercapnia, which may prolong apneas and deepen the oxygen desaturation. As a result, it is important to counsel patients with OSA about the adverse effects of alcohol and sedative medications.

Smoking Cessation

Data from the Wisconsin Sleep Cohort Study have demonstrated that cigaret smoking appears to be a risk factor for both snoring and OSA *(9)*. In this study, current smokers had a significantly higher risk of sleep-disordered breathing compared with never-smokers (odds ratio, 4.44). Heavy smokers (>40 cigarettes/day) seem to have a higher risk compared with those who smoke fewer cigarettes. The mechanism is uncertain, but likely the tobacco smoke results in inflammation and edema of the upper airway, which predisposes the airway to collapse. Therefore, smokers should be advised to discontinue smoking. Occasionally, heavy snoring will disappear with smoking cessation, but it is unlikely that smoking cessation itself is a cure for significant OSA.

Sleep Hygiene

It has been demonstrated in several studies that sleep deprivation reduces the ventilatory response associated with hypoxia and hypercapnia. This reduction of ventilatory response results in a decrease in upper airway muscle activity, which would be associated with an increase in the severity of OSA. Sleep deprivation increases the severity of mild-to-moderate sleep-disordered breathing. Even short-term sleep fragmentation appears to be associated with an increase in upper airway collapsibility. It is possible then that sleep fragmentation and sleep deprivation could exacerbate OSA, although few studies have actually looked at this. However, it is reasonable to counsel patients regarding improvements in sleep hygiene such as a regular sleep–wake schedule and avoidance of caffeine and other stimulants to improve sleep.

Positional Therapy

It is known that both snoring and OSA are worse in the supine position than in the nonsupine position. The upper airway seems to collapse more readily in the supine position than in the lateral position. Positional apnea is quite common and may occur in up to 56% of patients *(10)*. Patients with positional OSA tend to be younger and less obese and to have less severe OSA. Positional OSA may represent one point in the spectrum between snoring and severe OSA. That is the reason that during the polysomnogram, data are collected about the severity of OSA in the supine vs nonsupine position. In patients with positional OSA—i.e., when OSA is at least twice as severe in the supine position vs the nonsupine position—sleeping only in the nonsupine position does improve the AHI. One study showed that positional therapy improved hypertension in patients with OSA *(11)*. A prospective, randomized, single-blind, crossover study examined the effects of positional therapy. Compared with CPAP, positional therapy resulted in a similar improvement in sleep architecture, daytime alertness, quality of life, and performance on psychometric testing. These data suggest that advising patients to sleep in the nonsupine position is worthwhile and can result in significant improvements in the health consequences of OSA. A tennis ball T-shirt is fairly easy to construct. Three tennis balls can be placed into a sock, which can then be pinned onto the back of a T-shirt. Alternatively, a pocket can be sewn onto the back of a T-shirt and tennis balls placed into the pocket. Occasionally, a patient is capable of sleeping on three tennis balls, and the next step is to wear a backpack filled with towels or T-shirts. Such mechanical devices have been found to be very effective in promoting the lateral position *(1)*.

Pharmacological Treatment

Several drugs have been used in the treatment of OSA. An evidence-based review of all these drugs has been recently written by Hudgel *(12)*. Medroxyprogesterone acetate is known to increase central response to hypercapnia or hypoxemia, and is suggested to increase central drive to pharyngeal muscles *(13,14)*. It was thought that these properties might be useful in treating OSA. However, despite some individual responses in hypercapneic patients, thus far the literature indicates medroxyprogesterone is not useful in the treatment of OSA *(15)*. Acetazolamide produces a mild metabolic acidosis that stimulates a compensatory hyperventilation and respiratory alkalosis. The hypothesis is that if acetazolamide increased ventilatory drive by this mechanism, then there could be an improvement in OSA. Several studies have shown improvement in central sleep apnea, but most studies have not found a clinically important effect in OSA *(16,17)*.

Theophylline has been studied in several well-controlled studies. Theophylline appears to improve periodic breathing associated with congestive heart failure, but has not been shown to improve OSA *(18)*. Additionally, theophylline has been shown to adversesly affect nocturnal sleep, decreasing total sleep time, and sleep efficiency in one study. Various antidepressants have been tried as treatments for OSA. Protriptyline improves OSA primarily by decreasing the percentage of time in rapid eye movement (REM) sleep. Because OSA is often more severe in REM than non-REM sleep, by decreasing REM sleep, the overall severity of OSA is lessened *(19)*. Severity of OSA in non-REM sleep is not affected. Protriptyline may be effective in patients with OSA specific to REM sleep, but larger and better studies are needed. The serotonergic drugs have been tried in a small number of studies and generally found to have only a small effect in the treatment of OSA *(20)*.

Relief of Nasal Obstruction

Nasal obstruction is a frequent complaint among patients with OSA. Nasal obstruction may be caused by mucosal congestion from allergic or nonallergic rhinitis, or anatomical obstructions such as a deviated nasal septum or enlarged nasal turbinates. Acute nasal blockage can produce fragmented sleep and obstructive apneas during sleep. Nasal congestion can make using CPAP more difficult. Medical treatment of nasal obstruction can improve symptoms of snoring and daytime sleepiness, and may improve mild sleep-disordered breathing. However, it is uncommon for treatment of nasal congestion alone—for example, with inhaled nasal corticosteroids—to improve OSA significantly. Nevertheless, nasal congestion should be treated as one element of a treatment program for OSA, especially, if it appears that it is a major component interfering with CPAP therapy. Treatment options for reducing nasal obstruction include nasal decongestants, antihistamines, inhaled steroids, and immunotherapy in the case of allergic rhinitis. There are few studies of these agents in the treatment of OSA, and no evidence-based recommendations can be made about their use. Nasal dilator devices have been proposed and for each of these there is typically a very small number of studies that typically show a mild degree of improvement *(21)*.

Oxygen

Supplemental oxygen has been used frequently as treatment for OSA. OSA is associated with oxygen desaturation, and the recurrent episodes of desaturation may result in cardiac manifestations such as pulmonary hypertension and cardiac dysrhythmias. Repetitive hypoxemia may result in cognitive impairment. The evidence would indicate that supplemental oxygen does improve baseline oxygen saturation and reduces the lowest oxygen saturations observed. However, oxygen also increases apnea duration. Daytime sleepiness and fatigue do not seem to be reduced with the use of supplemental oxygen. Supplemental oxygen would be indicated primarily in patients with underlying lung disease or chronic heart disease who have significant low baseline oxygen saturations. Often, the use of CPAP for OSA will also improve baseline oxygen saturation. However, supplemental oxygen is often indicated in patients with cardiac or lung disease who have persistent low saturations despite the use of CPAP.

SURGICAL THERAPY OF OSA

Surgical procedures are frequently introduced into clinical practice without careful evaluation; surgical therapy for OSA has not been an exception to this rule. A detailed review of the literature regarding surgery for OSA was done by the Cochrane Airways Group Sleep Apnoea Randomised Controlled Trial Register in 2000 *(22)*. At that time, no randomized trials of surgical treatments for OSA could be identified. Hence, all the literature was graded as a C, level III, or -IV concatenating of only nonrandomized cohort studies and case series. Since then, there have been several randomized trials of surgical procedures but the numbers are still relatively small *(23)*.

Tracheostomy

Tracheostomy was the original treatment for OSA when the condition was initially identified in the early and mid-1970s. The original cases were mostly morbidly obese individuals with quite severe symptoms of OSA. Tracheostomy bypassed the site of obstruction quite effectively, and predictably relieved symptoms. Certainly patients with very severe OSA were good candidates for tracheostomy, but patients with milder forms were quite reluctant to undergo tracheostomy for the obvious cosmetic reasons. However, with the introduction of CPAP into medical practice, tracheostomy quickly became a much lesser used surgical operation. It is used now primarily as an emergency procedure to maintain airway access when there is upper airway obstruction. It is also used in patients with very severe cases of OSA who are admitted to the hospital, perhaps in severe left or right heart failure, and who are also unable to tolerate CPAP or bilevel positive airway pressure. Tracheostomy does work virtually 100% of the time and it is a fairly easy operation for a surgeon to accomplish. It has obvious undesirable morbidity on the part of the patient.

The Powell–Riley Protocol for Surgery for OSA

The current standard for the surgical approach to OSA surgery is the approach developed by Powell and Riley at Stanford University *(24,25)*. They have proposed and developed a two-phase approach for surgical treatment of OSA. Their approach is based on the philosophy that they are using surgical treatment to cure OSA, not simply to make it less severe. Their surgical approach is based on careful evaluation of the upper airway, based on physical examination and radiographic evaluation. Obstruction in any part of the upper airway is treated. Surgical management is done in a staged manner rather than an all-in-one approach. The rationale for the staged approach is that they believe this decreases the risk of doing too much surgery that is not necessary. Surgical treatment is done conservatively because they believe outcomes are often difficult to predict. The surgical staging also decreases hospital stay, limits postoperative risk, causes less pain and trauma, and is better accepted by most patients.

Phase 1 of the surgery is primarily surgery on the soft tissues of the upper airway. Nasal obstruction such as a deviated nasal septum or enlarged turbinates is approached first. The pharyngeal region of the upper airway can be surgically approached by uvulopalatopharyngoplasty (UPPP) or tonsillectomy if indicated. Obstruction in the hypopharyngeal region is based on advancing the genioglossus muscle forward and placing tension on the base of the tongue in order to increase pharyngeal space and prevent the genioglossus from collapsing into the airway during sleep. Techniques used here include laser midline glossectomy, lingualplasty, partial glossectomy, or temperature-controlled radiofrequency (TCRF) techniques.

A complete re-evaluation is done approx 4–6 months after phase 1 surgery is completed. Polysomnography and an assessment of symptoms and quality of life are done. If there is a need for further surgery, then phase 2 surgical procedures such as maxillomandibular advancement procedure are considered. The criteria used by Powell and Riley for a successful response are to reduce the respiratory disturbance index (RDI) to less than 20 or reduce it to ≤50% of the preoperative RDI, maintain oxygen saturations more than 90%, normalize sleep architecture, resolve complaints of excessive daytime sleepiness, and provide a response equivalent to CPAP.

The Powell–Riley staging of surgery into phase 1 and phase 2 surgeries appears to be the most rational approach and they have provided data on hundreds of patients on whom they have operated during the last 20 years at Stanford University. As a result, this is considered to be the standard approach. The following discussion will discuss each of the surgical procedures done as either phase 1 or phase 2 surgical procedures.

Nasal Reconstruction

Nasal obstruction is important in the pathophysiology of sleep-disordered breathing. Chronic nasal congestion or difficulty with nasal breathing are common complaints in the individual with OSA. Nasal obstruction increases upstream airway resistance, reduces inspiratory airflow, and predisposes the airway to collapse, acting as a resistor above the posterior pharynx. Nasal obstruction is often associated with increased snoring and the presence of obstructive apneas. Nasal obstruction has been demonstrated to increase the number of apneas and hypopneas. Complete nasal obstruction also produces marked sleep disturbance in normal individuals. Also, the presence of nasal obstruction increases the required CPAP pressure and has been shown to reduce tolerance of CPAP. In the absence of nasal breathing, oral breathing predominates. When oral breathing is the predominant route of breathing, typically the mandible rotates downward in order to open up the mouth and this results in the tongue being pushed posteriorly, which also predisposes to airway collapse.

Nasal reconstructive surgery may also improve CPAP tolerance. Radiofrequency treatment of turbinate hypertrophy has been shown in one study to improve tolerance of CPAP. A deviated nasal septum, enlarged turbinates, nasal valve or alar collapse, or external nasal deformities can all be addressed surgically. However, it is uncommon for nasal surgery alone to be an effective treatment for either snoring or OSA. However, it makes sense that nasal obstruction may impair the use of CPAP, and specific abnormalities such as a grossly deviated nasal septum or large nasal polyps would warrant treatment, including surgery, to improve the patient's ability to use CPAP. Also, humidifiers attached to a CPAP device can be effective at improving nasal breathing, as humidity would attenuate the mucosal blood flow flux that is associated with irritation that occurs with the use of CPAP.

Uvulopalatopharyngoplasty

It is understood that excessive tissue in the area of the palate and the lateral pharyngeal areas are prone to collapse with inspiration and are important in the pathogenesis of OSA. For years, surgeons have attempted to treat snoring and OSA by surgically removing excessive soft tissue in the pharyngeal area and shortening the soft palate. Several studies have shown that UPPP increases space in the posterior pharyngeal airway by removing tonsillar tissue and redundant soft tissue. The literature on UPPP has been unclear for many years. The reason is that there are many different variations on the surgical procedure of UPPP and evaluation of this surgery is impaired by the use of different techniques, patient selection, patient anatomy, and severities of sleep-disordered breathing. Also, the definition of a successful response has varied in the past, although articles in the last 10 years have had a fairly uniform definition of success.

A review paper by the American Sleep Disorders Association published in 1996 surveyed all the literature up to that time on UPPP. If all studies were combined, there appeared to be approx 40% success rate, again depending on the definition of improvement. Review of the information showed that success in treating sleep apnea depended on the level of obstruction. In the classification initially proposed by Fujita, type 1 obstruction was pharyngeal obstruction only; type 2 was base of tongue obstruction; and type 3 was obstruction both in the pharyngeal area and in the base of the tongue. The literature shows that in type 1 obstruction (pharyngeal only), the improvements were approx 75% reduction in apnea index (AI), a 57% reduction in RDI, and a 25% improvement in the lowest reported saturation.

Again in this area, success depended on the criteria used to define success. If the criteria for improvement were a 50% reduction in RDI and postoperative RDI of less than 20, or a 50% reduction in the AI and postoperative AI of less than 10, then 52% of type 1 patients improved, but only 5% of type 2 patients improved. If the type of obstruction was unknown, the overall improvement rate was about 45%. This makes sense in that if the pathophysiology of obstructive apnea is the tongue collapsing into the posterior pharyngeal airspace, then there is no rationale for believing that removing tissue from the pharynx would reverse this pathophysiology.

However, several studies have shown interesting improvements. One study done at a variety of Veterans Affairs hospitals showed a survival advantage to UPPP over CPAP therapy. Another study showed a reduction in cardiovascular mortality after UPPP compared with CPAP. Another study showed that the incidence of automobile accidents was lower in patients treated with UPPP compared with CPAP. Lateral pharyngoplasty was reported by Cahali et al. *(26)* to result in better clinical results and sleep outcomes compared with conventional UPPP. Apparently this surgical procedure also has less morbidity than conventional UPPP. Another variation on the standard UPPP is a procedure known as a uvulopalatal flap. This is an alternative that reduces the pain associated with the surgery and reduces the chance of nasopharyngeal incompetence and nasal regurgitation. There are no suture lines along the free edge of the soft palate, which lessens the pain associated with the procedure. The procedure can be reversed in the early preoperative period if there is evidence of nasal regurgitation. There were no significant differences in outcomes with this procedure compared with conventional UPPP.

A Friedman classification system has been proposed that appears to be highly effective at identifying patients who will benefit from UPPP. This Friedman system appears to predict UPPP outcome as well as the earlier Fujita system and is also easier to apply.

Laser-Assisted Uvuloplasty

In the early 1990s laser-assisted uvuloplasty (LAUP) was introduced. The major benefit of this procedure was, it was primarily an office-based procedure using a carbon dioxide laser to remove the uvula and to shorten the soft palate. A study by Walker showed favorable outcomes with this procedure in treating snoring and mild sleep apnea; however, many patients also experienced worsening of sleep-disordered breathing after this procedure. A recent randomized trial of LAUP showed that LAUP surgery is effective in some subjects with mild OSA for the treatment of snoring, but the reduction in AHI and the level of symptomatic improvement were minor overall *(27)*. Forty-five subjects with mild OSA were randomly assigned to receive LAUP or no treatment (control group). The AHI post-LAUP was reduced by 21% overall and to ≤10 per hour in 5 of 21 subjects (24%). Four of 24 subjects in the control group (16.7%) had an AHI of less than 10 per hour at outcome. The AHI decreased in the LAUP group, compared with no change in AHI for the control group at outcome. Ten LAUP subjects (48%) reported significantly improved snoring. There was no reduction in excessive daytime sleepiness, but there was a small improvement in quality of life *(27)*. This procedure has gradually diminished in popularity, and is used primarily as a snoring operation, and is not typically used as a treatment for true OSA.

Tongue Reduction Surgery

Because a large tongue and the propensity of the tongue to collapse against the posterior pharynx were significant in the pathophysiology of OSA, it stood to reason that reducing the size of the tongue should produce improvements in OSA. Laser midline glossectomy and lingualplasty were procedures designed to reduce the bulk of the tongue and increase posterior pharyngeal airspace. One series reported by Woodson reported a 77% response rate in improving sleep-disordered breathing. However, the popularity of this surgical procedure was limited markedly by the significant morbidity associated with the procedure, which included postoperative bleeding and airway edema. As a result, this procedure is seldom used anymore. The airway compromise associated with doing one of these procedures often necessitates a tracheostomy and a prolonged hospital stay.

Genioglossus Advancement

Hyoid Myotomy and Suspension

Because posterior collapse of the tongue is important in the pathophysiology of OSA, there have been efforts to stabilize the tongue or even pull the tongue forward in the pharynx in order to increase posterior pharyngeal space. Advancement of the tongue base by advancing the genial tubercle and the hyoid bone results in forward movement of the tongue base and does result in increased posterior pharyngeal space. This seems to stabilize the tongue base and also improves function of the pharyngeal dilator muscles, and results in an effective "jaw thrust." This is part of the phase 1 surgery as proposed by Riley and Powell at Stanford and is used successfully there. Genioglossus advancement and hyoid advancement are typically adjunctive procedures done in association with UPPP. Reports by Riley and Powell show that mild-to-moderate cases of OSA may have a success rate as high as 77%, whereas more severe cases have a success rate of 42%. A variety of case series report a success rate between 23 and 69%.

Advancing the hyoid bone can improve the outcome of genioglossus advancement. The hyoid bone and the hyoid complex are important in maintaining patency of the upper airway. Moving the hyoid bone forward increases posterior pharyngeal space. The hyoid advancement is not typically done at the same time as the genioglossus advancement in the Riley and Powell system, as the morbidity of the combined procedure is difficult for patients. One report from Riley and Powell indicates that hyoid advancement following UPPP and genioglossus advancement significantly improves sleep-disordered breathing.

Temperature-Controlled Radiofrequency

Radiofrequency ablation technology is used in a variety of areas in medicine. In the field of cardiology, radiofrequency ablation is used successfully in the treatment of supraventricular tachycardia such as Wolff-Parkinson-White syndrome or other re-entrant tachycardias. This type of technology is used in the treatment chronic atrial fibrillation. Also, radiofrequency ablation is used in urology for the treatment of benign prostatic hypertrophy. Radiofrequency can be delivered to a localized area and is fairly easy to use compared with laser procedures. Radiofrequency temperatures are lower than with typical lasers or electrocautery devices. The typical temperature of radiofrequency is 60–90°C, whereas electrocautery and laser can be 750–900°C. The lower temperatures are important in decreasing morbidity.

TCRF has been used to reduce snoring and improve upper airway resistance syndrome in a small group reported by Riley and Powell with a 77% reduction in subjective snoring. In this study, there was evidence of shrinkage of the midpalate area and there was improvement in quality of life and the Epworth sleepiness scale. TCRF can also be used to treat turbinate hypertrophy at the nasal level. By treating turbinate hypertrophy and reducing nasal obstruction, nasal resistance is decreased; this improves sleep-disordered breathing, lessens the amount of pressure required for CPAP, and improves CPAP tolerance.

Several studies using TCRF to reduce the volume of the tongue base have shown promising results. Combining UPPP with TCRF can be effective at improving sleep-disordered breathing. A randomized trial of TCRF of the tongue base and the palate compared with CPAP and placebo showed significant improvements in subjective symptoms of OSA without significant improvement in the objective measurements of OSA *(28)*. However, this surgical procedure appeared to be similar to the use of CPAP in improving quality of life and daytime sleepiness. Also, a very small number of side effects were observed, making this procedure an attractive alternative for treating cases of mild-to-moderate OSA.

Several observers in this area have noted that TCRF results are dependent on surgical skill and training and may not be generalized to the entire population of either patients or otolaryngology surgeons. There are learning curves associated with doing this procedure, and surgeons who have done dozens to hundreds of these procedures will likely have better results than surgeons doing only a handful of procedures.

Bimaxillary Advancement or Maxillomandibular Advancement Procedure

This is considered phase 2 surgery in the Riley and Powell system. Patients who have persistent obstructive apneas after phase 1 surgical procedures, as discussed above, are considered to be candidates for bimaxillary advancement or the procedure otherwise known as maxillomandibular advancement. This surgery should not be used as a primary surgery because many people can experience improvement with phase 1 surgery and hence would not need this other procedure. In the experience reported by Riley and Powell, patients who progressed through both phase 1 and phase 2 surgery had a cure rate of more than 90%. Long-term outcome is equally positive, with a 90% rate of long-term improvement.

ORTHODONTIC TREATMENT

The observation that in many patients OSA is associated with a narrow maxillary anatomy and a high arch to the hard palate have resulted in efforts at orthodontic treatment. Orthodontic treatment has proven to be the most successful in children and young adults. Pirelli et al. *(29)* reported that rapid maxillary expansion in children with OSA can be quite effective. Guilleminault and Li *(30)* have reported that maxillomandibular expansion can be effective in patients who have a narrow maxilla and a very high arch to the hard palate. In this study, six patients with maxillary and mandibular constriction were treated with orthodontics, which resulted in an improvement of OSA from an AHI of 13–4.5 per hour and a significant improvement in daytime symptoms. This is clearly an option that bears further investigation to outline its role in the treatment of OSA.

CONCLUSIONS

A variety of surgical procedures are used in the treatment of OSA. There is no ideal or optimal surgical treatment at the current time. UPPP can be effective in carefully selected patients. Patients who have obstruction primarily at the pharyngeal area and do not have a tongue-base obstruction are optimal candidates. The results of UPPP can be enhanced by genioglossus advancement procedures and hyoid myotomy and advancement as well. These surgical procedures are typically considered to be phase 1 surgical procedures in the Riley and Powell scheme. Phase 2 in the Riley and Powell scheme entails bimaxillary advancement or maxillomandibular advancement. In the hands of skillful surgeons, the combination of phase 1 and phase 2 surgery is associated with a more than 90% chance of cure of sleep apnea in carefully selected patients. TCRF procedures are increasing in popularity. TCRF therapy of the soft palate and/or the base of tongue can improve sleep-disordered breathing in a certain number of patients and is an important option. Orthodontic treatment in certain individuals is another method of improving the pharyngeal anatomy.

REFERENCES

1. Ryan CF (2005) Sleep x 9: an approach to treatment of obstructive sleep apnoea/hypopnoea syndrome including upper airway surgery. Thorax 60:595–604.
2. Stradling J, Crosby J (1991) Predictors and prevalence of obstructive sleep apnoea and snoring in 1001 middle aged men. Thorax 46:85–90.
3. Strobel R, Rosen R (1996) Obesity and weight loss in obstructive sleep apnea: a critical review. Sleep 19:104–115.
4. Schwartz A, Gold A, Schubert N, et al. (1991) Effect of weight loss on upper airway collapsibility in obstructive sleep apnea. Am Rev Respir Dis 144:494–498.
5. Sampol G, Munoz X, Sagales M, et al. (1998) Long-term efficacy of dietary weight loss in sleep apnoea/hypopnoea syndrome. Eur Respir J 12:1156–1159.
6. Charuzi I, Lavie P, Peiser J, et al. (1992) Bariatric surgery in morbidly obese sleep-apnea patients: short- and long-term follow-up. Am J Clin Nutr 55:594S–596S.
7. Scheuller M, Weider D (2001) Bariatric surgery for treatment of sleep apnea syndrome in 15 morbidly obese patients: long-term results. Otolaryngol Head Neck Surg 125:299–302.
8. Balsiger B, Murr M, Poggio J, et al. (2000) Bariatric surgery: surgery for weight control in patients with morbid obesity. Med Clin North Am 84:477–484.
9. Wetter D, Young T, Bidwell T, et al. (1994) Smoking as a risk factor for sleep-disordered breathing. Arch Intern Med 154:2219–2224.
10. Oksenberg A, Khamaysi I, Silverberg D, et al. (1997) Positional vs nonpositional obstructive sleep apnea patients: anthropomorphic, nocturnal polysomnographic, and multiple sleep latency test data. Chest 112:629–639.

11. Berger M, Oksenberg A, Silverberg D, et al. (1997) Avoiding the supine position during sleep lowers 24 h blood pressure in obstructive sleep apnea (OSA) patients. J Hum Hypertension 11:657–664.
12. Hudgel DW, Thanakitcharu S (1998) Pharmacological treatment of sleep-disordered breathing. Am J Respir Crit Care Med 158:691–699.
13. Skatrud JB, Dempsey JA, Kaiser DG (1978) Ventilatory response to medroxyprogesterone acetate in normal subjects: time course and mechanism. J Appl Physiol 44:939–944.
14. Zwillich CW, Natalino MR, Sutton FD, et al. (1978) Effects of progesterone on chemosensitivity in normal men. J Lab Clin Med 92:262–269.
15. Strohl KP, Hensley MJ, Saunders NA, et al. (1981) Progesterone administration and progressive sleep apneas. JAMA 245:1230–1232.
16. White DP, Zwillich CW, Pickett CK, et al. (1982) Central sleep apnea: improvement with acetazolamide therapy. Arch Intern Med 142:1816–1819.
17. Sharp JT, Druz WS, D'Souza V, et al. (1985) Effect of metabolic acidosis upon sleep apnea. Chest 87:619–624.
18. Javaheri S, Parker TJ, Wexler L, et al. (1996) Effect of theophylline on sleep-disordered breathing in heart failure. N Engl J Med 335:562–567.
19. Conway WA, Zorick F, Piccione P, et al. (1982) Protriptyline in the treatment of sleep apnoea. Thorax 37:49–53.
20. Hanzel DA, Proia NG, Hudgel DW (1991) Response of obstructive sleep apnea to fluoxetine and protriptyline. Chest 100:416–421.
21. Bahammam AS, Tate R, Manfreda J, et al. (1999) Upper airway resistance syndrome: effect of nasal dilation, sleep stage, and sleep position. Sleep 22:592–598.
22. Bridgman SA, Dunn KM (2000) Surgery for obstructive sleep apnoea. Cochrane Database Syst Rev (2):CD001004.
23. Steward D, Weaver E, Woodson B (2005) Multilevel temperature-controlled radiofrequency for obstructive sleep apnea: extended follow-up. Otolaryngol Head Neck Surg 132:630–635.
24. Riley RW, Powell NB, Li KK, et al. (2000) Surgery and obstructive sleep apnea: long-term clinical outcomes. Otolaryngol Head Neck Surg 122:415–421.
25. Powell N, Riley R, Guilleminault C (2005) Surgical management of sleep-disordered breathing. In: *Principles and Practice of Sleep Medicine.* 4th ed. (Kryger MH, Roth T, Dement WC, eds.) WB Saunders, Philadelphia, PA, pp. 1081–1097.
26. Cahali M, Formigoni G, Gebrim E, et al. (2004) Lateral pharyngoplasty versus uvulopalatopharyngoplasty: a clinical, polysomnographic and computed tomography measurement comparison. Sleep 27:942–950.
27. Ferguson K, Heighway K, Ruby R (2003) A randomized trial of laser-assisted uvulopalatoplasty in the treatment of mild obstructive sleep apnea. Am J Respir Crit Care Med 167:15–19.
28. Woodson B, Steward D, Weaver E (2003) A randomized trial of temperature-controlled radiofrequency, continuous positive airway pressure, and placebo for obstructive sleep apnea syndrome. Otolaryngol Head Neck Surg 128:848–861.
29. Pirelli P, Saponara M, Guilleminault C (2004) Rapid maxillary expansion in children with obstructive sleep apnea syndrome. Sleep 27:761–766.
30. Guilleminault C, Li K (2004) Maxillomandibular expansion for the treatment of sleep-disordered breathing: preliminary result. Laryngoscope 114:893–896.

12 Positive Airway Pressure Therapy for Obstructive Sleep Apnea/Hypopnea Syndrome

Neil S. Freedman, MD, FCCP

CONTENTS

INTRODUCTION

Continuous positive airway therapy (CPAP) remains the mainstay of therapy for obstructive sleep apnea syndrome (OSAS). CPAP therapy has been demonstrated to resolve sleep-disordered breathing events and improve several clinical outcomes. The first part of this review will concentrate on conventional fixed-pressure CPAP therapy with the second portion of this chapter focussing on newer technological advancements in the delivery of positive pressure therapy.

Nasal CPAP therapy was initially described as a treatment for sleep apnea by Sullivan et al. *(1)* in 1981. As the initial description, nasal CPAP therapy has become the mainstay of treatment for patients with OSAS *(2)*. CPAP is conventionally delivered through a nasal mask at a fixed pressure that remains constant throughout the respiratory cycle. CPAP therapy exerts its beneficial effects by acting as a pneumatic splint to prevent the upper airway soft tissue from collapsing. It does not exert its effects by increasing upper airway muscle activity *(3)*.

INDICATIONS FOR CPAP THERAPY

CPAP therapy is indicated for the treatment of moderate-to-severe OSAS and for patients who have mild OSAS and associated symptoms and/or underlying cardiovascular disease *(2,4)*. The Centers for Medicare and Medicaid Services (CMS), based on recommendations from the Practice Parameters Committee from the American Academy of Sleep Medicine (AASM) *(4)*, recently reconfirmed its position on the requirements for CPAP therapy in patients with OSAS *(5)*. Specifically, the Practice Parameters Committee and CMS stated that:

From: *Current Clinical Practice: Primary Care Sleep Medicine: A Practical Guide*
Edited by: J. F. Pagel and S. R. Pandi-Perumal © Humana Press Inc., Totowa, NJ

1. A diagnosis of OSAS must be made by polysomnography (PSG) performed in a sleep laboratory. Unattended studies and studies performed at home or in a mobile facility are not considered reasonable;
2. In order to qualify for CPAP therapy by these standards, adults with moderate-to-severe OSAS must meet one of the following criteria using the apnea-hypopnea index (AHI):
   a. AHI ≥15 events/hour, or
   b. AHI ≥5 events/hour and ≤14 events/hour with documented symptoms of excessive daytime sleepiness, impaired cognition, mood disorders, or insomnia, or documented hypertension, ischemic heart disease, or history of stroke.

Per the CMS and AASM Committee criteria, the AHI must be based on a minimum of 2 hours of sleep recorded by PSG using actual recorded hours of sleep (the AHI may not be extrapolated or projected).

DETERMINING THE OPTIMAL CPAP SETTING

The optimal CPAP settings for home use may be defined as the minimal pressure required to resolve all apneas, hypopneas, snoring, and arousals related to these events in all stages of sleep and in all positions *(2,4)*. Simply, the optimal CPAP setting should resolve all sleep-disordered breathing in supine rapid eye movement sleep, to account for the effects of gravity and changes in muscle tone that may occur in different sleep stages and positions *(6–8)*. The recent review by the Practice Parameters Committee of the AASM currently recommends a full night of CPAP titration based on the criteria outlined previously *(4)*. A repeat CPAP titration need only be performed if symptoms of OSAS reappear despite compliance with CPAP therapy or if a patient sustains a significant weight loss through either diet or bariatric surgery.

A split-night sleep study, in which the initial portion of the study is used to objectively document an individual's sleep-disordered breathing followed by a CPAP titration during the second portion of the night may be indicated in certain situations *(4)*. A split-night sleep study may be indicated when the following criteria have been met:

1. An AHI of ≥40 events/hour is recorded during the initial 2 hours of the PSG.
2. At least 3 hours remain during the PSG to conduct an adequate CPAP titration.

A second full night of CPAP titration should be performed if an optimal CPAP pressure setting cannot be achieved during the second portion of the split-night study. Split-night studies can also be considered for individuals who demonstrate an AHI of 20–40 events/hour during the initial 2 hours of a sleep study, although data suggest that CPAP titrations in this subgroup of patients may be less accurate when performed in the split-night protocol setting. Also, although split-night studies potentially reduce waiting times to initiate home CPAP therapy, especially in areas with long sleep laboratory waiting times, a significant portion of patients with OSAS will undergo suboptimal CPAP titrations using this format *(9)*.

Although current recommendations warrant that CPAP titrations occur during a full overnight in-laboratory PSG, some data suggest that conventional fixed-pressure CPAP as well as auto-CPAP (APAP) therapy can be successfully initiated in an unattended home setting *(10–12)*. Masa et al. *(11)* recently demonstrated in a large ($n = 360$), randomized, controlled study that both APAP and CPAP (set by a prediction formula) initiated in the unattended home setting were equivalent to conventional fixed CPAP therapy that was initiated after titration of pressures in a monitored sleep laboratory setting. Specifically, they demonstrated no significant differences in objective compliance and improvements in clinical outcomes such as daytime sleepiness and quality of life. Other studies also confirm that CPAP therapy initiated in an unattended home setting can be successful in most uncomplicated OSAS patients when CPAP settings are determined either by a clinical prediction formula *(13)*, by CPAP self-adjusted to resolve snoring *(10)*, or by APAP therapy *(12)*.

As results such as these continue to be reproduced in future studies, positive pressure therapy for uncomplicated OSAS may be initiated in the home. It is also possible that in the future, in-laboratory CPAP titrations may be reserved for patients with OSAS and concomitant cardiac and/or respiratory disease, those with obesity-hypoventilation syndrome and for those who are having difficulty with CPAP initiated in an unattended setting. If this mode of CPAP treatment comes to fruition, patients with OSAS will benefit by realizing shorter waiting times to CPAP therapy and health care dollars should be saved by reducing the need for unnecessary PSGs *(11,12,14)*.

Benefits of CPAP Therapy

CPAP Treatment and Daytime Sleepiness

Several studies have repeatedly shown that CPAP therapy significantly improves or resolves symptoms of daytime sleepiness in OSAS patients who suffer from this complaint *(11,15–20)*. The minimal and optimal amounts of nocturnal use necessary to improve symptoms of daytime sleepiness are not well defined, as even partial nocturnal use (as little as 4 hour per night) has been associated with significant improvements in daytime symptoms. Although the minimal amount of time required on a nightly basis to improve symptoms of daytime sleepiness is not well established, it is clear that CPAP therapy is required for a least a portion of each night, as symptoms of daytime sleepiness reappear when CPAP therapy is discontinued for as little as one night *(21)*.

Although most patients with daytime sleepiness related to OSAS will achieve significant improvements in symptoms after CPAP therapy has been instituted, this is not the case for all patients. There remains a subgroup of OSAS patients that continue to have symptoms of residual daytime sleepiness despite adequate compliance with CPAP therapy *(22)*. The actual prevalence of residual daytime sleepiness in CPAP-compliant patients remains undefined. The mechanisms responsible for this syndrome of residual daytime sleepiness also remain unclear, but may be related to the oxidative injury effects of long-term intermittent hypoxemia on sleep–wake regions in the brain *(23)*.

CPAP Treatment and Neurocognitive/Psychological Functioning

Numerous studies have assessed the effects of sleep-disordered breathing on neurocognitive/psychological functioning *(20,24–33)*. Altered memory, concentration, and reaction time may occur, but the levels of cognitive dysfunction vary over a wide range of performance areas in patients with different degrees of OSAS. Few studies on the effect of treatment for OSAS on neurocognitive function are robust. One small prospective study evaluating the effects of CPAP therapy on 20 patients with severe OSAS (mean respiratory disturbance index [RDI], 67 ± 16 events/hour) found that most patients demonstrated a significant improvement in cognitive function at 3 months and 12 months after CPAP therapy was instituted *(32)*. Treatment with CPAP demonstrated significant improvements in concentration and in recent verbal, visual, and spatial memory. Munoz et al. *(34)* prospectively studied 80 patients with severe OSAS (mean RDI, 60 ± 21 events/hour) and compared them with 80 control patients matched for age and sex. Baseline data demonstrated that the patients with OSAS were significantly more somnolent ($p < 0.001$) and had longer reaction times ($p < 0.05$) and poorer vigilance ($p < 0.01$) than control subjects. After 12 months of therapeutic nasal CPAP treatment, significant improvements occurred in levels of daytime somnolence ($p < 0.0002$) and vigilance ($p < 0.01$), whereas changes in reaction times were relatively minor.

Several small randomized, placebo-controlled trials have evaluated the effect of CPAP therapy on the reversibility of neurocognitive deficits in patients with OSAS *(20,24–26)*. A total of 98 patients were evaluated in these trials, with 50 of the 98 patients having relatively mild OSA with an AHI between 5 and 15 events/hour of sleep (mean AHI, 26 ± 28 events/hour). All patients had an AHI of ≥5, two or more symptoms related to OSA, and no coexisting illnesses or sleep disorders. Patients were treated with 1 month of CPAP treatment and 1 month of oral placebo treatment. Compared with the placebo arm of the study, all cognitive performance scores demonstrated either trends or significant improvements with CPAP. Significant improvements ($p < 0.05$) with CPAP therapy vs placebo were seen in the Trailmaking B test, WAIS-R Digit Symbol Substitution test, the Performance IQ Decrement test, and the PASAT 2s test. Trends toward significant improvement with CPAP therapy were seen with WAIS-R Block Design subtest and the SteerClear test. Although there were several statistically significant improvements with CPAP therapy, the effect size of these changes was relatively small.

This last finding—concerning the relatively small effect size—may be secondary to a significant proportion of the study patients having relatively mild sleep apnea. Another possible explanation is that 1 month of CPAP therapy may be insufficient to reverse changes that have accumulated during long periods of time (months to years). Also, the mean nocturnal CPAP usage was only 3.3 hour per night, which is less than the typical average of 4.5 hour per night. Finally, it is possible that some of the cognitive deficits seen in patients with OSAS are irreversible, possibly related to repeated episodes of nocturnal hypoxemia *(23,35)*.

Further research is required to better define the mechanisms responsible for the neurocognitve deficits observed in some patients with OSAS and to clarify the potential reversibility of these deficits. In addition, larger and more long-term studies will be required to better address these questions in patients with varying degrees of OSAS severity.

CPAP Treatment, Mood, and Depression

The relationship of OSAS with psychiatric disease is also unclear and controversial. Several studies link OSA with major depression and subclinical depressive symptoms *(8,36–42)*. Currently, however, no large-scale prospective data accurately estimate the prevalence of depression and other mood symptoms and disorders these patients. Although the actual prevalence of depression and other mood disorders is unknown, they are estimated to occur in up to 20% of all patients with OSAS *(40–42)*. The 5-year prevalence of major depressive disorder is estimated at 58% *(41)*, a figure three times higher than depression prevalence rates in the general population *(43)*. Eleven percent of patients with OSAS report previous treatment for depression *(39)*. Finally, although higher rates of depressive symptoms are present in patients with OSAS, patients with major depression do not demonstrate an increased incidence of OSAS *(42)*.

Assuming that OSAS adversely affects mood parameters, data concerning treatment with CPAP are also variable. Borak et al. *(32)* showed that although significant early improvements were seen in cognitive function, no significant improvements were seen in any emotional status parameters after 3 months and 12 months of CPAP therapy in 20 patients with severe OSAS. Ramos Platon and Espinar Sierra *(44)* prospectively followed 23 patients with severe OSAS before, during, and after 1 year of CPAP therapy. They found a progressive reduction of psychopathological signs along with a generalized improvement in psychosocial adaptation. The most significant changes were seen for depression ($p < 0.01$) and total adjustment degree ($p < 0.01$) after 1 year of treatment, suggesting that improvements in psychosocial function may take place gradually with proper therapy.

Munoz et al. *(34)* prospectively studied 80 patients with severe OSAS (mean RDI, 60 ± 21 events/hour of sleep) and 80 control patients matched for age and sex. OSAS patients were significantly more somnolent ($p < 0.001$), anxious ($p < 0.01$), and depressed ($p < 0.001$) than control subjects at baseline. After 12 months of therapeutic nasal CPAP treatment, significant improvements were seen in levels of daytime somnolence ($p < 0.0002$) and vigilance ($p < 0.01$), but no significant changes were demonstrated in levels of anxiety or depression.

Yu et al. *(45)* studied mood changes in 24 patients with OSAS using the profile of mood states questionnaire. Patients were randomly assigned to receive treatment with therapeutic-CPAP or placebo-CPAP for 1 week. After treatment, both groups showed significant improvement in mood states. The authors concluded that the effect of CPAP therapy on mood symptoms could represent a placebo effect. They also concluded that CPAP treatment may be an effective treatment for improving mood states, but only in those patients with severe depressive symptoms secondary to sleep apnea.

As is the case with the potential association between neurocognitive dysfunction and OSAS, the relationship linking psychiatric disease and OSAS and its potential improvement, and reversibility with CPAP treatment are variable. In addition to depressive symptoms being common in some patients with OSAS, a diversity of other psychological and behavioral problems may also be present. Depressive symptoms may occur in patients with all degrees of severity of OSAS, even in those with normal oxygen saturations and less severe OSAS. The mechanisms underlying changes in mood and personality in patients with OSAS are unclear, but are likely related to a combination of factors including chronic partial sleep deprivation induced by sleep fragmentation, chronic nocturnal hypoxemia, and other factors yet to be defined. Thus, the therapeutic effect of CPAP treatment on mood is variable as noted above. Further research is required to clearly identify the mechanisms and risk factors underlying psychiatric disease related to OSAS and the potential role of CPAP therapy in alleviating these symptoms.

CPAP Treatment and Quality of Life

As opposed to the controversial data concerning the effects of OSAS on mood and neurocognitive dysfunction, the adverse effects of OSAS on quality of life have been more strongly demonstrated in large-scale population-based studies *(46,47)*. These negative effects on quality of life are more common in those patients with more severe disease. Despite these data, insufficient evidence exists to accurately state whether the changes related to quality of life in patients with OSAS are partially or totally reversible with adequate CPAP therapy. Data obtained from several randomized, placebo-controlled trials by Engleman et al. *(20,24–26)* which primarily evaluated the affect of CPAP therapy on neurocognitive function, demonstrated significant improvements in many aspects of quality of life as assessed by the SF-36 questionnaire and the Nottingham

Health Profile Part 2 evaluation. These data should be interpreted cautiously, however, as the total sample size was small (98 patients) and many of the patients had relatively mild OSAS. In a randomized parallel controlled trial of 101 male patients with OSA, Stradling and Davies *(48)* demonstrated that the Vitality and Energy Scale for the SF-36 significantly ($p < 0.0001$) improved after 1 month of nasal CPAP treatment at therapeutic levels when compared with control patients using CPAP at subtherapeutic levels. In a follow-up study on this same group of patients, Jenkinson et al. *(49)* demonstrated that these improvements in quality-of-life measures were sustained after 5 months of therapy. Also, those patients who had initially been randomized to the subtherapeutic arm of the study demonstrated scores similar to the active group after receiving therapeutic CPAP therapy during the following 4-month period.

In summary, there is good evidence that symptoms of daytime sleepiness that result from OSAS are improved or completely reversed in the majority of patients who are compliant with CPAP therapy. Little can be said about the therapeutic effects of CPAP therapy on neurocognitive dysfunction and psychiatric disease that may occur as a result of OSAS. Given the weak association in the literature between OSAS, neurocognitve deficits, and psychiatric disease as well as the paucity of robust data objectively evaluating the effects of CPAP on these parameters, few conclusions can be made in regards to CPAP's effects on these measures. Finally, insufficient evidence exists to accurately state whether the changes related to quality of life in patients with OSAS are partially or totally reversible with adequate CPAP therapy.

Problems and Compliance With CPAP Therapy

In a perfect world, all patients with OSAS would use their CPAP therapy all night every night. Unfortunately, just like many therapies for other chronic diseases, compliance with CPAP therapy for OSAS is far from perfect. Although there are no formal definitions of what constitutes compliance with CPAP therapy, most studies have defined compliance as use for more than 4 hours per night for 70% of the observed nights. When patients are asked about their CPAP use, subjective compliance ranges between 65 and 90%. Objective measures of CPAP compliance have demonstrated that patients usually overestimate their CPAP usage *(50,51)*. Short-term follow-up of OSAS patients demonstrate that CPAP usage patterns fall into two groups: (1) those who use their CPAP for more than 90% of the nights with an average usage time of more than 6 hours per night; and (2) those who use their CPAP intermittently, with an average usage of less than 3.5 hours per night *(52)*. Long-term objective follow-up has demonstrated that approx 68% of patients with OSAS continue to use their CPAP therapy after 5 years *(50)*.

A pattern of CPAP compliance can usually be determined within the first few days and certainly by 3 months of therapy *(50,52,53)*. Weaver et al. *(52)* showed that a pattern of nightly CPAP use could be determined as early as day 4 of treatment. Overall, most of the studies have not been able to demonstrate factors that consistently predict compliance with CPAP therapy *(16,51,54–56)*. With that in mind, some studies have suggested certain parameters that may predict short- and long-term usage. Predictors of long-term CPAP compliance have included symptoms of subjective sleepiness (Epworth sleepiness scale >10), severity of OSAS (AHI >30 events/hour), and average nightly use within the first 3 months of therapy *(50)*. Patients reporting problems during their initial night with CPAP therapy are typically less likely to use CPAP on a regular basis *(53)*. Interestingly, the level of CPAP pressure has not been shown to be a predictor of CPAP utilization.

Typical problems that may lead to reduced compliance with CPAP therapy include claustrophobia, nasal congestion, and poor mask fit leading to leaks and skin irritation. Several interventions have been proposed and instituted in an attempt to improve CPAP compliance. Several studies have demonstrated that the addition of heated humidification improves symptoms of nasal congestion and increases objective CPAP use *(57–59)*. Patient education has been shown to improve CPAP compliance in many, but not all studies *(51,60,61)*. Simple interventions such as weekly phone calls and mailings may improve compliance, especially when performed in the initial weeks of therapy *(61)*. Although proper initial mask fit is key to CPAP acceptance, changing masks once a problem has developed has not been shown to improve long-term compliance. Changing a patient to bilevel therapy once a problem has developed with CPAP therapy has also not been shown to improve long-term use of positive airway pressure *(62)*. Although a ramp feature that slowly increases pressure to a therapeutic level is common on most of the current CPAP devices, there is no peer-reviewed literature evaluating the effect of ramp on compliance with CPAP therapy.

Technological Advances in the Treatment of OSAS: APAP and Beyond

As reviewed previously, CPAP therapy is difficult for many patients to tolerate despite its clinical efficacy. Clinicians, patients, and industry are continually evaluating better methods to make CPAP therapy more acceptable. The next part of this review will summarize new advances in technology related to treating OSAS, specifically focussing on advances in the delivery of positive airway pressure.

AUTO-CPAP

Automatic (also known as auto-, automated, autoadjusting, or autotitrating) APAP further advances CPAP therapy with the ability to detect and respond to changes in upper airway resistance in real time *(63)*. Although this technology may be used to detect and diagnose patients with OSAS, this review will focus on the literature related to APAP's ability to treat patients in whom OSAS has already been diagnosed. APAP noninvasively detects variations of upper airway obstruction and airflow limitation including snoring, hypopneas, and apneas. Sensors used to detect the spectrum of upper airway obstruction vary among the different APAP machines. Most currently available machines have the ability to detect snoring through mask pressure vibration and apneas/hypopneas through changes in airflow detected through a pneumotachograph, nasal pressure monitor, or alterations in compressor speed. Some units detect flow limitation through an algorithm utilizing a flow-vs-time profile. Fewer units utilize the forced oscillation technique method, which is an alternative method that noninvasively detects changes in upper airway resistance or impedance *(64–66)*.

Once upper airway flow limitation has been detected, the APAP devices automatically increase the pressure until the flow limitation has been resolved. Once a therapeutic pressure has been achieved, the APAP devices reduce pressure until flow limitation resumes. Each APAP device follows different algorithms to increase and decrease pressure in response to changes in airway flow and resistance during a set period of time. Most devices have a therapeutic pressure range between 3 and 20 cm H_2O, with the ability to adjust the upper and lower pressure limits based on the clinical conditions. Because pressures changes occur throughout the sleep period, some have postulated that APAP devices may actually increase sleep fragmentation *(67)*. In general, the frequency of microarousals and sleep fragmentation induced by APAP devices appears to be small

(68). Also, clinical outcomes related to subjective sleepiness also show no significant differences from conventional CPAP therapy.

Is There One Best APAP Method to Detect Airflow Limitation? This question is difficult to answer as there have been few peer-reviewed studies that have compared different APAP devices in a head-to-head fashion. Senn et al. *(69)* compared two APAP devices with conventional CPAP in a clinical trial of 29 patients with OSAS. The APAP devices utilized different algorithms to assess airflow limitation:

1. The DeVilbiss AutoAdjust LT (Sunrise Medical; Somerset, PA), which responds to apnea/hypopnea and snoring.
2. The AutoSet T (Resmed; North Ryde, Australia), which responds to changes in inspiratory flow contour in addition to apnea/hypopnea and snoring. They evaluated patients during three consecutive 1-month periods in random order and found that all three treatment modalities significantly improved daytime symptoms, quality-of-life domains, and AHIs to a similar degree. Pevernagie et al. *(70)* demonstrated that the flow-guided Autoset T and an impedence-guided APAP provided a similar reduction in the AHI, although the flow-guided APAP more significantly resolved snoring. Alternatively, Kessler et al. *(71)* found that AutoSet and the SOMNOsmart predicted significantly different therapeutic pressures for fixed CPAP therapy based on one night of APAP titration. Thus, the literature remains inconclusive in determining if any APAP technology is superior for detecting and responding to airflow limitation.

Do All APAP Machines Respond Equally to Different Types of Airflow Limitation? As noted previously, few clinical studies have compared different APAP devices in a head-to-head fashion. Abdenbi et al. *(72)* and Farre et al. *(73)* conducted unique bench studies in which they separately subjected five different commercially available APAP devices to simulated breathing patterns that would typically be encountered in patients with OSAS. Farre et al. *(73)* demonstrated that the response of the devices to apneas, hypopneas, flow limitation, and snoring were considerably different. In some devices, the response was modified by air leaks similar to ones found in patients. Remarkably, two devices did not respond at all when subjected to a pattern of repetitive apneas. Also, not all devices responded when subjected to different patterns of hypopneic and flow limitation events. Abdenbi's group *(72)* demonstrated that although all devices responded to apneas appropriately, responses to mask leak, hypopneas, and snoring were different in different devices. These results raise the question of whether the conclusions derived from clinical studies using various APAP machines are valid as it is difficult to evaluate the effectiveness of various APAP devices if the procedure is not well-defined.

In a clinical trial independent of manufacturer financial support, three different APAP devices—AutoSet, Horizon, and Virtuoso—were compared with conventional CPAP. All devices reduced the AHI, but only two of three APAP devices reduced the AHI to less than 5 events/hour in all patients. The mean pressure was lower with two APAP devices and higher in the other APAP device compared with conventional CPAP *(74)*. Taken together, it is clear from both the bench and clinical literature that all APAP devices are not created equally and data derived from one device can not necessarily be extrapolated to another APAP device.

Is APAP as Good as, Better Than, or Worse Than Conventional CPAP for the Treatment of OSAS? A meta-analysis by Ayas et al. *(75)* compared the effectiveness of APAP against standard CPAP regarding several clinical parameters and outcomes.

A total of nine randomized clinical trials studying a total of 282 patients were reviewed *(12,66,76–82)*. The meta-analysis concluded that compared with standard CPAP, APAP is almost always associated with a reduction in mean pressure. Aside from this difference, APAP and standard CPAP were similar in objective compliance, their ability to eliminate respiratory events, and their ability to improve subjective daytime sleepiness. Based on these findings, the recommendations by the committee were that APAP not be used as first-line therapy in all patients with OSAS given the added cost of APAP devices compared with standard CPAP devices. It was also suggested that APAP could be considered in other situations such as home titrations or other subgroups of patients with OSAS. More recent randomized controlled trials comparing various APAP devices to conventional CPAP *(11,70,83,84)* confirm the findings of the meta-analysis by Ayas et al. *(75)*. It should be noted that these results and recommendations apply to patients with uncomplicated moderate-to-severe OSAS. No recommendations can be made for more mild OSAS and/or OSAS associated with underlying chronic lung disease, obesity-hypoventilation syndrome, and/or concomitant congestive heart failure with associated central apneas as there is a relative absence of peer-reviewed literature assessing APAP in these patient groups.

Currently available machines still have several limitations. Most APAP devices are somewhat limited in their ability to distinguish between central and obstructive apneas. Also, the ability of the APAP devices to respond to sustained hypoventilation in the absence of upper airway obstruction is unclear, as most APAP studies have excluded patients at high risk, including those patients with obesity-hypoventilation syndrome and/or chronic respiratory diseases. Given these limitations, a report from the AASM regarding APAP use recommended that APAP devices not be used in the following groups of patients:

1. Those with congestive heart failure;
2. Those with lung diseases such as chronic obstructive pulmonary disease; and
3. Patients expected to have nocturnal arterial oxyhemoglobin desaturation because of conditions other than OSAS (e.g., obesity-hypoventilation syndrome).

Finally, patients who do not snore (either naturally or as a result of palatal surgery) should not be titrated with an APAP device that relies on vibration or sound in the device's algorithm *(85,86)*. The same report recommended that APAP devices not be used for split-night titrations given the lack of data to support such a practice.

Can Unattended APAP Titrations be Used to Determine a Therapeutic Pressure Setting for Conventional Fixed CPAP Devices? A common scenario in clinical practice is that of the patient who either is having problems while using conventional CPAP or does not want to go back to the sleep laboratory for an initial or retitration study. Currently, there are not enough data to support the use of unattended APAP titrations to determine a fixed CPAP setting. The 2002 AASM Report on APAP devices stated that the use of unattended APAP either to initially determine pressure for fixed CPAP or for self-adjusting APAP treatment in CPAP-naive patients was not established at the time of the report *(86)*. The best device and the best method of determining the best effective pressure for CPAP therapy remain unknown.

Studies since the 2002 AASM report continue to confirm that unattended APAP titration data cannot be used to determine optimal treatment pressures for conventional CPAP use. Kessler et al. *(71)* used two different APAP devices (AutoSet and SOMNOsmart) in random order on two consecutive nights to determine an optimal fixed CPAP setting. The AutoSet device utilizes analysis of flow and the SOMNOsmart uses a forced oscillation algorithm to determine upper airway resistance to flow. They defined the therapeutic pressure as the 95th percentile of airway pressure over time. They observed significant differences between the two devices in this variable, with a mean difference of 2.9 cm H_2O ($p = 0.005$). In summary, they found that the two devices predicted significantly different therapeutic pressures for fixed CPAP therapy based on one night of APAP titration *(71)*.

Patients being treated with fixed CPAP on the basis of an APAP titration or who are currently being treated with APAP must be followed up to determine treatment efficacy and safety. A re-evaluation and, if necessary, a standard CPAP titration should be performed if symptoms do not resolve or the CPAP or APAP treatment seems to lack efficacy *(86)*.

Can Unattended Home APAP be Used as the Sole Treatment for Patients With OSAS Without the Use of PSG? Until recently, there was minimal evidence to support unattended APAP use as the sole treatment for OSAS without objectively confirming treatment efficacy through PSG. Since the 2002 AASM report, several randomized controlled trials have evaluated APAP in CPAP-naïve patients with OSAS in this unmonitored setting *(11,12,83)*. All of these studies demonstrated that APAP and conventional CPAP therapy result in similar treatment outcomes. Specifically, these studies demonstrated no significant differences in objective compliance, and similar improvements in daytime sleepiness and quality of life. If these results continue to be demonstrated in future studies, home treatment of OSAS with APAP could potentially reduce waiting times to positive airway pressure treatment and save health care dollars.

In summary, APAP technology appears to be as effective as conventional fixed CPAP therapy when used in an attended setting in patients with uncomplicated OSAS. Recent controlled trials also support its use in the unattended setting at home. Although it reduces the mean pressure, it appears to result in similar compliance rates and effects on clinical outcomes. Although APAP therapy has demonstrated some shortcomings in the peer-reviewed literature, the technology is rapidly advancing. It is possible that APAP therapy may take the place of the standard in-laboratory CPAP titration in the not-so-distant future. Although currently APAP devices are somewhat more expensive that standard CPAP, their cost is rapidly declining. APAP's main benefits in the future will likely be their ability to provide more rapid treatment to patients with OSAS and possibly the saving of health care dollars by eliminating unnecessary sleep studies *(11,12,83)*.

Bilevel Positive Pressure Therapy

Bilevel therapy's potential benefits in treating patients with OSAS were first described in 1990 *(87)*. As opposed to CPAP therapy, which allows a fixed pressure throughout the respiratory cycle, bilevel therapy allows the independent adjustment of the expiratory positive airway pressure (EPAP) and the inspiratory positive airway pressure. In its initial description, bilevel therapy demonstrated that obstructive events could be eliminated at a lower EPAP compared with conventional CPAP pressures *(87)* Although intuitively one would predict that bilevel would increase compliance by reducing unwanted pressure-related side effects, there is no convincing data to date that bilevel therapy improves compliance *(62)*. Bilevel therapy remains a viable option for CPAP-intolerant patients with OSAS, OSAS with concurrent respiratory disease, and/or obesity-hypoventilation syndrome *(2)*. The role of bilevel therapy in otherwise uncomplicated OSA remains unclear *(88)*.

Newer bilevel systems have been introduced by several companies. Respironics introduced a novel bilevel device that differs from conventional bilevel systems in two major respects. First, the inspiratory pressure is reduced slightly near the end of inspiration and the expiratory pressure is slightly reduced near the beginning of expiration. Second, the magnitude of change of the inspiratory positive airway pressure and EPAP is proportional to patient effort. In a randomized study of 27 patients with OSAS during a 1-month period, this novel bilevel system was as effective as conventional nasal CPAP. There were no differences in compliance or measures of subjective sleepiness and quality of life *(89)*. This report again confirms the findings of previous studies that the role of bilevel therapy in otherwise uncomplicated OSA remains unclear.

C-Flex

A common complaint in many patients with OSAS is the uncomfortable feeling of exhaling against positive pressure. This is one potential major barrier to long-term CPAP therapy acceptance and compliance. C-Flex (Respironics) is a relatively new technology that allows pressure relief during exhalation in an attempt to make CPAP therapy more comfortable. In simple terms, the C-Flex technology briefly reduces the CPAP pressure during exhalation before returning the pressure to its baseline CPAP setting before the initiation of inspiration. The C-Flex technology monitors the patient's airflow during exhalation and reduces expiratory pressure in response to the airflow. The amount of pressure relief varies on a breath-by-breath basis, depending on the actual patient airflow. The amount of pressure relief is also dictated by patient preference. Patients can choose from three C-Flex settings, corresponding to the amount of expiratory pressure relief they desire. C-Flex setting 1 allows the least amount of pressure relief (1 cm H_2O), whereas setting 3 allows the most pressure relief (3 cm H_2O). It would be akin to a modified bilevel device, without the increase in pressure during inhalation.

Currently there is only one peer-reviewed study comparing the C-Flex technology and conventional CPAP therapy *(90)*. In a nonrandomized study that followed CPAP-naive patients with OSAS during a 3-month period, C-Flex compliance was higher by an average of 1.7 hour per night when compared with compliance in conventional CPAP users. Subjective sleepiness and objective outcomes were similar in the two groups. Although these results imply that C-Flex technology may improve CPAP compliance, further randomized controlled trials will be necessary to confirm these findings. Based on the paucity of data currently available on C-Flex technology, no recommendations can be made regarding its use in clinical practice.

New Interfaces (Masks)

CPAP treatment for patients with OSAS is typically delivered through a nasal mask. Full-face masks remain an option for CPAP users, although they are usually less well tolerated than nasal masks *(58,91)*. Although there are several types of nasal masks currently on the market, there does not appear to be any specific mask that is accepted more than any of the others. In general, proper mask fit is more important to acceptance of CPAP therapy than the type of mask used.

Nasal pillows offer a variation to the typical nasal mask. There is only one report in the peer-reviewed literature comparing nasal pillows vs standard nasal masks for the delivery of CPAP therapy in the treatment of OSAS *(92)*. Massie and Hart *(92)* demonstrated that nasal pillows (Breeze; Mallinckrodt Corp; Minneapolis, MN) were a well-tolerated and effective interface for CPAP therapy for patients requiring pressures of ≤14 cm H_2O (higher CPAP pressures were not required in this study population) during the 3-week study period. Although patients reported less air leak with nasal pillows, there was no significant differences in mean daily use, Epworth Sleepiness Scale scores, or quality of life as assessed by the Functional Outcomes of Sleep Questionnaire between the nasal pillows and the standard nasal mask group.

The newest interface for the delivery of CPAP therapy is the Oracle™ oral device (Fisher & Paykel). The Oracle interface allows positive pressure therapy to be delivered through the mouth. The Oracle is constructed with a rigid plastic framework that is encased by two separate silicon components. The first component, the SoftSeal, rests inside the mouth and incorporates a tongue guide designed to keep the tongue from blocking the flow of air. The second component, the SnapFlap, rests on the outer cheek and provides a secondary pressure seal. This portion of the mask keeps the device in the patient's mouth without the need for headgear *(93)*.

Several studies have evaluated the Oracle interface for the delivery of CPAP therapy in OSAS *(93–96)*. These studies demonstrated that delivery of CPAP therapy through the oral route with the Oracle device is relatively equivalent to standard nasal CPAP therapy. In general, there were no significant differences in ability to improve polysomnographic variables of OSAS, compliance, or Epworth sleepiness scale scores. Side effects specifically related to the Oracle included upper airway dryness and gum pain.

Can I Switch My Patient to an Oral Device Using the Same Pressures Determined During a Sleep Study That Utilized a Nasal Mask? From a clinical standpoint, one might question whether similar pressures are required to optimally treat OSAS through the oral route vs the standard nasal route. Smith et al. *(96)* evaluated the individual pressure-flow curves during the application of nasal and oral CPAP. They found comparable pressure-flow relationships with pressure applied through either the oral or nasal routes. Thus, the application of comparable positive pressure through either the nose or the mouth is equally effective in overcoming the upper airway collapse seen in OSAS. Based on these initial findings, it may be possible to prescribe a treatment pressure using either route at the initial titration. Because the study group was relatively small ($n = 7$), further studies will be necessary to determine if retitration would be necessary, should a patient wish to switch to an alternative device after a period of time.

CONCLUSIONS

CPAP therapy remains the mainstay of treatment for OSAS. Despite its potential to improve several clinical outcomes, long-term compliance remains suboptimal. Newer technologies, specifically auto-CPAP, have the potential to improve treatment for OSAS by reducing the waiting times currently observed before instituting positive airway pressure therapy and thus potentially reducing health care spending.

REFERENCES

1. Sullivan C, Issa F, Berthon-Jones M, et al. (1981) Reversal of obstructive sleep apnea by continuous positive airway pressure applied through the nares. Lancet 1:862–865.
2. Loube DI, Gay PC, Strohl KP, et al. (1999) Indications for positive airway pressure treatment of adult obstructive sleep apnea patients: a consensus statement. Chest 115:863–866.

3. Strohl K, Redline S (1986) Nasal CPAP therapy, upper airway muscle activation and obstructive sleep apnea. Am Rev Respir Dis 134:555–558.
4. Kushida C, Littner M, Morgenthaler T, et al. (2005) Practice parameters for the indications for polysomnography and related procedures: an update for 2005. Sleep 28:499–421.
5. Center for Medicare and Medicaid Services. Continuous positive airway pressure (CPAP) for obstructive sleep apnea (OSA), 2005.
6. Pevernagie D, Shepard J (1992) Relations between sleep stage, posture and effective nasal CPAP levels in OSA. Sleep 15:162–167.
7. Series F, Marc I (2001) Importance of sleep stage and body position-dependence of sleep apnoea determining benefits of auto-CPAP therapy. Eur Respir J 18:170–175.
8. Oksenberg A, Silverberg D, Arons E, et al. (1999) The sleep supine position has a major effect on optimal nasal continuous positive airway pressure. Chest 116:1000–1006.
9. Sanders M, Kern N, Costantino J, et al. (1993) Adequacy of prescribing positive airway pressure therapy by mask for sleep apnea on the basis of a partial night trial. Am Rev Respir Dis 147: 1169–1174.
10. Fitzpatrick MF, Alloway CED, Wakeford TM, et al. (2003) Can patients with obstructive sleep apnea titrate their own continuous positive airway pressure? Am J Respir Crit Care Med 167:716–722.
11. Masa JF, Jimenez A, Duran J, et al. (2004) Alternative methods of titrating continuous positive airway pressure: a large multicenter study. Am J Respir Crit Care Med 170:1218–1224.
12. Planes C, D'Ortho M, Foucher A, et al. (2003) Efficacy and cost of home-initiated auto-nCPAP versus conventional nCPAP. Sleep 26:156–160.
13. Oliver Z, Hoffstein V (2000) Predicting effective continuous positive airway pressure. Chest 117:1061–1064.
14. Hukins CA (2005) Arbitrary-pressure continuous positive airway pressure for obstructive sleep apnea syndrome. Am J Respir Crit Care Med 171:500–505.
15. Engleman HM, Douglas NJ (2004) Sleep 4: sleepiness, cognitive function, and quality of life in obstructive sleep apnoea/hypopnoea syndrome. Thorax 59:618–622.
16. Douglas NJ, Engleman HM (1998) CPAP therapy: outcomes and patient use. Thorax 53:47S–48S.
17. Douglas NJ (1998) Systematic review of the efficacy of nasal CPAP. Thorax 53:414–415.
18. Jenkinson C, Davies R, Mullins R, et al. (1999) Comparison of therapeutic and subtherapeutic nasal continuous airway pressure for obstructive sleep apnea: a randomized prospective parallel trial. Lancet 353:2100–2105.
19. Ballester E, Badia JR, Hernandez L, et al. (1999) Evidence of the effectiveness of continuous positive airway pressure in the treatment of sleep apnea/hypopnea syndrome. Am J Respir Crit Care Med 159:495–501.
20. Engleman H, Martin S, Kingshott R, et al. (1998) Randomised, placebo-controlled trial of daytime function after continuous positive airway pressure therapy for the sleep apnoea/hypopnoea syndrome. Thorax 53:341–345.
21. Kribbs N, Pack A, Kline L, et al. (1993) Effects of one night without nasal CPAP treatment on sleep and sleepiness in patients with obstructive sleep apnea. Am J Respir Crit Care Med 147:1162–1168.
22. Black J, Hirshlowitz M (2005) Modafinil for the treatment of residual excessive sleepiness in nasal continuous positive airway pressure-treated obstructive sleep apnea/hypopnea syndrome. Sleep 28:464–471.
23. Veasey S, Davis C, Fenik P, et al. (2004) Long-term intermittent hypoxia in mice: protracted hypersomnolence with oxidative injury to sleep-wake brain regions. Sleep 27:194–201.
24. Engleman H, Martin S, Deary I, et al. (1994) The effect of continuous positive airway pressure therapy on daytime function in the sleep apnoea/hyponoea syndrome. Lancet 343:572–575.
25. Engleman H, Martin S, Deary I, et al. (1997) Effect of CPAP therapy on daytime function in patients with mild sleep apnoea/hypopnoea syndrome. Thorax 52:114–119.
26. Engleman H, Kingshott R, Wraith P, et al. (1999) Randomized placebo-controlled crossover trial of CPAP for mild sleep apnea/hypopnea syndrome. Am J Respir Crit Care Med 159:461–467.
27. Engleman H, Kingshott R, Martin S, et al. (2000) Cognitive function in the sleep apnea/hyponea syndrome (SAHS). Sleep 23:S102–S108.
28. Greenberg G, Watson R, Deptula D (1987) Neuropsychological dysfunction in sleep apnea. Sleep 10:254–262.
29. Redline S, Strauss ME, Adams N, et al. (1997) Neuropsychological function in mild sleep-disordered breathing. Sleep 20:160–167.

30. Kim H, Young T, Matthews C, et al. (1997) Sleep-disordered breathing and neuropsychological deficits: a population-based study. Am J Respir Crit Care Med 156:1813–1819.
31. Bedard M, Montplaisir J, Richer F, et al. (1991) Obstructive sleep apnea syndrome: pathogenesis of neuropsychological deficits. J Clin Exp Neuropsychol 13:950–964.
32. Borak J, Cieslicki J, Koziej M, et al. (1996) Effects of CPAP treatment on psychological status in patients with severe obstructive sleep apnea. J Sleep Res 5:123–127.
33. Naegele B, Thouvard V, Pepin J, et al. (1995) Deficits of cognitive executive functions in patients with sleep apnea syndrome. Sleep 18:43–52.
34. Munoz A, Mayoralas L, Barbe F, et al. (2000) Long-term effects of CPAP on daytime functioning in patients with sleep apnoea syndrome. Eur Respir J 15:676–681.
35. Kingshott R, Engleman H, Deary I, et al. (1998) Does arousal frequency predict daytime function? Eur Respir J 12:1264–1270.
36. Aikens J, Caruana-Montaldo B, Vanable P, et al. (1998) Depression and general psychopathology in obstructive sleep apnea. Sleep 21(Suppl):71.
37. Aikens J, Caruana-Montaldo B, Vanable P, L, et al. (1999) MMPI correlates of sleep and respiratory disturbance in obstructive sleep apnea. Sleep 22:362–369.
38. Aikens J, Mendelson W (1999) A matched comparison of MMPI responses in patients with primary snoring or obstructive sleep apnea. Sleep 22:355–361.
39. Mendelson W (1992) Depression in sleep apnea patients. Sleep Res 21:230.
40. Millman R, Fogel B, McNamara M, et al. (1989) Depression as a manifestation of obstructive sleep apnea: reversal with nasal continuous positive airway pressure. J Clin Psychiatry 50:348–351.
41. Mosko S, Zetin M, Glen S, et al. (1989) Self-reported depressive symptomatology, mood ratings and treatment outcome in sleep disorders. J Clin Psychol 45:51–60.
42. Reynolds C, Kupfer D, McEachran A, et al. (1984) Depressive psychopathology in male sleep apneics. J Clin Psychiatry 45:287–290.
43. American Psychiatric Association (1995) *Diagnostic and Statistical Manual of Mental Disorders*. 4th ed. American Psychiatric Association,Washington, DC.
44. Ramos Platon M, Espinar Sierra J (1992) Changes in psychopathological symptoms in sleep apnea patients after treatment with nasal continuous airway pressure. Int J Neurosci 62(3–4):173–195.
45. Yu B, Ancoli-Israel S, Dimsdale J (1999) Effect of CPAP treatment on mood states in patients with sleep apnea. J Psychiatr Res 33:427–432.
46. Baldwin C, Griffith K, Nieto F, et al. (2001) The association of sleep-disordered breathing and sleep symptoms with quality of life in the Sleep Heart Health Study. Sleep 24:96–105.
47. Finn L, Young T, Palta M, et al. (1998) Sleep-disordered breathing and self-reported general health status in the Wisconsin Sleep Cohort. Sleep 21:701–706.
48. Stradling J, Davies R (2000) Is more NCPAP better? Sleep 23:S150–S153.
49. Jenkinson C, Davies R, Mullins R, et al. (2001) Long-term benefit in self-reported health status of nasal continuous airway pressure therapy for obstructive sleep apnoea. QJM 94:95–99.
50. McArdle N, Devereux G, Heidarnejad H, et al. (1999) Long-term use of CPAP therapy for sleep apnea/hypopnea syndrome. Am J Respir Crit Care Med 159:1108–1114.
51. Kribbs N, Pack A, Kline L, et al. (1993) Objective measurement of patterns of nasal CPAP use by patients with obstructive sleep apnea. Am Rev Respir Dis 147:887–895.
52. Weaver T, Kribbs N, Pack A, et al. (1997) Night to night variability in CPAP use over the first three months of treatment. Sleep 20:278–283.
53. Lewis K, Seale L, Bartle I, et al. (2004) Early predictors of CPAP use for the treatment of obstructive sleep apnea. Sleep 27:134–138.
54. Reeves-Hoche M, Meck R, Zwillich C (1994) Nasal CPAP: an objective evaluation of patient compliance. Am J Respir Crit Care Med 149:149–154.
55. Rauscher H, Formanek D, Popp W, et al. (1993) Self-reported vs measured compliance with nasal CPAP for obstructive sleep apnea. Chest 103:1675–1680.
56. Engleman H, Martin S, Douglas N (1994) Compliance with CPAP therapy in patients with the sleep apnoea/hypopnoea syndrome. Thorax 49:263–266.
57. Massie CA, Hart RW, Peralez K, et al. (1999) Effects of humidification on nasal symptoms and compliance in sleep apnea patients using continuous positive airway pressure. Chest 116:403–408.
58. Martins de Araujo MT, Vieira SB, Vasquez EC, et al. (2000) Heated humidification or face mask to prevent upper airway dryness during continuous positive airway pressure therapy. Chest 117: 142–147.

59. Rakotonanahary D, Pelletier-Fleury N, Gagnadoux F, et al. (2001) Predictive factors for the need for additional humidification during nasal continuous positive airway pressure therapy. Chest 119:460–465.
60. Wiese H, Boethel C, Phillips B, et al. (2005) CPAP compliance: video education may help. Sleep Med 6:171–174.
61. Chervin R, Theut S, Bassetti C, et al. (1997) Compliance with nasal CPAP can be improved by simple interventions. Sleep 20:284–289.
62. Reeves-Hoche M, Hudgel D, Meck R, et al. (1995) Continuous versus bilevel positive airway pressure for obstructive sleep apnea. Am J Respir Crit Care Med 151:443–449.
63. Roux FJ, Hilbert J (2003) Continuous positive airway pressure: new generations. Clin Chest Med 24:315–342.
64. Randerath WJ, Parys K, Feldmeyer F, et al. (1999) Self-adjusting nasal continuous positive airway pressure therapy based on measurement of impedance: a comparison of two different maximum pressure levels. Chest 116:991–999.
65. Randerath WJ, Schraeder O, Galetke W, et al. (2001) Autoadjusting CPAP therapy based on impedance: efficacy, compliance and acceptance. Am J Respir Crit Care Med 163:652–657.
66. Randerath WJ, Galetke W, David M, et al. (2001) Prospective randomized comparison of impedence-controlled auto-continuous positive airway pressure (APAP(FOT)) with constant CPAP. Sleep Med 2:115–124.
67. Marrone O, Insalaco G, Bonsignore MR, et al. (2002) Sleep structure correlates of continuous positive airway pressure variations during application of an autotitrating continuous positive airway pressure machine in patients with obstructive sleep apnea syndrome. Chest 121:759–767.
68. Fuchs F, Wiest G, Frank M, et al. (2002) Auto-CPAP for obstructive sleep apnea: induction of microarousals by automatic variations of CPAP pressure? Sleep 25:514–518.
69. Senn O, Brack T, Matthews F, et al. (2003) Randomized short-term trial of two AutoCPAP devices versus fixed continuous positive airway pressure for the treatment of sleep apnea. Am J Respir Crit Care Med 168:1506–1511.
70. Pevernagie DA, Proot PM, Hertegonne KB, et al. (2004) Efficacy of flow- vs impedance-guided autoadjustable continuous positive airway pressure: a randomized cross-over trial. Chest 126:25–30.
71. Kessler R, Weitzenblum E, Chaouat A, et al. (2003) Evaluation of unattended automated titration to determine therapeutic continuous positive airway pressure in patients with obstructive sleep apnea. Chest 123:704–710.
72. Abdenbi F, Chambille B, Escourrou P (2004) Bench testing of auto-adjusting positive airway pressure devices. Eur Respir J 24:649–658.
73. Farre R, Montserrat JM, Rigau J, et al. (2002) Response of automatic continuous positive airway pressure devices to different sleep breathing patterns: a bench study. Am J Respir Crit Care Med 166:469–473.
74. Stammnitz A, Jerrentrup A, Penzel T, et al. (2004) Automatic CPAP titration with different self-setting devices in patients with obstructive sleep apnoea. Eur Respir J 24:273–278.
75. Ayas N, Patel S, Malhotra A, et al. (2004) Auto-titrating vs standard continuous positive airway pressure for the treatment of obstructive sleep apnea: results of a meta-analysis. Sleep 27:249–253.
76. Massie CA, McArdle N, Hart RW, et al. (2003) Comparison between automatic and fixed positive airway pressure therapy in the home. Am J Respir Crit Care Med 167:20–23.
77. Teschler H, Wessendorf T, Farhat A, et al. (2000) Two months auto-adjusting versus conventional nCPAP for obstructive sleep apnoea syndrome. Eur Respir J 15:990–995.
78. Meurice J, Marc I, Series F (1996) Efficacy of auto-CPAP in the treatment of obstructive sleep apnea/hypopnea syndrome. Am J Respir Crit Care Med 153:794–798.
79. Series F, Marc I (1997) Efficacy of automatic continuous positive airway pressure therapy that uses an estimated required pressure in the treatment of the obstructive sleep apnea syndrome. Ann Intern Med 127:588–595.
80. Hudgel DW, Fung C (2000) A long-term randomized cross-over comparison of auto-titrating and standard nasal continuous positive airway pressure. Sleep 23:1–4.
81. D'Ortho M-P, Grillier-Lanoir V, Levy P, et al. (2000) Constant vs automatic continuous positive airway pressure therapy: home evaluation. Chest 118:1010–1017.
82. Konermann M, Sanner B, Vyleta M, et al. (1998) Use of conventional and self-adjusting nasal continuous positive airway pressure for treatment of severe obstructive sleep apnea syndrome: a comparative study. Chest 113:714–718.

83. Hukins CA (2004) Comparative study of autotitrating and fixed-pressure CPAP in the home: a randomized, single-blind crossover trial. Sleep 27:1512–1517.
84. Noseda A, Kempenaers C, Kerkhofs M, et al. (2004) Constant vs auto-continuous positive airway pressure in patients with sleep apnea hypopnea syndrome and a high variability in pressure requirement. Chest 126:31–37.
85. Berry R, Parish J, Hartse K (2002) The use of auto-titrating continuous positive airway pressure for the treatment of adult obstructive sleep apnea. Sleep 25:148–173.
86. Littner M, Hirshkowitz M, Davilla D, et al. (2002) Practice parameters for the use of autotitrating continuous positive airway pressure devices for titrating pressures and treating adult patients with obstructive sleep apnea syndrome. Sleep 25:143–147.
87. Sanders M, Kern N (1990) Obstructive sleep apnea treated by independently adjusted inspiratory and expiratory positive airway pressures via nasal mask: physiologic and clinical implications. Chest 98:317–324.
88. Consensus Conference. Clinical indications for noninvasive positive pressure ventilation in chronic respiratory failure due to restrictive lung disease, COPD, and nocturnal hypoventilation: a consensus conference report. (1999) Chest 116:521–534.
89. Gay P, Herold D, Olson E (2003) A randomized, double-blind clinical trial comparing continuous airway pressure with a novel bilevel pressure system for the treatment of obstructive sleep apnea. Sleep 26:864–869.
90. Aloia MS, Stanchina M, Arnedt JT, et al. (2005) Treatment adherence and outcomes in flexible vs standard continuous positive airway pressure therapy. Chest 127:2085–2093.
91. Mortimore IL, Whittle AT, Douglas NJ (1998) Comparison of nose and face mask CPAP therapy for sleep apnoea. Thorax 53:290–292.
92. Massie CA, Hart RW (2003) Clinical outcomes related to interface type in patients with obstructive sleep apnea/hypopnea syndrome who are using continuous positive airway pressure. Chest 123:1112–1118.
93. Anderson F, Kingshott R, Taylor R, et al. (2003) A randomized crossover efficacy trial of oral CPAP (Oracle) compared with nasal CPAP in the management of obstructive sleep apnea. Sleep 26:721–726.
94. Beecroft J, Zanon S, Lukic D, et al. (2003) Oral continuous positive airway pressure for sleep apnea: effectiveness, patient preference, and adherence. Chest 124:2200–2208.
95. Khanna R, Kline L (2003) A prospective 8 week trial of nasal interfaces vs. a novel oral interface (Oracle) for the treatment of obstructive sleep apnea hypopnea syndrome. Sleep Med 4:333–338.
96. Smith PL, O'Donnell CP, Allan L, et al. (2003) A physiologic comparison of nasal and oral positive airway pressure. Chest 123:689–694.

13 Oral Appliances for the Treatment of Obstructive Sleep Apnea

Donald A. Falace, DMD

CONTENTS

INTRODUCTION

The principal methods of treatment for obstructive sleep apnea (OSA) include behavioral modification, continuous positive airway pressure (CPAP), oral appliances, and various types of upper airway surgery. CPAP is the gold standard for treatment of OSA, but many patients are unable to tolerate or refuse to use CPAP. In these instances, oral appliances are an acceptable treatment alternative. Current guidelines developed by the American Academy of Sleep Medicine (formerly the American Sleep Disorders Association) recommend that oral appliances are indicated for the treatment of patients with snoring or mild OSA who do not respond to weight loss or sleep position change, and for patients with moderate-to-severe OSA who are intolerant of or who refuse treatment with CPAP *(1)*. Oral appliances are also used as a supplement to CPAP and in patients who have failed surgery or who refuse surgery.

TYPES OF ORAL APPLIANCES

Oral appliances were first described for use in the treatment of OSA in 1982 and involved the use of a tongue-retaining device *(2)*. Since that time, many different types and designs of oral appliances have been developed. Currently, there are more than 50 different appliances, but the Food and Drug Administration (FDA) has approved only 30 of them for the treatment of OSA, with the remainder approved only for the treatment of

From: *Current Clinical Practice: Primary Care Sleep Medicine: A Practical Guide*
Edited by: J. F. Pagel and S. R. Pandi-Perumal © Humana Press Inc., Totowa, NJ

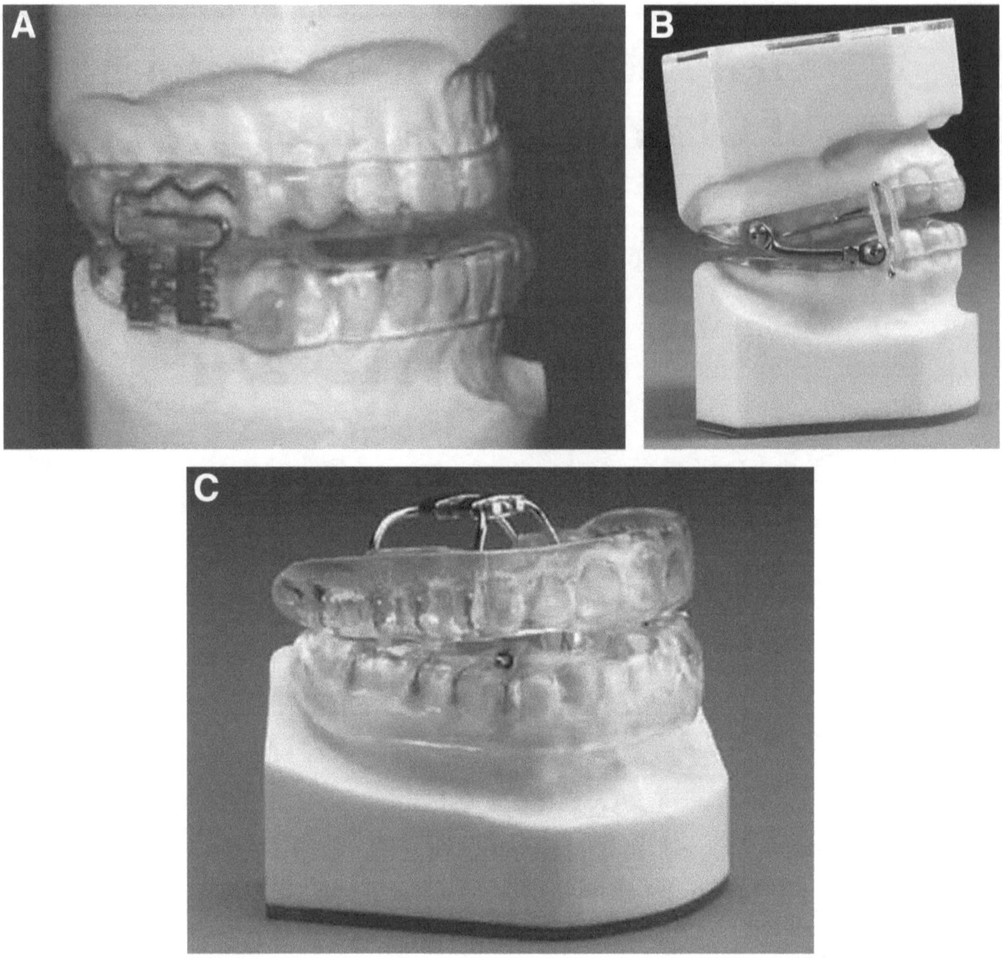

Fig. 1. (A) Adjustable PM positioner (Courtesy of Jonathan Parker, DDS, Minneapolis, MN). **(B)** Herbst appliance (Great Lakes Orthodontics; Tonowanda, NY). **(C)** Klearway (Great Lakes Orthodontics, Tonowanda, NY).

snoring. They are all variations on a theme, however, and basically accomplish the same outcome, namely to mechanically open the airway by lifting and maintaining the tongue away from the posterior oropharynx. This movement is analogous to the jaw thrust technique used in basic life support. There are two basic types of oral appliances:

1. Mandibular repositioners that engage the mandible and reposition it (and indirectly the tongue) in an anterior or forward direction.
2. Tongue-retaining devices that directly engage the tongue by suction and hold it in a forward or anterior position.

Mandibular repositioning appliances are the most common types of appliances used to treat OSA. Typically, they are custom-made of acrylic resin and consisting of upper and lower portions that cover the dental arches and then are connected together. The upper and lower portions can be fused together to form a rigid (monoblock) appliance that does not allow any movement of the mandible or adjustment capability. Conversely, the portions can be attached together by a rod, wire, strap, hook, or screw assembly, allowing for varying degrees of movement of the lower jaw as well as providing anterior–posterior, and sometimes vertical, adjustment capability (Fig. 1). Some appliances are a single-arch

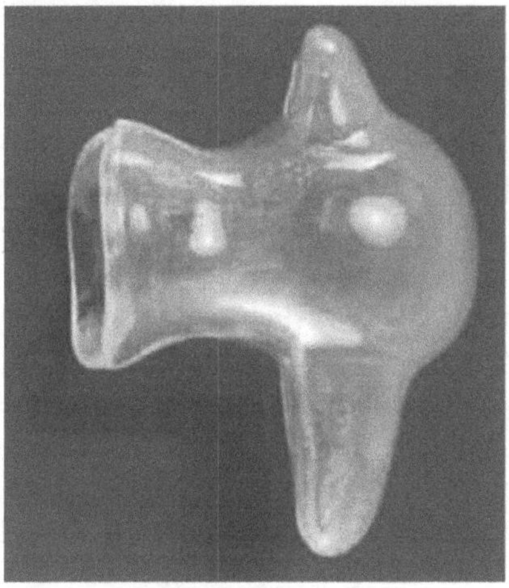

Fig. 2. Tongue-stabilizing device (Great Lakes Orthodontics; Tonowanda, NY).

appliance fitted only to the upper teeth with a ramp that extends lingually and inferiorly behind the incisors. It functions only as the patient closes the mouth, when the mandibular teeth make contact with the ramp and the mandible is guided forward as it closes. This type of appliance is effective only when the patient's mouth is closed during sleep. The single-arch appliances are not FDA-approved for treatment of OSA.

Tongue-retaining devices are typically made of medical-grade silicone in the shape of a bulb or cavity. The tongue is stuck into the bulb and the bulb is then squeezed slightly and released. The resulting suction holds the tongue in place in the bulb with the remaining portion of the device being maintained on the outside of the mouth by a flange or frame (Fig. 2). These devices can be used for patients in whom a mandibular repositioner is contraindicated; however, it has been reported that tongue-retaining devices are less effective than a titratable mandibular repositioner *(3,4)*. Furthermore, many patients do not tolerate tongue-retaining devices as well as mandibular repositioners *(5)*. Tongue-retaining devices are not FDA-approved for the treatment of OSA.

MECHANISM OF ORAL APPLIANCES

The exact mechanism by which oral appliances exert their effect most likely involves their effect on tongue position and the oropharyngeal anatomy. A recent Medline review concluded that the most common site of obstruction detected in studies of patients with OSA was at the level of the oropharynx *(6)*. Furthermore, it has been shown that a major risk factor for the development of OSA in normal-weight snorers is hypertrophy of the tongue base *(7)*. It has further been shown that with the use of oral appliances there is a clear increase in upper airway volume, and a decrease in the collapsibility of the airway *(8–10)*. There also appears to be an enhancement in resting genioglossus muscle activity, which may contribute to a decrease in pharyngeal collapsibility *(11)*.

EFFICACY OF ORAL APPLIANCES

Numerous uncontrolled studies have been published that report varying degrees of success with different types of oral appliances, ranging from 76% for mild OSA to 40% for more severe OSA *(12–17)*. Two large prospective studies of patients with a broad spectrum of severity both reported overall 1-year success rates as defined by a reduction of the apnea–hypopnea index (AHI) to less than 10/hour of 54% *(17,18)*.

Three randomized, crossover, controlled trials comparing oral appliances and placebo appliances in patients with a wide range of severity have demonstrated that oral appliances improve the AHI as well as hypoxemia in patients with OSA. Two of these studies, with a total of 97 subjects, used adjustable appliances and had the same strict criteria for success, with complete success defined as a reduction of the AHI to less than 5/hour and partial success defined as a reduction of the AHI by more than 50% but still more than 5/hour *(19,20)*. In both studies, complete success was attained by 37% of subjects and partial success attained by another 26% of subjects. Thus, complete or partial success was realized by 63% of subjects. In a third study with 20 subjects, a nonadjustable monoblock appliance was used and success was defined as a reduction of the AHI to less than 10/hour combined with an hourly rate of arterial oxygen desaturations of less than 10/hour *(21)*. Thirty-five percent of the subjects had a successful outcome. It was noted that six of the subjects who did not meet the criteria for success had a pretreatment AHI of more than 50/hour.

Long-term compliance data for oral appliances is lacking, but the compliance rate for oral appliances after 1 year, ranges from 48 to 84% *(22,23)*. Available data suggest that this figure decreases somewhat over time, with compliance at 4 years or more reported to be 62–76% *(18,24)*. A recent study reported on the long-term compliance of a group of 251 patients for whom an oral appliance had been prescribed for treatment of OSA a mean of 5.7 years previously *(5)*. The investigators found that 64% were still using the appliance, 93.7% of these wore it for more than 4 hour per night, and 95% were satisfied with their treatment. The most frequent reasons cited for discontinuation was discomfort, little or no effect, or switched to CPAP. The nonusers had a higher incidence of side effects than did the users. There was no difference in baseline severity of disease between users and those who discontinued use.

ORAL APPLIANCES COMPARED WITH CPAP AND UVULOPALATOPHARYNGOPLASTY

There have been several uncontrolled, randomized, crossover studies comparing oral appliances and CPAP *(25–30)*. These have consistently found that both CPAP and oral appliances were effective treatments, with CPAP being superior to oral appliances in correcting the AHI and sleepiness, but with subjects preferring the use of oral appliances over CPAP. A recent randomized, controlled, crossover study comparing the efficacy of CPAP, oral appliances, and placebo tablet in 114 subjects with AHI scores between 5 and 30/hour similarly found that both CPAP and oral appliances effectively treated sleep-disturbed breathing and sleepiness, with the oral appliance having a lesser therapeutic effect, but being the treatment modality preferred by patients *(31)*. Of particular interest are two recent studies reporting that oral appliances and CPAP have similar beneficial effects on blood pressure and improved oxygen desaturation *(31,32)*.

There are very few studies comparing oral appliances with upper airway surgery in patients with OSA. A prospective study of 95 patients with OSA compared 49 patients who underwent uvulopalatopharyngoplasty (UPPP) and 46 patients who were given an oral appliance and then followed up for 1 year *(33)*. The success rate (>50% reduction in the apnea index [AI]) for the oral appliance group was 95% vs 70% for the UPPP. Normalization (AI <5 or AHI <10) was achieved by 78% of the oral appliance group and by 51% of the UPPP group. Another prospective study compared UPPP and oral appliances in patients with OSA *(34)*. Seventy-two patients with mild–moderate OSA were randomly assigned to treatment with either UPPP or with an oral appliance and then followed up for 4 years. Success was defined as at least a 50% reduction in the AI, which was attained by 81% of the oral appliance group and 53% of the UPPP group. Normalization (AI of <5 or an AHI <10) was observed in 63% of the oral appliance group and only 33% of the UPPP group. The compliance rate for the oral appliance group was 62%. Significant postoperative complaints of nasopharyngeal regurgitation and difficulty swallowing were reported by 8 and 10%, respectively, of the UPPP group.

Two large reviews summarizing the use of oral appliances for treating OSA have recently been published. A Cochrane Database Review *(35)* concluded that there was evidence that oral appliances improved subjective sleepiness and sleep-disordered breathing compared with control subjects, but that CPAP was the more effective of the two treatment modalities. It also suggested that until more evidence becomes available, it would seem appropriate to limit the use of oral appliances to patients who are unwilling or unable to use CPAP. A similar extensive review concluded that

1. Oral appliances are more effective than control interventions for treating OSA, and possibly more effective than UPPP;
2. Oral appliances are less effective than CPAP, but patients generally preferred oral appliance therapy; and
3. Oral appliances are a viable treatment for mild-to-moderate OSA *(36)*.

SIDE EFFECTS OF ORAL APPLIANCES

Oral appliances are generally well tolerated, but side effects are common *(5,37,38)*. Fortunately, most side effects are minor and transient and resolve quickly on removal of the appliance. Common side effects include dry mouth, increased salivation, tooth soreness, and jaw muscle or jaw joint discomfort. On occasion, pain can be severe enough that patients discontinue the use of the appliance *(22,38)*.

Bite changes are another side effect seen with oral appliances. These are most frequently described as an inability to close on the back teeth (posterior open bite) combined with heavy contact of the front teeth upon removal of the appliance in the morning. This is caused by continued protrusion of the mandible without the appliance in place. The cause of this is unclear, but is likely a factor of persistent shortening effects of the lateral pterygoid muscles and/or perhaps the accumulation of fluid in the posterior compartment of the temporomandibular joint capsule. In any event, these changes quickly resolve within a few seconds or minutes after removal of the appliance. Empirically, this may be accelerated by jaw stretching exercises or by forcefully biting on the molars.

It has been observed that about 10–15% of patients will experience more persistent or even permanent changes to the occlusion such as retroclination of the maxillary incisors, proclination of the mandibular incisors, and posterior open bite *(5,39,40)*. It is interesting that many patients in whom an occlusal change occurs are unaware of its presence until their dentist brings it to their attention *(37)*. If it does occur and is problematic for the patient, correction can necessitate orthodontic treatment, restorative dental treatment, or surgery. It has been suggested that cephalometrically measured gonial angles and mandibular plane angles may be predictors of two different types of occlusal changes *(40)*. The significance of occlusal changes should be kept in perspective. That is, oral appliances are being used to treat OSA, a significant medical problem with potentially serious consequences if left untreated. Many patients who are being treated with an oral appliance are those who are unable or unwilling to use CPAP and thus may otherwise go untreated. Therefore, the benefits of using an appliance must be weighed against the small risk of a change in the bite.

TREATMENT PROTOCOL

On referral of a patient from the physician for an oral appliance, the dentist obtains a thorough history. This includes a history of the OSA, its impact on the patient's life, a review of the polysomnogram report, and outcomes of previous treatment attempts. A complete dental history including a history of bruxism and temporomandibular disorders, is also recorded. A thorough examination of the oral and maxillofacial region is performed including oral and paraoral soft tissues, teeth, restorations, periodontal tissues, occlusion, masticatory musculature, temporomandibular joints, and range of mandibular motion. Radiographs are also taken, which may include intraoral films as well as a panogram and cephalogram. Any significant dental needs should be addressed before fabrication of an appliance.

A determination is then made concerning whether or not the patient is a candidate for an oral appliance. Contraindications for a mandibular repositioning appliance include the following:

1. Too few teeth.
2. Teeth with short clinical crowns.
3. Moderate-to-severe periodontal disease.
4. Moderate-to-severe temporomandibular disorders.
5. A severe gag reflex.

Predictors for successful outcome include female sex, mild sleep apnea in both men and women, supine-dependent apnea in men, and a higher amount of mandibular advancement *(18)*. The likelihood of successful outcome is decreased in patients with more severe OSA, increasing obesity, and nasal obstruction. Selection of a particular appliance is largely subjective and based on a variety of factors including comfort, ease of use, adjustability, jaw movement capability, presence of bruxism, number and distribution of sound teeth, desire of the patient, and experience of the dentist.

Once an appliance is selected, impressions of the dental arches are taken and plaster models are made. A bite registration is obtained with the patient in the desired protruded position; this will determine the position of the mandible with the appliance in place. If an adjustable appliance is used, this position will be a reference position from which increases or decreases in protrusion can be made. The models and bite registration are then sent to the laboratory for fabrication of the appliance. Once the appliance is made, the patient returns for the initial try-in and adjustment. If the appliance is adjustable, there will then be a period of several weeks during which time the appliance is titrated to the optimum treatment position. This is determined by the patient's report of improvement in snoring, sleep quality, waking more rested, and being less sleepy during the day. Occasionally, oximetry, respiratory flow monitors, or other devices may be used to aid in this determination. When the final treatment position is attained, the physician is notified in the event that a repeat sleep study with the appliance in place is desired. Regular follow-up monitoring by the dentist is important to ensure the ongoing effectiveness of the appliance and to identify and correct any developing problems. One suggested approach is to see the patient every 6 months for the first 2 years, and then yearly thereafter.

CONCLUSIONS

Oral appliances are an effective and viable treatment for patients with mild OSA, and for patients with moderate-to-severe sleep apnea who are intolerant of or who refuse treatment with CPAP. They are also more effective than some forms of upper airway surgery. Oral appliances are generally well-tolerated and although they are not as effective as CPAP in correcting the AHI, they are preferred by patients. The effectiveness of oral appliances decreases with the severity of disease and with increasing obesity. Side effects are common, but are usually minor and transient in nature.

REFERENCES

1. American Sleep Disorders Association (1995) Practice parameters for the treatment of snoring and obstructive sleep apnea with oral appliances. Sleep 18:511–513.
2. Cartwright RD, Samelson CF (1982) The effects of a nonsurgical treatment for obstructive sleep apnea: the tongue-retaining device. JAMA 248:705–709.
3. Barthlen GM, Brown LK, Wiland MR, et al. (2000) Comparison of three oral appliances for treatment of severe obstructive sleep apnea syndrome. Sleep Med 1:299–305.
4. Ono T, Lowe AA, Ferguson KA, et al. (1996) A tongue retaining device and sleep-state genioglossus muscle activity in patients with obstructive sleep apnea. Angle Orthod 66:273–280.
5. De Almeida FR, Lowe AA, Tsuiki S, et al. (2005) Long-term compliance and side effects of oral appliances used for the treatment of snoring and obstructive sleep apnea syndrome. J Clin Sleep Med 1:143–149.
6. Rama AN, Tekwani SH, Kushida CA (2002) Sites of obstruction in obstructive sleep apnea. Chest 122:1139–1147.
7. Marchioni D, Ghidini A, Dallari S, et al. (2005) The normal-weight snorer: polysomnographic study and correlation with upper airway morphological alterations. Ann Otol Rhinol Laryngol 114:144–146.
8. Hiyama S, Tsuiki S, Ono T, et al. (2003) Effects of mandibular advancement on supine airway size in normal subjects during sleep. Sleep 26:440–445.
9. Kato J, Isono S, Tanaka A, et al. (2000) Dose-dependent effects of mandibular advancement on pharyngeal mechanics and nocturnal oxygenation in patients with sleep-disordered breathing. Chest 117:1065–1072.
10. Kyung SH, Park YC, Pae EK (2005) Obstructive sleep apnea patients with the oral appliance experience pharyngeal size and shape changes in three dimensions. Angle Orthod 75:15–22.
11. Tsuiki S, Ono T, Kuroda T (2000) Mandibular advancement modulates respiratory-related genioglossus electromyographic activity. Sleep Breath 4:53–58.
12. Lowe AA, Sjoholm TT, Ryan CF, et al. (2000) Treatment, airway and compliance effects of a titratable oral appliance. Sleep 23(Suppl 4):S172–S178.
13. Marklund M, Franklin KA, Sahlin C, et al. (1998) The effect of a mandibular advancement device on apneas and sleep in patients with obstructive sleep apnea. Chest 113:707–713.
14. Menn SJ, Loube DI, Morgan TD, et al. (1996) The mandibular repositioning device: role in the treatment of obstructive sleep apnea. Sleep 19:794–800.
15. Pancer J, Al-Faifi S, Al-Faifi M, et al. (1999) Evaluation of variable mandibular advancement appliance for treatment of snoring and sleep apnea. Chest 116:1511–1518.
16. Pellanda A, Despland PA, Pasche P (1999) The anterior mandibular positioning device for the treatment of obstructive sleep apnoea syndrome: experience with the Serenox. Clin Otolaryngol Allied Sci 24:134–141.
17. Yoshida K (2000) Effects of a mandibular advancement device for the treatment of sleep apnea syndrome and snoring on respiratory function and sleep quality. Cranio 18:98–105.
18. Marklund M, Stenlund H, Franklin KA (2004) Mandibular advancement devices in 630 men and women with obstructive sleep apnea and snoring: tolerability and predictors of treatment success. Chest 125:1270–1278.

19. Gotsopoulos H, Chen C, Qian J, et al. (2002) Oral appliance therapy improves symptoms in obstructive sleep apnea: a randomized, controlled trial. Am J Respir Crit Care Med 166:743–748.
20. Mehta A, Qian J, Petocz P, et al. (2001) A randomized, controlled study of a mandibular advancement splint for obstructive sleep apnea. Am J Respir Crit Care Med 163:1457–1461.
21. Johnston CD, Gleadhill IC, Cinnamond MJ, et al. (2002) Mandibular advancement appliances and obstructive sleep apnoea: a randomized clinical trial. Eur J Orthod 24:251–262.
22. Clark GT, Sohn JW, Hong CN (2000) Treating obstructive sleep apnea and snoring: assessment of an anterior mandibular positioning device. J Am Dent Assoc 131:765–771.
23. Fransson AM, Tegelberg A, Leissner L, et al. (2003) Effects of a mandibular protruding device on the sleep of patients with obstructive sleep apnea and snoring problems: a 2-year follow-up. Sleep Breath 7:131–141.
24. Ringqvist M, Walker-Engstrom ML, Tegelberg A, et al. (2003) Dental and skeletal changes after 4 years of obstructive sleep apnea treatment with a mandibular advancement device: a prospective, randomized study. Am J Orthod Dentofacial Orthop 124:53–60.
25. Clark GT, Blumenfeld I, Yoffe N, et al. (1996) A crossover study comparing the efficacy of continuous positive airway pressure with anterior mandibular positioning devices on patients with obstructive sleep apnea. Chest 109:1477–1483.
26. Engleman HM, McDonald JP, Graham D, et al. (2002) Randomized crossover trial of two treatments for sleep apnea/hypopnea syndrome: continuous positive airway pressure and mandibular repositioning splint. Am J Respir Crit Care Med 166:855–859.
27. Ferguson KA, Ono T, Lowe AA, et al. (1997) A short-term controlled trial of an adjustable oral appliance for the treatment of mild to moderate obstructive sleep apnoea. Thorax 52:362–368.
28. Ferguson KA, Ono T, Lowe AA, et al. (1996) A randomized crossover study of an oral appliance vs nasal-continuous positive airway pressure in the treatment of mild-moderate obstructive sleep apnea. Chest 109:1269–1275.
29. Randerath WJ, Heise M, Hinz R, et al. (2002) An individually adjustable oral appliance vs continuous positive airway pressure in mild-to-moderate obstructive sleep apnea syndrome. Chest 122:569–575.
30. Tan YK, L'Estrange PR, Luo YM, et al. (2002) Mandibular advancement splints and continuous positive airway pressure in patients with obstructive sleep apnoea: a randomized cross-over trial. Eur J Orthod 24:239–249.
31. Barnes M, McEvoy RD, Banks S, et al. (2004) Efficacy of positive airway pressure and oral appliance in mild to moderate obstructive sleep apnea. Am J Respir Crit Care Med 170:656–664.
32. Gotsopoulos H, Kelly JJ, Cistulli PA (2004) Oral appliance therapy reduces blood pressure in obstructive sleep apnea: a randomized, controlled trial. Sleep 27:934–941.
33. Wilhelmsson B, Tegelberg A, Walker-Engstrom ML, et al. (1999) A prospective randomized study of a dental appliance compared with uvulopalatopharyngoplasty in the treatment of obstructive sleep apnoea. Acta Otolaryngol 119:503–509.
34. Walker-Engstrom ML, Tegelberg A, Wilhelmsson B, et al. (2002) 4-year follow-up of treatment with dental appliance or uvulopalatopharyngoplasty in patients with obstructive sleep apnea: a randomized study. Chest 121:739–746.
35. Lim J, Lasserson TJ, Fleetham J, et al. (2004) Oral appliances for obstructive sleep apnoea. Cochrane Database Syst Rev (4):CD004435.
36. Hoekema A, Stegenga B, De Bont LG (2004) Efficacy and co-morbidity of oral appliances in the treatment of obstructive sleep apnea-hypopnea: a systematic review. Crit Rev Oral Biol Med 15:137–155.
37. Fritsch KM, Iseli A, Russi EW, et al. (2001) Side effects of mandibular advancement devices for sleep apnea treatment. Am J Respir Crit Care Med 164:813–818.
38. Pantin CC, Hillman DR, Tennant M (1999) Dental side effects of an oral device to treat snoring and obstructive sleep apnea. Sleep 22:237–240.
39. Robertson CJ (2001) Dental and skeletal changes associated with long-term mandibular advancement. Sleep 24:531–537.
40. Monteith BD (2004) Altered jaw posture and occlusal disruption patterns following mandibular advancement therapy for sleep apnea: a preliminary study of cephalometric predictors. Int J Prosthodont 17:274–280.

14 Medicolegal Aspects of Obstructive Sleep Apnea/Hypopnea Syndrome

Brian A. Boehlecke, MD, MSPH, FCCP

CONTENTS

INTRODUCTION

Despite frequent speculation by speakers at national medical meetings that physicians may be held legally liable for accidents caused by patients with obstructive sleep apnea/hypopnea syndrome (OSAHS) who have not been promptly diagnosed and treated, very little has been published on the topic. A patient involved in a drowsy driving accident resulting in serious injury or death is the most likely situation in which physicians could face charges of legal negligence in relation to management of a patient with OSAHS. State regulations for physician reporting of patients with medical conditions that may render them unfit for driving safely vary from "no requirement" to mandatory reporting of all patients with a diagnosis listed as reportable. In two instances in Ontario, Canada, physicians were found liable because of failure to report potentially medically unfit patients to authorities before the patient had automobile crashes *(1)*. In New Jersey, falling asleep at the wheel and driving while "fatigued" can be considered reckless driving (Maggie's Law), with fatigued defined as *having had no sleep for more than 24 conservative hours*. American Medical Association policy H-15.958 (Fatigue, Sleep Disorders, and Motor Vehicle Crashes) states that physicians should "inform patients about the personal and societal hazards of driving or working while fatigued and advise patients about measures they can take to prevent fatigue-related and other unintended injuries." It also states they should "become familiar with the laws and regulations concerning drivers and highway safety in the state(s) where they practice" *(2)*.

From: *Current Clinical Practice: Primary Care Sleep Medicine: A Practical Guide*
Edited by: J. F. Pagel and S. R. Pandi-Perumal © Humana Press Inc., Totowa, NJ

A task force of the European Respiratory Society on public health and medicolegal implications of sleep apnea concluded that " ... whatever the legislation, the clinician has a responsibility to inform his *(sic)* patients of the risks related to sleepiness and to discourage him from driving as long as he is not effectively treated" *(3)*. It is clear that physicians have an ethical, if not legal, responsibility to inform a patient with OSAHS about the increased risk of automobile crashes associated with this condition and to counsel him or her to refrain from drowsy driving. Information regarding the medical aspects of the impact of OSAHS on the risk of automobile crashes and the effect of continuous positive airway pressure (CPAP) therapy on that risk, as well as suggestions for a practical approach to the medicolegal risk of managing patients with OSAHS, follows.

HAZARDS OF DROWSY DRIVING

Evidence that drowsy drivers are at risk for motor vehicle crashes comes from data using self-reported crashes, state motor vehicles driving records, and experimental studies on driving simulators. Patients with OSAHS have been reported to be two to seven times as likely to have a motor vehicle crashes as control subjects, with an overall estimated risk from a meta-analysis of six studies of 2.5% *(4)*. Retrospective study of insurance company data for 60 patients with OSAHS and 60 control subjects showed that the patients had a higher rate of crashes in a 3-year period (OR = 2.6) and a higher proportion had two or more crashes than control subjects *(5)*. However, the number of crashes was not related to the self-rated sleepiness score on the Epworth sleepiness scale (ESS), apnea/hypopnea index, or time with saturation less than 90% on polysomnogram. Nor was the number related to performance on a driving simulator, but there was a trend of increased number of crashes in those with the longest reaction time. Stutts and colleagues *(6)* interviewed approx 1000 people who had been in automobile accidents *(crashers)* who were reported by law officers as having been asleep, fatigued, or neither at the time of the crash, and approx 400 people who had not been in automobile accidents *(noncrashers)*.

Only 1.3% of those classified as "asleep at the time of the crash" had been previously diagnosed as having a sleep disorder, despite 25% of them admitting to having driven more than 10 times while drowsy and 91% admitting to having fallen asleep driving at least once. Mean ESS score for these subjects was 7.6, whereas that for crashers classified as neither asleep nor fatigued at the time of the crash was 5.6. Noncrasher control subjects had a mean score of 5.1. Thus, most crashers with probable drowsy driving crashes had not been medically diagnosed and did not perceive themselves to be excessively sleepy. Despite the elevated risk of crashing that most patients with OSAHS have, many patients have not had a crash, so which patients should be restricted and how much benefit would accrue from restrictions is not clear *(7)*.

PHYSICIAN RESPONSIBILITY

The physician has a responsibility to detect conditions that may impair driving and cause increased risk of harm to the patient or the public. Legal requirements for reporting such patients to authorities vary by state. Some states require physicians to report all patients with any listed conditions, regardless of impairments (mandatory reporting). Other states require that physicians report patients with a listed condition, only if the physician considers the condition to cause significant impairment of driving capacity (functional reporting). Yet, other states do not require any reporting but do allow it if the physician considers the patient or the public to be at significant risk of harm (permissive reporting). North Carolina has a statute giving physicians *limited* immunity from civil and criminal liability "as long as he *(sic)* was acting in good faith and without malice." If we practice in a *permissive* reporting state, factors bearing on a decision for our policy include the ethical standards and beliefs we and our medical community hold regarding the following:

1. The importance of patients' privacy.
2. The amount of responsibility for public health that should be born by physicians vs patients.
3. The effectiveness of reporting in reducing overall risk.

There is some evidence that patients may hide symptoms if they fear loss of driving privileges. Findley *(8)* found that 21 of 30 patients being evaluated for OSAHS stated that they would avoid medical evaluation if there were mandatory reporting to the division of motor vehicles (DMV).

PATIENT RESPONSIBILITY

Can a physician rely on trustworthy and motivated patients to restrict their driving when feeling sleepy? This depends on whether such patients have an accurate perception of their level of drowsiness, i.e., their propensity to fall asleep. Unfortunately, many individuals with OSAHS do not accurately perceive their level of drowsiness, as indicated by the poor correlation of self-reported sleepiness on ESS and an objective measurement of sleep propensity, the mean sleep onset latency during four to five nap opportunities in a multiple sleep latency test (MSLT) in the laboratory. This inaccuracy of perception of sleepiness was also demonstrated in the *real world* findings on drowsy driving crashes, reported by Stutts and colleagues *(6)*. Another *real world* study of drowsy driving was performed by Philip and coworkers *(9)*. They had 10 young men drive 600 miles on a French expressway after an average of breaks never taken 8.25 hours of sleep (RD1) and after an average of only 1.8-hour sleep (RD2). Breaks were taken every 105 minutes for testing, which included self-rating of sleepiness on the Karolinska sleepiness scale and measurement of reaction time. Subjects reported being more sleepy and more fatigued at all times of the day during RD2, but, surprisingly, reaction time remained quite constant throughout the drive, even during the sleep-deprived drive. There was an increase in reaction time at 5 PM on the sleep-deprived drive, suggesting an effect from fatigue. The authors reported that, "In the rested condition, the experimenter never had to take control of the car. In the sleep-restricted condition, 7 out of 10 subjects had to be assisted by the experimenter." A sleep-deprived person's perception of his or her sleepiness and functional impairment is further impaired by alcohol. The addition of small amounts of alcohol (blood alcohol concentration of approx 0.04%) to sleep restriction worsened performance on a driving simulator and the electroencephalography manifestation of sleepiness increased, but the subjects did not perceive increased sleepiness *(10)*.

OBJECTIVE TESTS OF SLEEPINESS

Self-related sleepiness does not correlate closely with the propensity for sleep measured on MSLT in the laboratory, but the objective results on the MSLT do not correlate closely with the frequency of sleep-related adverse incidents in the *real world*. Aldrich *(11)* found that MSLT results were not predictive of self-reported previous crash history in 424 patients with OSAHS. Sleep latency on MSLT has been shown to correlate with crash frequency on driving simulator *(12)*, but it is recognized that subjects are aware that no dire consequences occur if they fall asleep on the simulator, in contrast to the situation for the actual driving, the latter, therefore, providing move-motivation to resist falling asleep. Patients may be able to maintain alertness when motivated to do so, despite a high propensity to fall sleep when allowed to do so (MSLT instructions are to "try to fall asleep"). MSLT results do not correlate closely with the ability to stay awake when asked to do so in the laboratory setting, as measured by the maintenance of wakefulness test (MWT), for which instructions are to "try to stay awake." However, results on MWT after sleep deprivation have not been shown to correlate closely with performance on a driving simulator. Sleep latency on MWT explained only 20–30% of the variance of driving performance after 5 hours of sleep restriction *(13)*. However, it did correlate with number of crashes on the simulator when alcohol ingestion (mean blood alcohol intent 0.004 g/dL) was combined with sleep restriction.

Simulator performance is also not highly predictive of crash history for patients with OSAHS. Turkington and colleagues *(14)* found that the respiratory disturbance index on polysomnogram was not associated with earlier driving events or performance on the driving simulator. The authors also stated, "Patients who performed well on the simulator were unlikely to have had an accident in the previous year, but there was no relationship between those who performed poorly and accident history." However, Hack and colleagues *(15)* did find that the performance of untreated patients with OSAHS (>10/hour, 4% desaturations) was similar to that of control subjects, with 24 hours of sleep deprivation or with blood alcohol content of 0.072 g/dL.

EFFECT OF TREATMENT

Does treatment of OSAHS with CPAP reduce the risk of crashing? George *(16)* derived crash rates from DMV data for 210 patients with OSAHS over a 3-year period before and after CPAP therapy. Crash rate was 0.18 while untreated, but fell to 0.06 with treatment. A beneficial effect of CPAP treatment on simulator performance of patients with OSAHS was demonstrated by Hack and colleagues *(17)*. Off-road events decreased from 17.8–9 after 1 month on effective CPAP pressure but showed no change after a month of "ineffective" pressure set at 1 cm of water. An early beneficial effect of CPAP treatment was demonstrated by Turkington and coworkers *(18)*. There was "marked improvement" in "off-road" events by day 3 and significant improvement in tracking errors and reaction time by day 7.

PUBLISHED GUIDELINES

What are reasonable guidelines for physicians for dealing with the issue of drowsy driving in their patients? Recommendations for physicians were published by the American Thoracic Society in 1994 *(19)*. They included the following statement: "learn about applicable state laws, be alert for symptoms of excessive daytime somnolence or others symptoms of OSAHS especially in commercial drivers, assess risk of impaired driving in patients with OSAHS (risk is increased if patient has had recent accidents or "near misses," or has severe OSAHS or severe excessive daytime sleepiness), report high-risk drivers to DMV if they insist upon during before treatment initiated or fail to comply with treatment. High-risk truck, bus, or other occupational drivers may be considered for reporting."

CONCLUSIONS

OSAHS is associated with an increase risk of crashing, but absolute risk is still relatively low. A high apnea/hypopnea index is probably associated with higher risk, but other factors highly modify the risk for individual patients. Patient's perception of his or her sleepiness is often inaccurate. Propensity to fall asleep quickly when asked to do so (MSLT) does not accurately predict an inability to stay awake when motivated to do so. No current, clinically available test is highly predictive of crash risk. CPAP treatment can effectively reduce excessive daytime sleepiness and crash risk.

WHAT TO DO?

Try to be fair to your patients while avoiding legal and moral liability, i.e., follow the law and your conscience. Make a clinical assessment of the patient's overall risk for unsafe driving, his or her perception of that risk, and his or her willingness to take appropriate measures to minimize risk. Strongly consider reporting a patient to DMV if your assessment of the factors discussed indicates a high risk and low likelihood of adequate reduction in risk without this intervention, especially for commercial drivers. The author uses the MWT if asked to make a specific statement of fitness to drive for commercial drivers. This is, admittedly, a maneuver to legally protect oneself from all angles.

REFERENCES

1. Weaver T, George C Cognition and performance in patients with obstructive sleep apnea. in: *Principles and practice of sleep medicine.* 4th ed. (Kryger M, Roth T, Dement W, eds.) Elsevier, Burlington, MA, 2005, p. 1030.
2. American Medical Association. Fatigue, Sleep Disorders, and Motor vehicle crashes. H-15.958. Available at: www.ama-assn.orgapps/pf_new/pf_online. Last accessed Dec. 2006.
3. McNicholas W, Krieger J, Task Force Members (2002) Public health and medicolegal implications of sleep apnoea. Eur Respir J 20:1594–1609.
4. Sassani A, Findley L, Kryger M (2004) Reducing motor-vehicle collisions, costs, and fatalities by treating obstructive sleep apnea syndrome. Sleep 27:453–458.
5. Barbe F, Pericas J, Araceli M (1998) Automobile accidents in patients with sleep apnea syndrome. Am J Respir Crit Care Med 158:18–22.
6. Stutts JC, Wilkins JW, Vaughn BV (1999) Why do people have drowsy driving crashes? Input from drivers who just did [AAA Foundation for Traffic Safety Web site]. Available at: www.aaafoundation.org/pdf/Sleep.pdf. Accessed Oct. 2006.
7. Pack A, Pien G (2004) How much do crashes related to obstructive sleep apnea cost? Sleep 27:369–370.
8. Findley L (2002) The threat of mandatory reporting to a driver's license agency discourages sleepy drivers from being evaluated for sleep apnea. Am J Respir Crit Care Med 165:A513.
9. Philip P, Sagaspe P, Taillard J (2003) Fatigue, sleep restriction, and performance in automobile drivers: a controlled study in a natural environment. Sleep 26:277–280.
10. Horne J, Reyner L, Barrett P (2003) Driving impairment due to sleepiness is exacerbated by low alcohol intake. Occup Environ Med 60:689–692.
11. Aldrich M (1989) Automobile accidents in patients with sleep disorders. Sleep 12:487–494.
12. Pizza P, Contardi S, Mustachio B, et al. (2004) A driving simulation task: correlations with multiple sleep latency test. Brain Res Bull 63:423–426.
13. Banks S, Catcheside P, Lack L, et al. Does the MWT relate to driving simulator performance? Abstract presented at Annual Meeting of the American Academy of Sleep Medicine, 2004.

14. Turkington P, Sircar M, Allgar V, et al. (2001) Relationship between obstructive sleep apnoea, driving simulator performance, and risk of road traffic accidents. Thorax 56:800–805.
15. Hack M, Choi S, Vijayapalan P, et al. (2001) Comparison of the effects of sleep deprivation, alcohol, and obstructive sleep apnoea (OSA) on simulated steering performance. Respir Med 95:594–601.
16. George C (2001) Reduction in motor vehicle collisions following treatment of sleep apnoea with nasal CPAP. Thorax 56:508–512.
17. Hack M, Davis R, Mullins R, et al. (2000) Randomised prospective parallel trial of therapeutic versus subtherapeutic nasal continuous positive airway pressure on simulated steering performance in patients with obstructive sleep apnoea. Thorax 55:224–231.
18. Turkington P, Sircar M, Saralaya D, et al. (2004) Time course of changes in driving simulator performance with and without treatment in patients with sleep apnoea hypopnoea syndrome. Thorax 59:56–59.
19. American Thoracic Society (1994) Sleep apnea, sleepiness, and driving risk: Am J Respir Crit Care Med 150:1463–1473.

15 Overview of the Treatment of Obesity

Neil S. Freedman, MD, FCCP

Contents

INTRODUCTION

Obesity is a chronic disease that has become more common in America during the last 20 years *(1)*. The prevalence of overweight adults in the United States is 65%, with obesity affecting at least 31% of American adult population *(1)*. These increases in overweight and obesity are observed in all ethnic groups and both sexes in this country *(1)*. Increases in the prevalence of obesity are also being seen among the children and adolescents *(2,3)*. Obesity is a known risk factor for several medical comorbidities and is the most common risk factor associated with obstructive sleep apnea syndrome (OSAS) *(4)*. Although the exact mechanisms linking excess body weight to the pathophysiology of OSAS are not totally clear, most population-based and cross-sectional studies have found a strong association between OSAS and excess body weight *(5–10)*. Whereas excess weight has been clearly linked to OSAS, there is presently no consensus that any particular body habitus phenotype is the most important in the pathophysiology of OSAS.

Although continuous positive airway pressure (CPAP) is the most commonly prescribed therapy for obstructive sleep apnea, in most cases it is only treating a symptom of obesity and not the underlying cause of OSAS. Although obesity is the most frequently identified risk factor in OSAS, there have been relatively few studies examining the effect of weight loss on outcomes in this syndrome *(9–17)*. Most of these studies have been limited in that they were observational and uncontrolled, and examined morbidly obese, predominantly male subjects. Even given the limitations of the literature, weight loss does appear to be an effective means of reducing OSAS severity in overweight persons with OSAS *(4)*. The amount of weight loss required to significantly reduce or cure OSAS also remains unclear. Data from the Wisconsin Sleep Cohort suggest that a 1% reduction in weight has been correlated with a 3% improvement in the severity of OSAS based on the apnea/hypopnea index (AHI). Also, for those with a

From: *Current Clinical Practice: Primary Care Sleep Medicine: A Practical Guide*
Edited by: J. F. Pagel and S. R. Pandi-Perumal © Humana Press Inc., Totowa, NJ

normal or mildly elevated AHI at baseline, a 10% increase in body weight has been associated with a sixfold increase in the chance of developing moderate/severe OSAS (AHI > 15 events/hour) *(10)*.

This chapter will review the literature regarding weight-loss therapies in general and their relationship to outcomes in patients with OSAS. Specific treatment options for obesity that will be reviewed include behavior modification, drug therapy, exercise, dietary modifications, and surgery.

DEFINITIONS

The World Health Organization (WHO) and the National Heart, Lung, and Blood Institute have uniformly defined obesity using the calculated body mass index (BMI) *(18,19)*. The BMI is a simple and practical way to calculate the degree to which a person is overweight. It is correlated with body fat and is relatively unaffected by height. BMI = body weight (kg) divided by height (m) squared. A normal BMI is less than 25 kg/m^2 and alone is typically not associated with increased risk of death or cardiovascular morbidity. *Overweight* is defined as a BMI between 25 and 29.9 kg/m^2, *obesity* as a BMI of more than 30 kg/m^2, and *morbid obesity* as either a BMI of more than 40 kg/m^2 or a BMI of more than 35 kg/m^2 in the presence of comorbidities. Obesity can be further subdivided into three classes: class 1 obesity (BMI 30–34.9 kg/m^2), class 2 obesity (BMI 35–39.9 kg/m^2), and class 3 obesity (BMI of more than 40 kg/m^2).

The BMI is a reliable and valid measurement for identifying adults at increased risk for weight-related morbidity and mortality *(20)*. The relationship between increasing body weight and health risks is curvilinear, with the lowest mortality associated with a BMI of 22 kg/m^2 *(21)*. Increased relative risk of mortality in both men and women increases as BMI increases more than 25 kg/m^2. At any given BMI, the health risk is increased by other factors, including more amounts of abdominal body fat, hyperlipidemia, hypertension, age of less than 40 years, and/or a strong family history of cardiovascular disease.

BEHAVIOR MODIFICATION

Behavior modification is the cornerstone of any successful weight-loss treatment plan. Because the majority of obesity is because of overeating and a sedentary lifestyle, the goals of behavioral therapy are to help individuals to modify their eating habits and to increase exercise and physical activity. The most effective interventions combine nutrition education, diet and exercise counseling, and behavioral strategies that help individuals to acquire the skills and supports needed to change eating patterns and to become more physically active *(20)*. In fact, without proper modification of harmful lifestyle behaviors, other interventions aimed at weight loss will likely fail.

The first reported study of behavior modification therapy for the treatment of obesity dates back to 1967 *(22)*. For individuals who remain compliant, the average weight loss associated with behavioral modification therapy alone ranges between 9 and 10% of the individual's initial body weight *(23)*. The US Preventive Services Task Force recommends that clinicians screen all adult patients for obesity and offer intensive counseling and behavioral interventions to promote sustained weight loss for obese adults *(20)*. This report found that there is fair to good evidence that high-intensity counseling about diet, exercise, or both, together with behavioral interventions aimed at skill development, motivation, and support strategies, produces modest sustained weight loss (typically 3–5 kg for 1 year or more) in adults who are obese *(20)*. Although the US Preventive Services Task Force did not find any direct evidence that intensive counseling alone reduces obesity-related mortality or morbidity, they did find that improvements in intermediate outcomes (blood pressure, lipids, glucose tolerance) from modest weight loss provided indirect evidence of health benefits. They concluded that the benefits of screening and behavioral interventions outweigh potential harms *(20)*. They also concluded that there is insufficient evidence to recommend for or against the use of counseling of any intensity and/or behavioral interventions to promote sustained weight loss in overweight (BMI 25–29 kg/m^2) adults.

There are only a couple of studies that specifically evaluated the role of behavioral therapy on weight loss in patients with OSAS. Individualized cognitive-behavioral therapy has been demonstrated to complement dietary treatment in patients with OSAS, although it is unclear if this form of therapy adds any benefit over that achieved by diet alone *(24)*. Hypnotherapy in addition to diet modification and CPAP therapy has been associated with a small but significant weight loss (1–3 kg at 18 months) *(25)*.

Behavioral treatments for obesity focus on several components. The *antecedents* of eating behavior focus on identifying food intake and settings in which eating occurs. The individuals are typically instructed to keep records of when, where, and how much they eat over time and then attempt to identify problems and change future behavior. Altering the *behavior of eating* itself is also a main goal of behavioral treatment. Separating the events that trigger eating from eating itself is a main goal of stimulus control therapy. Finally, the *consequences* of eating for self-reward are modified. Rewards for changes in good behaviors rather than changes in weight should be the focus. Importantly, food should not be used as a reward for successful changes in behavior *(26)*.

Weight loss and its maintenance are lifelong endeavors. Behavioral goals and the time frame for achieving them should be clearly defined. Goals with this and any type of obesity treatment need to be realistic. The ideal outcome of a return to normal body weight is unrealistic for most individuals. In fact, an initial weight loss of 5–10% of one's initial body weight during the first 3–6 months is a more realistic short-term goal. Support from family and friends can be a key component of weight-loss success or failure. Although data are limited, participation in a structured commercial weight-loss program (Weight Watchers) may result in more weight loss than independent self-help dieting *(27)*.

Exercise

Low levels of physical activity and recreation have been strongly linked to weight gain in both adult men and women as well as in children *(20,28,29)*. Although exercise is known to improve many cardiovascular risk factors, its role in weight-loss treatment is less dramatic. Exercise alone as the sole treatment for obesity has minimal effect on body weight (~0.1 kg/week), unless it is performed in a rigorous fashion *(30,31)*. The lack of significant weight reduction with exercise alone is likely related to an increase in muscle mass with a concomitant reduction in body fat. Although it seems unfair, men appear to lose more weight than women for a given amount of exercise. In fact, exercise added to caloric-restriction programs has little additional effect on weight loss *(32,33)*. It is thought, although there are conflicting reports that exercise in combination with a calorie-reduction diet reduces the loss of lean body mass during weight loss. Exercise likely does not add much to weight-loss therapy because of the relatively small amount of calories burned during an average individual's workout. Moderate exercise for 20–30 minutes daily burns only approx 100–150 calories per session. One can see that it is more efficient to reduce calorie intake as a means of weight reduction rather than increasing exercise. Although exercise alone or in combination with diet does not result in significant weight loss, it has an important role in the maintenance of weight loss in the long-term *(34)*.

Dietary Therapy

Human metabolism has evolved to store food energy as fat in times of excess and use this energy for survival in times of need *(35)*. Simply, weight loss will result when caloric intake is lesser than energy expenditure and *vice versa*. Although this concept appears to be relatively straightforward, no single weight-control diet has been found that is appropriate for all individuals *(35)*. Despite the present dietary guidelines of reducing dietary fat to less than 30% of the total calories consumed *(36)*, obesity in America continues to become more prevalent in all age groups.

Interestingly, although excess weight is the most identifiable risk factor for OSAS, relatively few studies have focused on the role of dietary weight loss as a treatment. Most studies have been limited to small sample sizes and short-term follow-up *(9,14,17,37–42)*. Only one study was randomized and had an adequate control group, and this study dates back to the mid-1980s *(11)*. To summarize the results of these studies, weight reduction was imposed through varying forms of calorie-restricted diets with weight reduction ranging from 8 to 24% of baseline body weight. Although most studies demonstrated a significant improvement in the AHI, almost all studies demonstrated residual moderate-to-severe sleep apnea after treatment (AHI, 14–62 events/hour).

Recommendations for dietary weight loss are not straightforward. Despite the current dietary guidelines, most Americans continue to gain excess weight. This syndrome may be more related to excess intake in general, rather than the actual components of dietary consumption. Although 29% of men and 44% of women in America describe themselves as trying to lose weight, only about 20% report restricting caloric intake *(18)*. The most commonly utilized diet plans can be separated into reduced-calorie or adjusted-component (low-carbohydrate/high-fat) plans.

Simple daily calorie reduction should lead to weight reduction for most people. Most studies demonstrate that obese individuals can lose approx 1 pound/week by decreasing their daily intake to 500–1000 kcal, lower than the caloric intake required to maintain their current weight *(43)*. Unfortunately, most individuals also have no concept of how many calories they consume in a day, underestimating intake by as much as 30% *(44)*.

Because most individuals have no idea of their current or an appropriate daily caloric intake, estimates can be made to help and guide them. The WHO recommends a method that allows for a direct estimate of resting metabolic rate and permits for different activity levels when calculating daily energy expenditure *(45)*. A simpler rule of thumb is that 22 kcal/kg ± 20% is required to maintain 1 kg of body weight in a normal adult. So for a 90-kg man, the calorie range for weight maintenance would be between 1584 and 2376 kcal/day. This wide variability in energy requirements is affected by several factors including sex, activity level, age, and genetics *(45)*. In general, when prescribing reduced-calorie diets for patients, start by prescribing a daily caloric intake that is based on the aforementioned formula minus 20% and adjust intake as needed over time. As an example, for the 90-kg male mentioned earlier, prescribe a diet of 1584 kcal/day to start. Adjust the caloric intake up or down depending on weight-loss results over time. Remember, a realistic weight-loss plan should result in a 5–10% weight loss during a 3–6-month period of time. Patients should also be counseled that caloric intake will have to be reduced as they lose weight to compensate for reduced calorie needs *(46)*.

The roles of dietary fats and carbohydrates in weight gain and loss remain controversial. The Seven Countries study, which investigated the relationship between diet and heart disease, demonstrated that the Netherlands has one of the lowest prevalence rates of obesity in Europe, yet has a diet that is made up of 48% fat *(47)*. Several studies evaluating an Atkins-type low-carbohydrate/high-fat diet have demonstrated weight loss equal to or more than traditional low-calorie diets over periods of up to 1 year *(48–50)*. These studies also demonstrated improvements in many components of the lipid profile, in spite of increased fat ingestion. Finally, improved insulin sensitivity was observed in many of the subjects. Based on these findings, the current consensus concerning low-carbohydrate diets is that they are effective for short-term weight loss and are not associated with deleterious changes in glucose metabolism or lipid profiles. Further studies are still required to determine their long-term efficacy and safety *(35)*.

Drug Therapy

Drug therapy can be used as part of a comprehensive weight-loss program. Changes in diet and behavior alone unfortunately donot produce sustained weight loss for most adults. As with other weight-loss treatments, drug therapy does not cure obesity and weight gain is common after weight-loss medications are discontinued *(51)*. Currently, drug therapy for obesity is approved for use in adults who have a BMI of more than 27 kg/m^2 and obesity-related comorbidities or a BMI of more than 30 kg/m^2 in the absence of such conditions *(52)*. Experts recommend that pharmacological treatment of obesity be used only as part of a more comprehensive program that also includes lifestyle modification interventions such as diet and/or exercise counseling *(20)*.

The Food and Drug Administration (FDA) has approved two medications for the short-term treatment of obesity. *Short-term* has been widely interpreted as treatment for up to 12 weeks *(52)*. Phentermine and diethylpropion are sympathomimetic agents that reduce food intake by causing early satiety. Both drugs have been demonstrated to lead to moderate improvements in weight loss (2–10 kg) compared with placebo *(53–55)*. Phentermine alone has not been independently associated with pulmonary hypertension or cardiac valvular abnormalities *(56)*. Other sympathomimetic agents such as phenylpropanolamine, ephedrine, and ephedra are currently not approved for weight loss and have been taken off the market because of potentially life-threatening side effects *(57)*. There are currently no data evaluating any of these agents as adjuncts to weight loss in patients with OSAS.

Sibutramine (Meridia, Reductil; Abbott Laboratories; Abbott Park, IL) is a specific inhibitor of both serotonin and norepinephrine reuptake that has been approved for long-term therapy for obesity in conjunction with a reduced-calorie diet. Its modes of actions include reduction in food intake and stimulation of thermogenesis (at least in animal studies). Several studies have demonstrated its effectiveness in both the short- and long-term (up to 2 years) treatment of obesity *(58–63)*. Weight loss related to sibutramine combined with a reduced-calorie diet has ranged from 5 to 9.5%, vs 1 to 4%

for the placebo groups. Weight loss with sibutramine appears to be dose-related, with the recommended initial dose being 10 mg daily. It can be titrated up or down depending on results and/or side effects and is approved by the FDA up to a maximum dose of 15 mg daily.

Potential side effects from sibutramine include increases in diastolic blood pressure and pulse, which cause discontinuation of the drug in approx 5% of patients. Other potential side effects include dry mouth, insomnia, headache, and constipation. It should also be noted that the FDA approved the use of the sibutramine as a diet drug against the wishes of its advisory committee that actually voted against its approval by a 5:4 vote. The concern of the committee was that the health risks associated with the use of sibutramine for the treatment of obesity outweighed the potential benefits. During the period from February of 1998 until September 2001, there had been 397 adverse reactions reported to the FDA, including 152 hospitalizations and 29 deaths.

Orlistat (Xenical; Roche Pharmaceuticals; Nutley, NJ) is the only FDA-approved medication for obesity that reduces nutrient absorption. Its mode of action is that of altering the breakdown and absorption of fat by inhibiting the action of pancreatic lipases, resulting in increased fecal fat excretion. Orlistat is minimally absorbed and tends not to interfere with metabolism of many commonly used medications. It may interfere with the absorption of the fat-soluble vitamins, and vitamin supplementation is recommended.

The recommended dose of orlistat is 120 mg with or 1 hour after meals three times a day. Trials have demonstrated that patients treated with orlistat for up to 2 years can lose and maintain up to 9% of their preintervention weight, compared with 5.8% in the placebo groups *(64–67)*. Improvements in lipid profiles, hypertension, and glycemic control have also been observed. Side effects are typically mild, but occur in 1–30% of patients. Side effects include flatulence, fecal incontinence, oily spotting, and increased frequency of defecation. Approximately 9% of individuals discontinue the use of orlistat secondary to side effects.

Surgery

For those individuals who are unable to lose a significant amount of weight by conventional means, surgery offers another potential treatment option. The National Institutes of Health consensus conference recommended that surgical intervention for the treatment of obesity be considered for adults with a BMI of more than 40 kg/m^2 or a BMI of more than 35 kg/m^2 with serious coexisting obesity-related conditions such as severe sleep apnea, cardiovascular disease, type 2 diabetes, and/or joint disease *(68)*. No recommendations were made for children or adolescents because of insufficient data.

Although various surgical procedures for the treatment of obesity exist, gastric bypass and gastric banding are the two most commonly performed procedures *(69)*. In gastric bypass, the stomach is partitioned and the proximal gastric pouch is anastomosed to a limb of small bowel. Gastric banding involves the creation of a small proximal gastric pouch by placement of a band near the upper portion of the stomach. In general, the Roux-en-Y gastric bypass procedure results in more weight loss than gastric banding and is more likely to reverse the medical problems associated with severe obesity *(69–71)*. Laparoscopic gastric bypass is currently the most commonly performed bariatric procedure. Weight loss resulting from these procedures is more dramatic than other therapies (20–50% of initial weight) with the majority of the weight loss occurring in the first 1–2 years after the procedure.

There is currently no comprehensive registry for bariatric surgery, so it is difficult to determine the incidence of minor and more serious complications. Postoperative mortality is estimated to range from 0.1 to 2% *(69–71)*. In 2003, the American Society for Bariatric Surgery issued guidelines for granting bariatric surgery privileges. The group is currently developing a "centers of excellence" program to better identify comprehensive programs. Also, the National Institute of Diabetes and Digestive and Kidney Diseases has established a clinical consortium, known as the Longitudinal Assessment of Bariatric Surgery that will study the risks and benefits as well as physiological effects of bariatric surgery during a 5-year period.

As is the case with bariatric surgery in general, quality systematic data regarding weight-loss surgery for the treatment of OSAS are sparse. Most data have been generated from uncontrolled studies and case series *(15,16,72–74)*. Study size has been generally small (*n* = 4–40), with long-term follow-up ranging from 2 months to 10 years. Most studies evaluated the gastric bypass procedure. Weight reduction ranged between 23 and 73% of initial body weight. All studies demonstrated a significant reduction in AHI, although most patients were not cured of their OSAS after their procedure (residual AHI, 1.4–26 events/hour).

DOES CPAP THERAPY IMPROVE WEIGHT LOSS?

Patients with OSAS are commonly chronically fatigued, which is thought in part to reduce their motivation for diet modification and exercise programs. Only two studies exist that specifically address the role of CPAP in weight loss in patients with OSAS. Kajaste et al. *(24)* randomly assigned 31 obese men with OSAS to 6 months of either CPAP therapy or no positive-pressure treatment in addition to cognitive-behavioral treatment and diet modification. The addition of CPAP therapy did not result in significantly more weight loss at 6 months or during the remaining 3 years of follow-up. This study had many limitations such as small sample size, male-only population, and lack of objective documentation of CPAP compliance. Ip and colleagues *(75)* demonstrated in a small group (*n* = 30) of patients with OSAS that although 6 months of CPAP therapy significantly reduced leptin resistance to the levels of matched control subjects, no significant change in weight was seen during that same period of time. Given the limited amount of objective data, the role of CPAP therapy in weight loss in patients with OSAS remains unclear.

CONCLUSIONS

In general, when discussing weight-loss options with your obese or overweight patients, the most effective interventions combine nutrition education, diet and exercise counseling, and behavioral strategies that help individuals acquire the skills and supports needed to change eating patterns and become more physically active *(20)*. When prescribing a reduced-calorie diet program, be specific in terms of the number of calories to be consumed on a daily basis. Having patients enroll in a more organized program such as Weight Watchers® may improve their chances of attaining a significant and sustained weight loss. Although exercise is an important component of any program aimed at improving cardiovascular health, exercise alone in general will not lead to significant weight loss. For those patients unable (or unwilling) to lose a significant amount of weight by more traditional means, the addition of prescription weight-loss medications or referral for bariatric surgery may be appropriate. Finally, make sure you provide your patients with realistic weight-loss expectations. Attaining ideal body weight (BMI < 25 kg/m^2) is not realistic for most people. Weight loss of approx 1–2 pounds/week or a 5–10% weight loss during the initial 3–6 months is more realistic.

Obesity is a common problem in this country and worldwide and is the most identifiable risk factor associated with OSAS. As compared with other therapies such as CPAP and upper airway surgery, there are relatively few studies related to weight loss as a primary therapy for OSAS. Hence, answers to questions such as, which is the best weight-loss treatment plan to recommend to patients and how much weight loss is required to improve or cure an individual's OSAS remain unclear. Clearly, more data from larger, more long-term, and properly controlled studies will be required in the future regarding the role of weight-loss therapies in the treatment of OSAS.

REFERENCES

1. Flegal KM, Carroll MD, Ogden CL, et al. (2002) Prevalence and trends in obesity among US adults, 1999-2000. JAMA 288:1723–1727.
2. Hedley AA, Ogden CL, Johnson CL, et al. (2004) Prevalence of overweight and obesity among US children, adolescents, and adults, 1999-2002. JAMA 291:2847–2850.
3. Ogden CL, Flegal KM, Carroll MD, et al. (2002) Prevalence and trends in overweight among US children and adolescents, 1999-2000. JAMA 288:1728–1732.
4. Young T, Peppard PE, Gottlieb D (2002) Epidemiology of obstructive sleep apnea. Am J Respir Crit Care Med 165:1217–1239.
5. Levinson P, McGarvey S, Carlisle C, et al. (1993) Adiposity and cardiovascular risk factors in men with obstructive sleep apnea. Chest 103:1336–1342.
6. Millman R, Carlisle C, McGarvey S, et al. (1995) Body fat distribution and sleep apnea severity in women. Chest 107:362–366.
7. Newman AB, Nieto FJ, Guidry U, et al. (2001) Relation of sleep-disordered breathing to cardiovascular disease risk factors: The Sleep Heart Health Study. Am J Epidemiol 154:50–59.
8. Mortimore IL, Marshall I, Wraith PK, et al. (1998) Neck and total body fat deposition in nonobese and obese patients with sleep apnea compared with that in control subjects. Am J Respir Crit Care Med 157:280–283.
9. Kiselak J, Clark M, Pera V, et al. (1993) The association between hypertension and sleep apnea in obese patients. Chest 104:775–780.
10. Peppard PE, Young T, Palta M, et al. (2000) Longitudinal study of moderate weight change and sleep-disordered breathing. JAMA 284:3015–3021.
11. Smith P, Gold A, Meyers D, et al. (1985) Weight loss in mildly to moderately obese patients with obstructive sleep apnea. Ann Intern Med 103:850–855.
12. Noseda A, Kempenaers C, Kerkhofs M, et al. (1996) Sleep apnea after 1 year domiciliary nasal-continuous positive airway pressure and attempted weight reduction: potential for weaning from continuous positive airway pressure. Chest 109:138–143.
13. Suratt P, McTier R, Findley L, et al. (1987) Changes in breathing and the pharynx after weight loss in obstructive sleep apnea. Chest 92:631–637.
14. Suratt P, McTier R, Findley L, et al. (1992) Effect of very-low-calorie diets with weight loss on obstructive sleep apnea. Am J Clin Nutr 56:182S–184S.
15. Harman E, Wynne J, Block A (1982) The effect of weight loss on sleep-disordered breathing and oxygen desaturation in morbidly obese men. Chest 82:291–294.
16. Pillar G, Peled R, Lavie P (1994) Recurrence of sleep apnea without concomitant weight increase 7.5 years after weight reduction surgery. Chest 106:1702–1704.
17. Aubert-Tulkens G, Culee C, Rodenstein D (1989) Cure of sleep apnea syndrome after long-term nasal continuous positive airway pressure therapy and weight loss. Sleep 12:216–222.
18. Clinical Guidelines on the Identification, Evaluation, and Treatment of Overweight and Obesity in Adults—The Evidence Report; National Institutes of Health. (1998) Obes Res 6(Suppl 2): 51S–209S.
19. *Obesity: Preventing and Managing the Global Epidemic*. World Health Organization, Geneva, Switzerland, 1997.

20. McTigue KM, Harris R, Hemphill B, et al. (2003) Screening and interventions for obesity in adults: summary of the evidence for the U.S. preventive services task force. Ann Intern Med 139:933–949.
21. Calle EE, Thun MJ, Petrelli JM, et al. (1999) Body-mass index and mortality in a prospective cohort of U.S. adults. N Engl J Med 341:1097–1105.
22. Stuart R (1967) Behavioral control of overeating. Behav Res Ther 5:357.
23. Foreyt JP, Goodrick GK (1993) Evidence for success of behavior modification in weight loss and control. Ann Intern Med 119:698–701.
24. Kajaste S, Brander P, Telakivi T, et al. (2004) A cognitive-behavioral weight reduction program in the treatment of obstructive sleep apnea syndrome with or without initial nasal CPAP: a randomized study. Sleep Med 5:125–131.
25. Stradling J, Roberts D, Wilson A, et al. (1998) Controlled trial of hypnotherapy for weight loss in patients with obstructive sleep apnoea. Int J Obes 28:278–281.
26. Bray G (2004) Behavior modification in the treatment of obesity. Up To Date 12:1–7.
27. Heshka S, Greenway F, Anderson J, et al. (2000) Self-help weight loss versus a structured commercial program after 26 weeks: a randomized controlled study. Am J Med 109:282–287.
28. Ravussin E, Lillioja S, Knowler W, et al. (1988) Reduced rate of energy expenditure as a risk factor for body-weight gain. N Engl J Med 318:467–472.
29. Robinson TN (1999) Reducing children's television viewing to prevent obesity: a randomized controlled trial. JAMA 282:1561–1567.
30. Slentz CA, Duscha BD, Johnson JL, et al. (2004) Effects of the amount of exercise on body weight, body composition, and measures of central obesity: STRRIDE; a randomized controlled study. Arch Intern Med 164:31–39.
31. Ross R, Dagnone D, Jones PJH, et al. (2000) Reduction in obesity and related comorbid conditions after diet-induced weight loss or exercise-induced weight loss in men: a randomized, controlled trial. Ann Intern Med 133:92–103.
32. Jakicic JM, Winters C, Lang W, et al. (1999) Effects of intermittent exercise and use of home exercise equipment on adherence, weight loss, and fitness in overweight women: a randomized trial. JAMA 282:1554–1560.
33. Jakicic JM, Marcus BH, Gallagher KI, et al. (2003) Effect of exercise duration and intensity on weight loss in overweight, sedentary women: a randomized trial. JAMA 290:1323–1330.
34. Miller W, Koceja D, Hamilton E (1997) A meta-analysis of the past 25 years of weight loss research using diet, exercise or diet plus exercise intervention. Int J Obes 21:941–947.
35. Acheson KJ (2004) Carbohydrate and weight control: where do we stand? Curr Opin Clin Nutr Metab Care 7:485–492.
36. Stamler J, Beard R, Connor W, et al. (1972) Report of inter-society commission for heart disease resources: prevention of cardiovascular disease; primary prevention of the atherosclerotic diseases. Circulation 42:A55–A95.
37. Schwartz A, Gold A, Schubert N, et al. (1991) Effect of weight loss on upper airway collapsibility in obstructive sleep apnea. Am J Respir Crit Care Med 144:494–498.
38. Rubenstein I, Colapinto N, Rotstein L, et al. (1988) Improvement in upper airway function after weight loss in patients with obstructive sleep apnea. Am Rev Respir Crit Care Med 138:1192–1195.
39. Rajala R, Partinen M, Sane T, et al. (1991) Obstructive sleep apnea in morbidly obese patients. J Intern Med 230:125–129.
40. Lojander J, Mustajoki P, Ronka S, et al. (1998) A nurse-managed weight reduction programme for obstructive sleep apnoea syndrome. J Intern Med 244:251–255.
41. Kansanen M, Vanninen E, Tuunainen A, et al. (1998) The effect of very-low calorie diet-induced weight loss on the severity of obstructive sleep apnea and autonomic nervous function in obese patients with obstructive sleep apnoea syndrome. Clin Physiol 18:377–385.
42. Pasquali R, Colella P, Cirignotta F, et al. (1990) Treatment of obese patients with obstructive sleep apnea syndrome (OSAS): effect of weight loss and interference of otorhinolaryngoiatric pathology. Int J Obes 14:207–217.
43. Wadden T, Foster G (2000) Behavioral treatment of Obesity. Med Clin North Am 84:441–461, vii.
44. Champagne CM, Bray GA, Kurtz AA, et al. (2002) Energy intake and energy expenditure: a controlled study comparing dietitians and non-dietitians. J Am Diet Assoc 102:1428–1432.
45. Lin P-H, Proschan MA, Bray GA, et al. (2003) Estimation of energy requirements in a controlled feeding trial. Am J Clin Nutr 77:639–645.
46. Leibel RL, Rosenbaum M, Hirsch J (1995) Changes in energy expenditure resulting from altered body weight. N Engl J Med 332:621–628.

47. Seidell J (2000) Obesity, insulin resistance and diabetes: a worldwide epidemic. Br J Nutr 83:S5–S8.
48. Samaha FF, Iqbal N, Seshadri P, et al. (2003) A low-carbohydrate as compared with a low-fat diet in severe obesity. N Engl J Med 348:2074–2081.
49. Foster GD, Wyatt HR, Hill JO, et al. (2003) A randomized trial of a low-carbohydrate diet for obesity. N Engl J Med 348:2082–2090.
50. Westman E, Yancy W, Edman J, et al. (2002) Effect of 6-month adherence to a very low carbohydrate diet program. Am J Med 113:30–36.
51. Yanovski SZ, Yanovski JA (2002) Obesity: drug therapy. N Engl J Med 346:591–602.
52. *The Physicians' Desk Reference*. 55th ed. Medical Economics, Montvale, NJ, 2004.
53. Inoue S (1995) Clinical studies with mazindol. Obes Res 3(Suppl 4):549S–552S.
54. Enzi G, Baritussio A, Marchiori E, et al. (1976) Short-term and long-term evaluation of a non-amphetaminic anorexiant (mazindol) in the treatment of obesity. J Int Med Res 4:305–318.
55. Steel J, Munro J, Duncan L (1973) A comparative trial of different regimens of fenfluramine and phentermine in obesity. Practitioner 211:232–236.
56. Connolly HM, Crary JL, McGoon MD, et al. (1997) Valvular heart disease associated with fenfluramine-phentermine. N Engl J Med 337:581–588.
57. Kernan WN, Viscoli CM, Brass LM, et al. (2000) Phenylpropanolamine and the risk of hemorrhagic stroke. N Engl J Med 343:1826–1832.
58. Fanghanel G, Cortinas L, Sanchez-Reyes L, et al. (2000) A clinical trial of sibutramine for the treatment of patients suffering essential obesity. Int J Obes Relat Metab Disord 24:144–150.
59. Bray G, Blackburn G, Ferguson J, et al. (1999) Sibutramine produces dose-related weight loss. Obes Res 7:189–198.
60. McMahon FG, Fujioka K, Singh BN, et al. (2000) Efficacy and safety of sibutramine in obese white and African American patients with hypertension: a 1-year, double-blind, placebo-controlled, multicenter trial. Arch Intern Med 160:2185–2191.
61. Ryan D (2000) Use of sibutramine and other noradrenergic drugs in the management of obesity. Endocrine 2:175–187.
62. James W, Astrup A, Finer N, et al. (2000) Effect of sibutramine on weight maintenance after weight loss: a randomized trial. Lancet 356:2119–2125.
63. Apfelbaum M, Vague P, Ziegler O, et al. (1999) Long-term maintenance of weight loss after a very-low calorie diet: a randomized blinded trial of the efficacy and tolerability of sibutramine. Am J Med 106:179–184.
64. Davidson MH, Hauptman J, DiGirolamo M, et al. (1999) Weight control and risk factor reduction in obese subjects treated for 2 years with orlistat: a randomized controlled trial. JAMA 281:235–242.
65. Hauptman J, Lucas C, Boldrin MN, et al. (2000) Orlistat in the long-term treatment of obesity in primary care settings. Arch Fam Med 9:160–167.
66. Rossner S, Sjostrom L, Noack R, et al. (2000) Weight loss, weight maintenance, and improved cardiovascular risk factors after 2 years treatment with orlistat for obesity. Obes Res 8:49–61.
67. Hill JO, Hauptman J, Anderson JW, et al. (1999) Orlistat, a lipase inhibitor, for weight maintenance after conventional dieting: a 1-y study. Am J Clin Nutr 69:1108–1116.
68. NIH conference: gastrointestinal surgery for severe obesity; Consensus Development Conference Panel. (1991) Ann Intern Med 115:956–961.
69. Steinbrook R (2004) Surgery for severe obesity. N Engl J Med 350:1075–1079.
70. Sjostrom CD, Peltonen M, Wedel H, et al. (2000) Differentiated long-term effects of intentional weight loss on diabetes and hypertension. Hypertension 36:20–25.
71. Sjostrom C, Lissner L, Wedel H, et al. (1999) Reduction in incidence of diabetes, hypertension and lipid disturbances after intentional weight loss induced by bariatric surgery: the SOS Intervention Study. Obes Res 7:477–484.
72. Peiser J, Lavie P, Ovnat A, et al. (1984) Sleep apnea syndrome in the morbidly obese as an indication for weight reduction surgery. Ann Surg 199:112–115.
73. Sugerman H, Fairman R, Sood R, et al. (1992) Long-term effects of gastric surgery for treating respiratory insufficiency of obesity. Am J Clin Nutr 55:597S–601S.
74. Charuzi I, Ovnat A, Peiser J (1985) The effect of surgical weight reduction on sleep quality in obesity related sleep apnea syndrome. Surgery 97:535–538.
75. Ip MS, Lam KS, Ho C, et al. (2000) Serum leptin and vascular risk factors in obstructive sleep apnea. Chest 118:580–586.

16 Sleep in Patients With Pulmonary Disease

Susan M. Harding, MD, FCCP

CONTENTS

INTRODUCTION

Sleep complaints are very prevalent in the patients with pulmonary disease. This review will examine sleep effects on respiration, explore ventilatory responses during sleep in normal individuals, and examine mechanisms of hypoxemia in patients with pulmonary disease. Sleep disorders in patients with obstructive pulmonary diseases, including chronic obstructive pulmonary disease (COPD), cystic fibrosis (CF), asthma, and restrictive parenchymal disease will be reviewed. A diagnostic evaluation and management plan are also suggested for these patients.

NORMAL VENTILATORY RESPONSES DURING SLEEP

Effects of Sleep on Respiration

Sleep is associated with a decrease in the responsiveness of the respiratory center to chemical and mechanical stimuli that is further decreased during rapid eye movement (REM) sleep. Furthermore, respiratory muscle responsiveness to respiratory controller output is decreased during sleep and is further decreased during REM sleep *(1)*. The discussion points will include control of breathing and hypoxic and hypercapnic ventilatory responses during sleep. Furthermore, upper airway muscle tone and arousal responses during sleep will be discussed and other factors will be examined, including drugs that influence ventilatory control.

From: *Current Clinical Practice: Primary Care Sleep Medicine: A Practical Guide*
Edited by: J. F. Pagel and S. R. Pandi-Perumal © Humana Press Inc., Totowa, NJ

With sleep onset and the loss of wakefulness stimuli, control of breathing becomes automatic. There are decreases in respiratory drive and upper airway muscle tone. $PaCO_2$ increases by 4–6 mmHg, leading to decreases in pH by 0.03–0.05 U. PaO_2 decreases by 3–8 mmHg in normal individuals. Despite these changes, there is only a 2% decrease in arterial oxygen saturation (SaO_2) with sleep onset in normal individuals *(2)*. There is a decrease in basal metabolic rate during sleep, but cerebral blood flow increases by 4–25% during non-REM (NREM) sleep and increases even more (up to 80%) during REM sleep *(3)*.

With stage 1 sleep, ventilatory instability ensues. Investigators report this as "unsteady" NREM sleep *(4)*. In the brain stem, respiratory control transitions between wakefulness and metabolic control influences. Minute ventilation decreases 1–10 L/minute during this time. The $PaCO_2$ may increase to the point of arousal, leading to hyperventilation past the wakefulness set point that, with sleep onset, triggers periodic breathing. Periodic breathing is present in approx 40–80% of normal individuals during unsteady NREM sleep. The set point for ventilation also fluctuates with the fluctuating level of wakefulness.

Unsteady NREM sleep transitions to steady NREM sleep during sleep stages 2, 3, and 4 *(4)*. Respirations are very regular with a regular rate and tidal volume. The "automatic pilot" of respiration is in full swing. Minute ventilation decreases 0.4–1.5 L/minute. Tidal volume decreases by about 10%, resulting in an increase in end tidal CO_2. Pulmonary artery pressure increases by 4–5 mmHg. Pulmonary function, including functional residual capacity, decreases by 10%, without significant changes in ventilation-perfusion relationships in normal individuals.

With the onset of REM sleep, ventilation becomes very erratic. Breathing becomes irregular and rapid, and respiratory rate may increase up to 150% of baseline *(5)*. Tidal volume decreases by as much as 44%. These changes are the most prominent during phasic REM (associated with eye movements), as compared with tonic REM sleep. Also, during the first eye movements of a REM period, there can be a sudden decrease in respiratory amplitude and airflow *(6)*. Pharyngeal muscle tone decreases and upper airway resistance increases during sleep *(7)*. Both phasic (with inspiration) and tonic muscle tone decrease during NREM sleep and further decrease during REM sleep.

There are also alterations in compliance of the chest wall and rib cage during sleep. Gravity and the supine position also influence respiratory function *(8)*. Muscles of respiration include the inspiratory muscles (diaphragm, external intercostals, scalenus, trapezius, and sternocleidomastoid) and the expiratory muscles (internal intercostals, pectus abdominus, internal and external obliques, and transverse abdominal muscle). During NREM sleep, the rib cage contribution to respiration is more than during wakefulness, as shown by increased electromyogram (EMG) signals of the external intercostals during inspiration *(4)*. Minimal EMG changes are noted in the diaphragm *(9)*. This leads to expansion of the rib cage and an increase in transdiaphragmatic pressure. During REM sleep, the rib cage contribution to respiration decreases when there is a marked decrease in intercostal EMG muscle activity. Diaphragmatic EMG activity increases during REM sleep; however, there is a decrease in transdiaphragmatic pressure, so that diaphragmatic efficiency decreases. This decrease in the rib cage and abdominal muscle contribution to respiration during REM sleep is because of supraspinal inhibition of the γ-motor neurons and, to a lesser extent, the α-motor neurons. There is presynaptic inhibition of the afferent terminals to the muscle spindles.

Note that the diaphragm contains primarily α-motor neurons with a very limited number of λ-motor neurons and muscle spindles, so that the diaphragm is less affected during REM sleep *(4)*.

Ventilatory and Arousal Responses During Sleep

The hypoxic ventilatory response is altered during sleep *(10)*. During NREM sleep, there is a 30–150% decrease in the hypoxic ventilatory response in men that is not present in women. Several theories exist regarding why this is true *(3)*. Men compared with women have a higher awake hypoxic ventilatory response, allowing for men to decrease this response even more with sleep, whereas in women this response is stable. During REM sleep in both sexes, there is an additional 50–75% decrease in the hypoxic ventilatory response. In conclusion, the hypoxic ventilatory response during sleep is depressed during NREM sleep in men and is even more depressed in REM sleep in both sexes.

The hypercapnic ventilatory response is depressed up to 50% during NREM sleep, and it is depressed even more during REM sleep *(11)*. There are no gender differences noted in this response, although there is some conflict about this in the literature. In general, the respiratory center has less sensitivity during sleep. Arousal responses to hypoxia and hypercapnia during sleep can be prolonged. Hypoxia, even when the SaO_2 is less than 70% or when the PaO_2 is 40 mmHg (with isocapnia), is a poor arousal stimulant *(12)*. Hypercapnia produces arousal responses more easily than hypoxia, with most normal individuals arousing when their $PaCO_2$ increases 15 mmHg higher than their wakefulness level. The normal arousal response to hypercarbia is increased when concomitant hypoxia is present. Arousal responses to an occluded airway and/or with bronchial irritation are also depressed during sleep. Arousal time from an occluded airway during REM sleep is quicker than during NREM sleep *(13)*. Sleep also suppresses the cough response to inhaled irritants. Coughing usually occurs during arousals.

Drug Effects on Ventilatory Control

Drugs, including alcohol, narcotics, benzodiazepines, and barbiturates depress ventilatory drive during sleep by suppressing upper airway muscle activity and tone, and by increasing upper airway resistance *(4)*. The arousal response is also impaired. Medroxyprogesterone is a respiratory stimulant that increases ventilatory drive, leading to decreases in $PaCO_2$ by 5 mmHg in normal individuals. Theophylline also increases the hypoxic ventilatory response. Acetazolamide inhibits carbonic anhydrase, thus increasing tissue CO_2 and central ventilatory drive. Acetazolamide causes a metabolic acidosis and blocks the lung's ability to excrete CO_2.

Summary

In conclusion, respiration changes during sleep. These changes may be exaggerated in patients with pulmonary disease. In normal individuals, there is a decrease in minute ventilation by 0.5–1.5 L/minute during sleep. There is a decrease in the metabolic rate, a decrease in chemosensitivity by 20–50%, and an increase in airway resistance. All of this leads to an increase of $PaCO_2$ by approx 2–8 mmHg, a PaO_2 decrease by 3–10 mmHg, and a 2% decrease in SaO_2 in normal individuals *(14)*. The impact of sleep on respiration includes changes in cortical inputs, changes in respiratory center sensitivity and chemoreceptor/mechanoreceptor sensitivity. Respiratory muscle contractility and thus, lung mechanics change along with functional residual capacity and airway resistance. In patients with pulmonary disease, these alterations may lead to ventilation-perfusion mismatch, hypoventilation, hypoxemia, and hypercapnia.

OBSTRUCTIVE PULMONARY DISEASE

Patients with obstructive pulmonary disease may have marked alterations in respiration during sleep *(14)*. Although COPD also includes CF and asthma, COPD will be discussed separately, including patients with emphysema and chronic bronchitis. In separate sections, CF and nocturnal asthma will be discussed.

Chronic Obstructive Pulmonary Disease

Sleep in Patients With COPD

COPD is potentially a preventable and treatable disease state, characterized by airflow limitation that is not fully reversible *(15)*. This airflow limitation is progressive and is associated with a heightened inflammatory response in the lungs. Cigarette smoking is the most common cause of COPD. COPD prevalence from the NHANES III Study is approx 14% in white male smokers, 7% in ex-smokers, and 3% of never smokers *(16)*. In white women, COPD is present in 13% of smokers, in 7% of ex-smokers, and in 3% of never smokers. COPD is associated with significant morbidity and mortality, with COPD being the fourth leading cause of death worldwide. Patients with COPD can have significant sleep disruption. They often complain of multiple arousals and insomnia. Furthermore, many patients have sleep-related hypoxemia that is more severe during REM sleep. Patients with COPD may also have obstructive sleep apnea (OSA) *(14)*.

Hypoventilation occurs during sleep leading to hypoxemia, which is most severe during REM sleep *(17,18)*. There is an increase in physiological dead space. Furthermore, there is a rapid, shallow breathing pattern noted during phasic REM bursts that significantly decreases minute ventilation. Although there is minimal data showing this, functional residual capacity also decreases. The flattened diaphragm also pulls in the flaccid lower chest wall during REM sleep. Ventilation-perfusion mismatch occurs with hypoventilation. Decreased oxygen in the lung may also be present. Furthermore, patients with COPD have lower baseline SaO_2 levels during wakefulness, so that the position of their baseline SaO_2 values on the oxyhemoglobin disassociation curve may predispose them to significant oxygen desaturation during sleep *(19)*. Aoki and colleagues *(20)* examined oxygen saturation during sleep in 26 stable patients with COPD who had an awakening oxygen SaO_2 of more than 90%. They defined significant oxygen desaturation during sleep as an SaO_2 of less than 90% for more than 10 minutes. Daytime arterial blood gases, pulmonary function tests, and 6-minute walk tests did not differentiate patients with COPD with sleep-related oxygen desaturation, from those without sleep-related oxygen desaturation. They noted four patterns of sleep-disordered breathing (SDB) in patients with COPD:

1. Hypoventilation (present 74% of the time).
2. Paradoxical respiratory movements (present 10% of the time).
3. Periodic breathing (present 12% of the time).
4. An unclassified type of breathing (present 5% of the time).

This study shows that multiple SDB patterns are present in patients with COPD, resulting in oxygen desaturation during sleep.

Other investigators, including Weitzenblum and colleagues *(19)* examined predictors of sleep-related hypoxemia in patients with COPD. The most important predictor was daytime SaO_2. Other predictors included daytime $PaCO_2$, a low ventilatory response to inhaled CO_2, and a patient being classified as a *blue bloater*. Also, patients with COPD with respiratory muscle dysfunction and those with a combination of OSA and COPD (called the "overlap" syndrome) were also more likely to have oxygen desaturation during sleep.

Examining differences between *pink puffers* and *blue bloaters*, Demarco and colleagues *(21)* examined SaO_2 during wakefulness and sleep. Blue bloaters had lower awake-sitting SaO_2 result; supine-awake SaO_2 result, and sleeping-supine SaO_2 result, compared with pink puffers. Blue bloaters had a 29% mean maximum fall in SaO_2 during sleep. They also had many more episodes of SaO_2 desaturation during sleep, compared with pink puffers. Furthermore, during sleep, SaO_2 was less than 80% for 120 minutes in the blue bloaters, compared with less than 1 minute in the pink puffers. Thus, blue bloaters are more likely to have significant oxygen desaturation during sleep, compared with pink puffers.

As part of the Sleep Heart Health Study, Sanders and colleagues *(22)* examined 1132 patients with mild COPD. OSA was *not* found to be more prevalent in patients with mild COPD, compared with subjects without COPD. However, sleep-related oxygen desaturation was more severe in patients with COPD and OSA, compared with patients with COPD and no OSA. Patients with COPD with an FEV_1/FVC ratio of less than 65% had an increased risk of having oxygen desaturation during sleep. When adjusting for age, sex, height, weight, smoking, and awake SaO_2, patients with an FEV_1/FVC ratio of less than 60% had an adjusted odds ratio of 3.36 for having oxygen desaturation during sleep. There are many consequences of sleep-related hypoxemia in patients with COPD, including disrupted sleep architecture, increased mean pulmonary artery pressure (especially during REM sleep), increased ventricular ectopy, and an increased myocardial blood flow demand.

Patients with COPD have alterations in their sleep architecture. They have prolonged sleep latency, decreased sleep efficiency, decreased total sleep time, and increased wake time after sleep onset *(23)*. Arousals are associated with oxygen desaturation. Furthermore, patients with COPD have decreased proportions of REM sleep and slow-wave sleep. Many factors contribute to this disruption of sleep architecture, including SDB, cough, dyspnea, oxygen desaturation, and medications, including theophylline and corticosteroids that can disrupt sleep. Sleep architecture findings in patients with COPD, as noted by Fleetham and colleagues *(24)*, included increased stage 1, decreased slow-wave sleep, and decreased REM sleep percentages. Saaresranta and colleagues *(25)* examined sleep variables in 15 postmenopausal women with COPD who had a mean FEV_1 of 0.73 L and daytime hypoxemia (with or without hypercapnia) and compared them to 20, age-matched, postmenopausal women. The women with COPD reported poor sleep, restlessness during sleep, and tiredness upon awakening almost every morning, more frequently than the control subjects. However, women with COPD did not complain of significant daytime sleepiness. The women with COPD also had higher proportions of stage 1 sleep and had delayed REM latencies, compared with the controls. Together, all of these investigations show that sleep architecture is disrupted in patients with COPD and that they often complain of poor sleep.

Sleep may impact pulmonary artery pressure in patients with COPD. Coccagna and colleagues *(26)* examined mean pulmonary artery pressure during sleep in 12 patients with severe COPD and wake time pulmonary arterial hypertension. Mean pulmonary artery pressure during wakefulness was 37 mmHg, which increased to 55 mmHg during REM sleep. The PaO_2 fell from 56 mmHg during wakefulness to 43 mmHg during REM sleep. The increases in pulmonary artery pressure were timely related to episodes of oxygen desaturation that occurred primarily during REM sleep. Patients with COPD and isolated sleep-related oxygen desaturation may not always have significant increases in pulmonary artery pressure during wakefulness. Chaouat and colleagues *(27)* examined mean pulmonary artery pressure during wakefulness in 76 patients with COPD and sleep-related oxygen desaturation and in 29 patients with COPD without sleep-related oxygen desaturation. Elevated pulmonary artery pressures during wakefulness were equally distributed between the two groups. These data do not support the hypothesis that isolated sleep-related hypoxemia fosters the development of persistent pulmonary arterial hypertension.

Patients with COPD may also have OSA. The presence of both COPD and OSA is called the "overlap syndrome." Chaouat and colleagues *(28)* and Bradley and colleagues *(29)* examined OSA in patients with COPD. Compared with patients with OSA without COPD, patients with OSA and COPD have more profound hypoxemia during sleep and have a higher risk of developing respiratory insufficiency, pulmonary arterial hypertension, and right heart failure. OSA prevalence was *not* increased in patients with COPD.

There is a debate concerning whether oxygen desaturation during sleep is associated with increased mortality. Fletcher and colleagues examined mortality during a 36-month period in patients with COPD who had a wake time PaO_2 of more than 60 mmHg *(30)*. Eleven of 38 patients with COPD and sleep-related oxygen desaturation died, compared with none of 13 patients with COPD and no sleep-related oxygen desaturation. Unfortunately, supplemental oxygen did not reduce mortality. Furthermore, Connaughton and colleagues *(31)* also examined sleep-related oxygen desaturation and survival in 97 patients with severe COPD, during a median follow-up period of 7–8 months. Mean nadir SaO_2 during sleep was related to survival. However, SaO_2 during sleep did not improve the prediction model for survival that was already obtained by using wake time values, including vital capacity and SaO_2. There was no difference in survival rates in patients with COPD and excessive oxygen desaturation during sleep and those without. The authors concluded that sleep time oxygenation does not add any prognostic information over that which can be obtained during wakefulness.

Management of COPD During Sleep

Douglas and colleagues *(32)* discuss sleep management issues for patients with COPD. All patients should be questioned about sleep difficulties. Also, ensure that patients have optimal COPD treatment, according to established current practice guidelines. Polysomnography is indicated in patients with COPD if they have symptoms of OSA or other primary sleep disorders that warrant diagnostic testing, according to current practice parameters. Also, consider performing polysomnography in patients with COPD who have excessive daytime sleepiness, polycythemia, pulmonary arterial hypertension, or cor pulmonale, despite having a wake time PaO_2 of 60–65 mmHg. Also, consider evaluation in patients with COPD who have a morning headache, despite using oxygen during sleep. Utilize 24-hour, long-term oxygen therapy if their diurnal

PaO_2 is less than 55–60 mmHg. Pulse oximetry during sleep is adequate to assess SaO_2 and to check adequacy of oxygen therapy during sleep. Many patients with COPD require a higher oxygen flow rate during sleep. Noninvasive intermittent positive pressure ventilation (NIPPV) is necessary in selected patients.

Patients with COPD should avoid hypnotics and excessive alcohol intake. Zolpidem may be used with caution, as there is minimal data available in patients with COPD *(33)*. Theophylline may improve sleep-time SaO_2 and the morning peak expiratory flow (PEF) rate; however, it may also disrupt sleep architecture. Inhaled anticholinergic therapy such as ipratropium or tiotropium may also improve sleep-time SaO_2. Inspiratory muscle training was helpful in a group study of patients with COPD who had sleep-related oxygen desaturation *(19)*.

Other medications that have been tried but are not recommended are almitrine, protriptyline, and medroxyprogesterone. Almitrine is a carotid body agonist that lessens hypoxemia, but this medication has significant toxicities, including pulmonary arterial hypertension, dyspnea, and neuropathy. Furthermore, it is not effective on a long-term basis and is not recommended. There is also minimal data in patients with COPD regarding use of protriptyline (which inhibits REM sleep). Protriptyline may cause significant urinary retention. Medroxyprogesterone has been evaluated for sleep-related oxygen desaturation *(34)*. Dolly and colleagues *(34)* examined patients with COPD and OSA who were randomized to receive either medroxyprogesterone or placebo. Patients on medroxyprogesterone had increases in wake-time PaO_2 and decreases in $PaCO_2$, but there was no change in SaO_2 nadir or OSA variables during sleep. Furthermore, Saaresvanta and colleagues *(35)* examined 13 postmenopausal women with an FEV_1 of less than 65% who were randomized to receive placebo or medroxyprogesterone. The treated group had a mean sleep-time SaO_2 increase of 1.7%, and the sleep-time SaO_2 nadir was improved by 3.9%. Medroxyprogesterone is associated with a hypercoagulable state and impotence, and it is not recommended. None of these three medications are Food and Drug Administration (FDA)-approved for COPD.

Inhaled anticholinergics are a cornerstone in COPD therapy. McNicholas and colleagues *(36)* examined tiotropium and sleep-time SaO_2 in 56 patients with COPD and an FEV_1 of less than 65% predicted, FEV_1/FVC ratio of less than 70%, and an awake PaO_2 of less than 75 mmHg. Tiotropium was given in the morning vs night time, vs bid, vs placebo, for 4 weeks. All treatment regimens were associated with a mild improvement in sleep-related oxygen desaturation by 2–3%, and there were no changes in sleep quality. This study underlines the importance of utilizing primary COPD treatments to improve SaO_2 during sleep. Oxygen therapy is indicated in patients with COPD who meet the criteria documented in Table 1 *(37)*. The most recent ATS/ERS guidelines on COPD report that nocturnal oxygen therapy is not recommended for isolated sleep-related hypoxemia, unless there are complications of hypoxemia present, including cor pulmonale or polycythemia that is not explained by wake-time PaO_2 *(15)*. They recommend measuring sleep-time SaO_2 in these patients, even if their wake time PaO_2 is more than 55 mmHg.

Treatment of OSA in patients with COPD is similar to treatment in patients without COPD. Nasal continuous positive airway pressure (CPAP) improves arterial blood gas and pulmonary artery pressure more so than oxygen therapy alone in these patients. Oxygen can be added to CPAP for patients who meet criteria for oxygen therapy. Bilevel positive airway pressure is useful in patients having difficulty exhaling against

Table 1
Oxygen Therapy for COPD (Either I or II Fulfilled)

	Awake		Asleep
I.	PaO_2 ≤55 mmHg or SaO_2 ≤88%	OR	SaO_2 ≤89% for at least five continuous minutes, with a nadir of ≤85%
II.	PaO_2 of 55–59 mmHg or SaO_2 ≤89% at rest or with exercise	OR	SaO_2 decrease of more than 5% for at least five continuous minutes with a nadir of ≤85% during sleep

PLUS
One or more of the following:
Dependent edema as a result of congestive heart failure
Pulmonary hypertension or cor pulmonale (pulmonary artery pressure, gated blood pool scan, echo or *P. pulmonale* on ECG)
Erythrocythemia with hematocrit more than 56%

a positive pressure, in patients who have worsening oxygenation on CPAP, or in patients with COPD and hypoventilation during sleep. Automatic self-titrating CPAP (auto-CPAP) is *not* recommended for patients with COPD because these devices have not been adequately tested in patients with COPD. Patients may not have the ability to trigger the device.

NIPPV during sleep in *stable* patients with COPD may be useful in selected patients *(38)*. Wijkstra and colleagues *(39)* did a meta-analysis of randomized controlled trials utilizing NIPPV in stable patients with COPD. Sixty-seven patients were identified in four trials who used NIPPV for at least 3 months. There were no significant effects on lung function, gas exchange, or sleep efficiency. The 6-minute walk test improved with NIPPV. Selected subgroups of patients may improve, but further research is required. The National Association for Medical Directors of Respiratory Care and the American College of Chest Physicians examined outcomes data and provided a consensus statement concerning NIPPV for patients with severe, stable COPD *(40)*. They recommended NIPPV use for patients with COPD (without OSA) who are still symptomatic, despite optimal COPD therapy, and who have a $PaCO_2$ of more than 55 mmHg or if they have a $PaCO_2$ between 50 and 54 mmHg, with evidence of nocturnal hypoventilation, based on sleep-time oximetry showing SaO_2 of less than 9% for at least 5 minutes while the patient was on their usual FIO_2 prescription. Also recommended is NIPPV for patients who have repeated hospitalizations for respiratory failure. The CMS guideline for patients with COPD to receive NIPPV requires the presence of a $PaCO_2$ of more than 52 mmHg and evidence of sleep-time hypoventilation, based on sleep time oximetry showing a sustained SaO_2 of less than 89% for ≥5 minutes while the patient is on their usual FIO_2 *(41)*. Furthermore, OSA must be excluded clinically. They require a 3-month trial of bilevel positive airway pressure, without a backup rate, to see if there is clinical improvement. Hopefully, future research will provide better guidance.

SLEEP IN PATIENTS WITH CF

Patients with CF can have sleep disruption. With improved therapy, patients with CF have a mean survival of 33 years of age *(42)*. They have airflow obstruction with bronchiectasis, air trapping, hypoxemia, hypercapnia, and cor pulmonale. Furthermore, they often have chronic sinusitis and nasal polyposis that increase upper airway resistance, predisposing them to upper airway obstruction during sleep. Night time coughing and medications used to treat CF may also disrupt sleep. Patients with CF are also at risk for developing vitamin deficiencies.

Jankelowitz and colleagues examined sleep with wrist actigraphy and sleep logs for 14 days in 20, adult, stable patients with CF, and in 20 age-, sex-, and body mass index-matched controls *(43)*. The patients with CF, compared with controls, had higher scores on the Pittsburgh Sleep Quality Index but had similar total sleep time, sleep latencies, sleep efficiencies, sleep onset, and sleep offset times as the control subjects. The patients with CF had a higher sleep fragmentation index, with more night-to-night variability, compared with control subjects. There was a relationship between FEV_1 and the sleep fragmentation index. This study verifies that sleep is disrupted in patients with CF, especially in those with significant pulmonary dysfunction.

There are significant physiological changes that occur during sleep in patients with CF, including hypoventilation and ventilation-perfusion mismatch, which are more pronounced during REM sleep *(44)*. There is a decrease in functional residual capacity during sleep and worsened SaO_2 in the supine position. Upper airway obstruction is present in many patients with CF. Milross and colleagues *(45)* examined 15 patients with CF and moderate-to-severe lung disease with documented oxygen desaturation. Minute ventilation fell by approx 6% from wakefulness to sleep onset and 21% from wakefulness to REM sleep. This decrease in minute ventilation was because of decreased tidal volume and not because of changes in respiratory rate. Sleep-related hypoventilation was noted, especially during REM sleep.

Furthermore, acute CF exacerbations can impact sleep. There is worsening in SaO_2 and a decreased proportion of REM sleep; however, minimal data exist. Treatment of acute CF exacerbations results in an increased amount of REM sleep, improvement in sleep quality, and sleep-related SaO_2. Poor sleep quality can impact inflammation and host defenses. Predicting SDB in patients with CF has been examined by multiple investigators, including Milross and colleagues *(46)* and Frangolia and colleagues *(47)*. Evening PaO_2 and morning $PaCO_2$ were the most predictive of sleep-related events. Patients with an awake-resting SaO_2 less than 93% desaturated during sleep, but who also had SaO_2 more than 93% and an FEV_1 of more than 65% predicted, very rarely had oxygen desaturation during sleep. These findings may be helpful to clinicians.

Milross and colleagues *(44)* recommend identifying patients with CF and SDB and sleep-related hypoxemia by using the following criteria:

1. A resting daytime SaO_2 of less than 94% and an FEV_1 of less than 65% predicted.
2. The presence of polycythemia or cor pulmonale.
3. Headache upon awakening or excessive daytime sleepiness or sleep disruption.

Consider measuring sleep-time SaO_2 and, in selected patients, arterial blood gases in the evening before sleep onset and upon awakening. Management of SDB and sleep-related hypoxemia in patients with CF is very similar to patients with severe COPD. Nocturnal oxygen can be prescribed. Monitor sleep time SaO_2, and if possible, measure arterial blood gas upon awakening to identify hypercapnia. NIPPV can be used with the onset of respiratory failure; however, after respiratory failure is well-established, there are minimal data available for this recommendation *(45)*. Many times, these patients with CF are being evaluated for lung transplantation. Hopefully, future research will further delineate NIPPV use in patients with CF.

NOCTURNAL ASTHMA

Lung function has a circadian rhythm in normal individuals, displaying optimal function at 4 PM and the lowest function at 4 AM, with a peak to trough variation of approx 5–8%. Asthmatics can have marked variation in pulmonary function throughout the 24-hour period, where peak to trough variation may be as high as 50% *(48)*. Asthma affects approx 15 million people in the United States, and nocturnal asthma symptoms are often overlooked by patients and their physicians. There is a correlation between nocturnal asthma symptom frequency, asthma severity, and the number of asthma medications utilized. Patients may complain of nocturnal wheezing, cough, and dyspnea. Nocturnal asthmatics have at least a 10% drop in PEF rates during the nocturnal period.

The epidemiology of nocturnal asthma has been evaluated by Turner-Warwick *(49)*. She examined 7729 asthmatics from the United Kingdom and found that approx 40% of asthmatics had nocturnal awakenings every night, and that 94% of asthmatics had awakenings at least once a month. There is a debate as to whether these asthmatics with nocturnal symptoms represent a different asthma phenotype or whether these asthmatics have inadequate asthma management or more severe asthma *(50)*. Since this landmark study, longer-acting asthma medications are available for use that help control nocturnal asthma symptoms and improve pulmonary function.

Chronobiology of Nocturnal Asthma

Chronobiology of nocturnal asthma is important to understand. Peak asthma symptoms occur at approx 4 AM, peak airflow obstruction occurs between 3 and 4 AM, and 40% of physician calls for asthma are between the hours of 12 and 8 AM *(51)*. Most emergency department visits for asthma occur between 12 and 8 AM, and most asthma deaths occur between 12 and 8 AM *(52)*. There are alterations in bronchial reactivity, airway inflammation, parasympathetic tone, and hormones around the 24-hour clock that promote airflow obstruction during the night. Furthermore, allergens, airway cooling, airway secretions, decreased mucociliary clearance during sleep, and nonadrenergic, noncholinergic neuronal pathways may also impact night time airway function. The pathophysiology and chronobiology of nocturnal asthma is complex and multifactorial *(48)*.

There is a heightened bronchial reactivity during the night time hours, evidenced by inhalation provocation challenges utilizing histamine, methacholine, propranolol, saline, and acetylcholine provocative agents *(53,54)*. Furthermore, airway inflammation is more severe at 4 AM compared with 4 PM. Nocturnal asthmatics have higher total cell counts, leukocytes, eosinophils, lymphocytes, macrophages, and epithelial cells noted from BAL obtained at 4 AM as compared with 4 PM *(55)*. There are also higher levels of histamine, eosinophilic cationic protein, and cellular generation of superoxide noted from BAL obtained at 4 AM compared with 4 PM *(56)*. Furthermore, eosinophilic alveolar inflammation correlates with overnight fall in lung function *(57,58)*. CD_4-positive lymphocytes are thought to be the principle controller cells responsible for eosinophil and lymphocyte recruitment and influx into alveolar tissue *(59)*. These cells are higher in number at 4 AM.

Allergens also play a role. Bedroom dust mites can exacerbate allergic asthma. Allergen exposure during the evening hours results in a more severe and longer late allergic response than allergen exposure during the morning—so there is a circadian-rhythm process involved *(60)*. β_2-Adrenergic-receptor function and gene regulation changes throughout the 24-hour period. At 4 AM, there is about a 33% decrease in leukocyte β_2-adrenergic-receptor density. This is coupled with impairment of the cyclic adenosine monophosphate response to isoproterenol, without significant changes noted in receptor-binding activity *(61)*. This downregulation may be related to gene polymorphism. Glycine at position 16 is associated with an accelerated downregulation of this receptor. Future studies may examine the importance of this polymorphism.

Neurohormonal changes occur throughout the 24-hour period, which has an impact on airway tone and inflammatory mediators *(48,50)*. Bronchoconstrictive mediators, including plasma histamine levels, peak at 4 AM and nadir at 4 PM. Plasma cortisol levels that have an anti-inflammatory action peak at 7 AM and nadir at 12 AM. Furthermore, Sutherland and colleagues *(62)* noted that the adrenal response to corticotropin is reduced in nocturnal asthmatics, which may play a permissive role. There is clear evidence of altered corticosteroid signaling in nocturnal asthma *(63,64)*. Plasma epinephrine and cyclic adenosine monophosphate levels peak at 4 PM and nadir at 4 AM. Plasma leukotriene levels peak at 12 AM. All of these changes result in more intense airway inflammation and bronchoconstriction during the night *(48)*.

There are also alterations in endogenous melatonin secretion in nocturnal asthmatics. Sutherland and colleagues *(65)* measured serum melatonin levels at 2-hour intervals in 11 control subjects, 13 nonnocturnal asthmatics, and 7 nocturnal asthmatics—all of whom kept regular sleep–wake schedules. Nocturnal asthmatics had higher peak melatonin levels and a delayed melatonin acrophase. In the nocturnal asthmatics, there was an association between increasing melatonin levels and the overnight decrease in FEV_1.

Parasympathetic tone increases during the nighttime hours. An exaggerated diurnal heart rate variation and sinus arrhythmia is frequently noted in nocturnal asthmatics *(66)*. Furthermore, inhaled ipratropium and intravenous atropine decrease diurnal PEF variation and improve PEF at 4 AM, so parasympathetic tone and autonomic regulation may be important. Sympathetic tone appears to be less important. Nonadrenergic, noncholinergic function may also impact nocturnal airway tone *(67)*. Airway cooling may play a role in nocturnal asthma. A decrease in core body temperature of 0.7°C has the potential to trigger an asthma attack. During NREM sleep, thermoregulation is intact, but the set point drops by 1°C. Humans are poikilothermic during REM sleep, so core body temperature may further drop. In a small study, warm humidified air was shown to improve lung function in nocturnal asthmatics *(68)*. Airway secretions may also play a role in nocturnal asthma. During sleep, cough reflexes and mucociliary clearance decrease. Martin *(48)* noted more secretions in the airways of nocturnal asthmatics when he performed bronchoscopy at 4 AM compared with 4 PM.

Sleep Effects on Airway Function

Sleep itself may influence airway resistance, as noted by Catterall and colleagues *(69)*. Progressive increases in lower airway resistance occurred during the evening. Sleep enhanced this response by approximately twofold. Staying awake throughout the night decreased the bronchoconstriction, as noted by monitoring morning PEF rates. Specific sleep stages are not associated with an increased rate of asthma attacks, as noted by Kales and colleagues *(70)*. Ballard and colleagues *(71)* measured lung volumes and airway resistance during sleep. Decreases in functional residual capacity noted in the supine position were more pronounced in the asthmatics, especially during REM sleep. These alterations resulted in increases in airflow resistance with maldistribution of ventilation and perfusion and passive airway narrowing.

Irvin and colleagues *(72)* noted that asthmatics had higher than expected increase in airway resistance, more so than predicted with the reduced lung volumes. Furthermore, airway resistance remained high when the lung volumes were normalized. This supported the hypothesis that there is airway parenchymal uncoupling in nocturnal asthma that may be partially related to distal airway inflammation *(56)*. There is evidence of sleep disruption in nocturnal asthmatics. They have multiple arousals, night time asthma attacks, and impairment of daytime functioning, including neurocognitive effects *(73,74)*. Some investigators note a decrease in stage 4 sleep. Sleep is more fragmented. Fortunately, hypoxemia during sleep is rarely severe in nocturnal asthmatics.

Comorbid Disorders and Nocturnal Asthma

OSA can also impact nocturnal asthma. Neuroreceptors in the glottic inlet in the larynx can cause reflex bronchoconstriction activated by snoring or apnea *(75)*. Ciftci and colleagues *(76)* examined if treatment of OSA improved outcomes in asthmatics with OSA. After 2 months of nasal CPAP, the asthma night time symptom score improved significantly; however, pulmonary function (spirometry) was unchanged. Chan and colleagues *(77)* examined the same question and found that nasal CPAP improved night time and daytime asthma symptoms and decreased the use of rescue bronchodilators. Furthermore, they noted an improvement in morning and evening PEF rates. They concluded that CPAP decreases vagal tone and stabilizes nocturnal SaO_2. Furthermore, obliteration of OSA eliminates upper airway irritation and reflexes bronchoconstriction. Martin and colleagues *(78)* noted that CPAP use in nocturnal asthmatics without OSA *did not* improve nocturnal asthma symptoms and in fact, noted that CPAP *worsened* sleep architecture, increased awake time, and decreased REM sleep percentage.

Gastroesophageal reflux (GER) may impact nocturnal asthma *(79)*. Up to 50% of asthmatics have nocturnal heartburn. Twenty percent of asthmatics awaken from sleep with heartburn, and 81% of asthmatics with reflux have abnormal esophageal acid contact times during reported sleep times *(80)*. Furthermore, esophageal acid provokes airway responses during sleep. Hydrochloric acid infused during sleep and spontaneous acid GER events increased airway resistance in asthmatics *(81–83)*. Antireflux therapy improves night time symptoms and morning PEF rates *(84)*.

Strategies to Put Nocturnal Asthma at Rest

There is some debate whether nocturnal asthma is a separate asthma phenotype or whether nocturnal asthma symptoms are just a marker of inadequate asthma treatment *(50)*. Treat asthma according to the National Institutes of Health (NIH) guidelines *(85)*. Monitor asthma medication compliance and rescue use of inhaled β-agonists. Ask about nocturnal asthma awakenings and night time bronchodilator use. Furthermore, monitor morning and evening PEF rates, and note whether a drop of 10% or more is present between morning and evening PEF rates. Other strategies that can put nocturnal asthma to rest are as follows:

1. Screen for OSA and GER, and treat them if present—remember that GER may be clinically silent *(86)*.
2. Screen for allergic rhinitis and sinusitis because these disease processes may worsen asthma.
3. Recommend weight loss if the patient is obese. For instance, Hakala and colleagues *(87)* noted that weight loss in nocturnal asthmatics improved diurnal and day-to-day PEF rates, FEV_1, and airway resistance.

Other strategies include environmental control of potential allergens in the bedroom and beyond. Think about dust mites. Recommend that the bedroom be free of carpet. Add mattress and pillow covers to control dust mites, and keep cats and other animals out of the bedroom. Immune desensitization can be helpful in specific instances. Assess asthma severity and the need for controller agents, particularly inhaled corticosteroids (ICS).

If nocturnal asthma is still present after using these management strategies, then add chronotherapeutic principles into your treatment plan. Consider the use of long-acting β-agonists (LABAs), ICS, leukotriene-modifying agents, oral corticosteroids, sustained release theophylline, and/or oral β-agonists. Incorporate these medications, as recommended by the NIH guidelines. Chronotherapeutic principles ensure that adequate drug levels are present during the time when symptoms are most severe *(48)*. Sometimes drug formulation and/or dose timing can have a major impact.

Inhaled LABAs, including salmeterol, have a duration of action of approx 12 hours, with peak effects within 2–3 hours. In a double-blind, randomized, placebo-controlled, crossover trial, Fitzpatrick and colleagues examined the effects of 50 or 100 μg of salmeterol given twice daily in 20 nocturnal asthmatics *(88)*. A 50-μg dose, given twice daily, improved PEF rate (by 69 L/minute) and sleep quality. The 100-μg dose given twice daily caused disruption of sleep architecture with lower amounts of stage 4 sleep noted; however, both dosages decreased the number of nocturnal asthma awakenings. Another study by Lockey and colleagues *(89)* examined 474 nocturnal asthmatics in a randomized, double-blind, placebo-controlled trial and noted that 12 weeks of salmeterol improved asthma quality of life, FEV_1, PEF rates increased the number of symptom-free days and nights, and decreased albuterol rescue therapy. Kraft and colleagues *(90)* noted in a double-blind, placebo-controlled trial in nocturnal asthmatics that inhaled salmeterol decreased nocturnal awakenings and albuterol rescue therapy use. There was no change in airway hyperresponsiveness or distal lung inflammation. Inhaled LABAs should be considered in asthmatics with nocturnal symptoms.

Oral, pulse-released, β_2-adrenergic agonists can also be useful. Martin and colleagues *(91)* noted that oral, pulse-released, β_2-adrenergic agonists are less expensive than inhaled LABAs and are not used as frequently as LABAs. Oral sustained release albuterol (4 mg in the morning and 8 mg in the evening) or inhaled salmeterol had equivalent improvements in PEF rate and in FEV_1. Furthermore, Bogin and colleagues *(92)* noticed no difference in sleep latency, total sleep time, arousals, REM, and sleep stage 4 percentages, comparing with 8 mg of oral albuterol to placebo. Oral, pulse-released albuterol may be an alternative to inhaled LABAs, especially in patients who cannot afford LABAs.

ICS are a key asthma controller medication. If shorter-acting ICS are used, a single dose at 3 PM produces optimal night time asthma control, as noted by Pincus and colleagues *(93)*. ICS may also be useful. Weerskink and colleagues *(94)* compared fluticasone with inhaled LABA in a trial. Salmeterol 50 μg bid or fluticasone 250 μg bid had similar efficacy in asthma outcomes. If LABAs and ICS do not improve nocturnal asthma, then the addition of oral corticosteroids may be considered. Beam and colleagues *(95)* examined the optimal dosing schedule of prednisone in nocturnal asthmatics. They examined the effectiveness of dosing prednisone at 3 PM, compared with 8 AM or 8 PM, and noted that only the 3 PM dose improved FEV_1 and 4 AM BAL inflammatory cell counts. Furthermore, there was no increase in adrenal suppression noted with the 3 PM dose, compared with the morning dose. If corticosteroids are given to treat nocturnal asthma, the optimum dosing time appears to be 3 PM.

Leukotriene modifiers may also be useful *(96,97)*. Bjermen and colleagues *(98)* compared 10 mg montelukast at bedtime vs 50 μg salmeterol bid in asthmatics with uncontrolled asthma symptoms while taking fluticasone 100 μg bid. Both montelukast and salmeterol improved nocturnal awakenings similarly in this 52-week study. Theophylline in the controlled-release form can also be useful. It allows for consistent levels over a 24-hour period. Controlled-release theophylline, given at approx 6–7 PM, decreased the late phase allergic reaction and lung parenchymal neutrophil influx *(99)*. There are conflicting data regarding the theophylline effect on sleep architecture. Selby and colleagues *(100)* compared theophylline with salmeterol in nocturnal asthmatics in a crossover design. Theophylline and salmeterol had similar effects on PEF rates and psychometric variables. Salmeterol therapy resulted in improved quality of life measures and lowered the number of arousals and awakenings, compared with theophylline.

Anticholinergics also have the potential to improve asthma; however, there are no data examining this *(101)*. Tiotropium, a long-acting anticholinergic agent, is not FDA-approved for asthma treatment. Hopefully future studies will examine this possibility. In conclusion, nocturnal-asthma management strategies include examining for adequate asthma control, utilizing the NIH guidelines, and including asthma controller medications. If these strategies do not improve nocturnal asthma, then rule out the possibility of comorbid diseases, including OSA, GER, sinusitis, and allergic rhinitis. Also, control allergens. Dose medications by utilizing chronotherapeutic principles. For example, upon awakening, consider dosing with a LABA and long-acting inhaled corticosteroid; at 3 PM, consider dosing oral corticosteroids if required; at 6–7 PM, consider dosing slow-release theophylline and slow-release oral albuterol (if used instead of LABA); at bedtime, dose LABA, long-acting ICS, and leukotriene modifiers *(102)*. Not all medications will be required in most patients. Hopefully, with current therapeutic agents, nocturnal asthma can be controlled.

INTERSTITIAL LUNG DISEASE

There are more than 100 disorders of the pulmonary parenchyma, classified as interstitial lung diseases (ILDs). These diseases are characterized by alterations in the lung parenchyma with cellular infiltrates that often lead to fibrosis. There is a reduction in lung compliance, so the lung becomes stiffer with increased recoil, and lung volumes are reduced. Patients with ILD have a rapid, shallow breathing pattern, a dry cough, and dyspnea. Their level of ventilation is higher than their CO_2 production, so hypercapnia is often not present until the end-stages of the disease, when respiratory failure develops. These patients have a very high drive to breathe.

SLEEP IN PATIENTS WITH ILD

Sleep disruption can occur in patients with ILD. Patients have decreased sleep efficiency, increased numbers of arousals, and increased proportions of stage 1 sleep. There is a minor decrease in respiratory rate with sleep onset; however, their respiratory rate often remains rapid. They may have oxygen desaturation during sleep *(103)*. Patients with an SaO_2 of less than 90% during sleep have more disrupted sleep, compared with individuals with an SaO_2 of more than 90% during sleep. Patients with oxygen desaturation also complain of fatigue and excessive daytime sleepiness. As noted, patients with ILD have the potential for oxygen desaturation during sleep. Perez-Padilla and colleagues *(104)* noted three potential patterns of sleep-related oxygen desaturation:

1. Oxygen desaturation occurring primarily during REM sleep related to hypoventilation, which is the most common form.
2. Another pattern of oxygen desaturation is a sustained decrease during REM and NREM sleep.
3. The third pattern is oxygen desaturation associated with snoring or obstructive apneic events.

The presence of sleep-related oxygen desaturation in patients with ILD is related to the patient's wake-time PaO_2, age, and lung compliance. Predicted oxygen saturation is equal to (75.023) (PaO_2) – 0.2 × age. Oxygenation during sleep can be monitored with nocturnal pulse oximetry *(103,105)*. There is no need for nocturnal polysomnography unless another primary sleep disorder such as OSA, is suspected.

Turner and colleagues *(106)* noted that 17% of patients with sarcoidosis had OSA, compared with 3% of the control group. The authors also noted a higher rate of OSA in male patients with sarcoidosis and in those with lupus pernio skin findings. Although this study examined patients with sarcoidosis, screen for OSA in all patients with ILD.

SLEEP MANAGEMENT IN PATIENTS WITH ILD

Medications utilized for treatment of certain ILDs, including corticosteroids and interferon$_1$-β, may disrupt sleep. Interferon$_1$-β causes chills, fever, and flu-like symptoms. Perform nocturnal pulse oximetry to determine whether sleep-related oxygen desaturation is present, and screen for OSA. Consider oxygen therapy if the wake time PaO_2 is less than 55 mmHg, or less than 60 mmHg if peripheral edema or polycythemia is present or if prolonged oxygen desaturation during sleep is present. Monitor wake time arterial blood gas to observe if daytime hypoxia or hypercarbia are present *(103,104,107)*.

Unfortunately, there is no treatment that slows the progression of idiopathic pulmonary fibrosis. These patients develop progressive respiratory failure. NIPPV can be considered for patients with end-stage ILD and chronic respiratory failure. Patients have severe dyspnea with a high respiratory drive and rate, with increased work of breathing. Bilateral positive airway pressure can be beneficial. When setting up bilateral positive airway pressure, set a rapid respiratory rate as well as high-flow rates, small tidal volumes, with short inspiratory and expiratory times *(107)*. Often, a low respiratory sensitivity trigger setting is required. Examine delivered tidal volumes and titrate supplemental oxygen, as required to maintain adequate oxygenation. There is minimal data examining if NIPPV improves outcomes in chronic respiratory failure in patients with ILD *(108)*.

REFERENCES

1. McNicolas WT (1997) Impact of sleep in respiratory failure. Eur Respir J 10:920–933.
2. Phillipson EA (1978) Control of breathing during sleep. Am Rev Respir Dis 118:909–939.
3. Douglas NJ (1985) Control of ventilation during sleep. Clin Chest Med 6:563–575.
4. Krieger J (1985) Breathing during sleep in normal subjects. Clin Chest Med 6:577–594.
5. Tabachnik E, Muller NL, Bryan AC, et al. (1981) Changes in ventilation and chest wall mechanics during sleep in normal adolescents. J Appl Physiol 51:557–564.
6. Douglas NJ (1984) Control of breathing during sleep. Clin Sci 67:465–472.

7. Hudgel DW, Hendricks C (1988) Palate and hypopharynx sites of inspiratory narrowing of the upper airway during sleep. Am Rev Respir Dis 138:1542–1547.
8. Yap JC, Watson RA, Gilbey S, et al. (1995) Effects of posture on respiratory mechanics in obesity. J Appl Physiol 79:1199–1205.
9. Lopes JM, Tabachnik E, Muller NL, et al. (1983) Total airway resistance and respiratory muscle activity during sleep. J Appl Physiol 54:773–777.
10. Douglas NJ, White DP, Weil JV, et al. (1982) Hypoxic ventilatory response decreases during sleep in normal men. Am Rev Respir Dis 125:286–289.
11. Douglas NJ, White DP, Weil JV, et al. (1982) Hypercapnic ventilatory response in sleeping adults. Am Rev Respir Dis 126:758–762.
12. Hedemark LL, Kronenberg RS (1982) Ventilatory and heart rate responses to hypoxemia and hypercapnia during sleep in adults. J Appl Physiol 53:307–312.
13. Issa FG, Sullivan CE (1983) Arousal and breathing responses to airway occlusion in healthy sleeping adults. J Appl Physiol 55:1113–1119.
14. Mohsenin V (2005) Sleep in chronic obstructive pulmonary disease. Semin Respir Crit Care Med 26:109–116.
15. Celli BR, MacNee W (2004) American Thoracic Society/European Respiratory Society Task Force. Standards for the diagnosis and management of patients with COPD: a summary of the ATS/ERS position paper. Eur Respir J 23:932–946.
16. Mannino DM, Homa DM, Akinbami LJ, et al. (2002) Chronic obstructive pulmonary disease surveillance: United States 1971-2000. MMWR 51:1–16.
17. O'Donoghue FJ, Catcheside PG, Ellis EE, et al. (2003) Sleep hypoventilation in hypercapnic chronic obstructive pulmonary disease: prevalence and associated factors. Eur Respir J 21:977–984.
18. O'Donoghue FJ, Catcheside PG, Eckert DJ, et al. (2004) Changes in respiration in NREM sleep in hypercapnic chronic obstructive pulmonary disease. J Physiol 599:663–673.
19. Weitzenblum E, Chaouat A (2004) Sleep and chronic obstructive pulmonary disease. Sleep Med Rev 8:281–294.
20. Aoki T, Ebihara A, Yogo Y, et al. (2005) Sleep-disordered breathing in patients with chronic obstructive pulmonary disease. COPD: J Chronic Obstructive Pulmonary Dis 2:243–252.
21. Demarco FJ Jr, Wynne JS, Block AJ, et al. (1981) Oxygen desaturation during sleep as a determinant of the "blue and bloated" syndrome. Chest 79:621–625.
22. Sanders MH, Newman AB, Haggerty CL, et al. (2003) Sleep Heart Health Study: sleep and sleep-disordered breathing in adults with predominantly mild obstructive airway disease. Am J Respir Crit Care Med 67:7–14.
23. Bellia V, Catalano F, Scichilone N, et al. (2003) Sleep disorders in the elderly with and without chronic airflow obstruction: the SARA study. Sleep 26:318–323.
24. Fleetham J, West P, Mezon B, et al. (1982) Sleep, arousals, and oxygen desaturation in chronic obstructive pulmonary disease: the effect of oxygen therapy. Am J Respir Dis 126:429–433.
25. Saaresranta T, Irjala K, Aittokallio T, et al. (2005) Sleep quality daytime sleepiness and fasting insulin levels in women with chronic obstructive pulmonary disease. Respir Med 99:856–863.
26. Coccagna G, Lugaresi E (1978) Arterial blood gases and pulmonary and systemic arterial pressure during sleep in chronic obstructive pulmonary disease. Sleep 1:117–124.
27. Chaouat A,Weitzenblum E, Kessler R, et al. (1997) Sleep-related O_2 desaturation and daytime pulmonary haemodynamics in COPD patients with mild hypoxaemia. Eur Resp J 10:1730–1735.
28. Chaouat A, Weitzenblum E, Krieger J, et al. (1995) Association of chronic obstructive pulmonary disease and sleep apnea syndrome. Am J Respir Crit Care Med 151:82–86.
29. Bradley TD, Rutherford R, Grossman RF, et al. (1985) Role of daytime hypoxemia in the pathogenesis of right heart failure in the obstructive sleep apnea syndrome. Am Rev Respir Dis 131:835–839.
30. Fletcher EC, Luckett RA, Goodnight-White S, et al. (1992) A double-blind trial of nocturnal supplemental oxygen for sleep desaturation in patients with chronic obstructive pulmonary disease and a daytime Pao_2 above 60 mm Hg. Am Rev Respir Dis 145:1070–1076.
31. Connaughton JJ, Catterall JR, Elton RA, et al. (1988) Do sleep studies contribute to the management of patients with severe chronic obstructive pulmonary disease? Am Rev Respir Dis 138:341–344.
32. Douglas NJ, Flenley DC (1990) Breathing during sleep in patients with obstructive lung disease. Am Rev Respir Dis 141:1055–1570.
33. George CF, Bayliff CD (2003) Management of insomnia in patients with chronic obstructive pulmonary disease. Drugs 63:379–387.

34. Dolly FR, Block AJ (1983) Medroxyprogesterone acetate and COPD: effect on breathing and oxygenation in sleeping and awake patients. Chest 84:394–398.
35. Saaresvanta T, Aittokallio T, Utriainen K, et al. (2005) Medroxyprogesterone improves nocturnal breathing in postmenopausal women with chronic obstructive pulmonary disease. Respir Res 6:28.
36. McNicholas WT, Calverley PM, Lee A, et al. (2004) Long-acting inhaled anticholinergic therapy improves sleeping oxygen saturation in COPD. Eur Respir J 23:825–831.
37. Gay PC (2004) Chronic obstructive pulmonary disease. Sleep Respir Care 49:39–51.
38. Hill NS (2004) Noninvasive ventilation for chronic obstructive pulmonary disease. Respir Care 49:72–87.
39. Wijkstra PJ, Avendano MA, Goldstein RS (2003) Inpatient chronic assisted ventilatory care: a 15-year experience. Chest 124:850–856.
40. Clinical indications for noninvasive positive pressure ventilation in chronic respiratory failure due to restrictive lung disease, COPD, and nocturnal hypoventilation: a consensus conference report. (1999) Chest 116:521–534.
41. www.cms.hhs.gov/manuals/pm_trans/R1744233.pdf. Accessed Oct. 2006.
42. Ramsey BW (1996) Management of pulmonary disease in patients with cystic fibrosis. N Engl J Med 335:179–180.
43. Jankelowitz L, Reid KJ, Wolfe L, et al. (2005) Cystic fibrosis patients have poor sleep quality despite normal sleep latency and efficiency. Chest 127:1593–1599.
44. Milross MA, Piper AJ, Dobbin CJ, et al. (2004) Sleep-disordered breathing in cystic fibrosis. Sleep Med Rev 8:295–308.
45. Milross MA, Piper AJ, Norman M, et al. (2001) Low-flow oxygenated bilevel ventilatory support: effects on ventilation during sleep in cystic fibrosis. Am J Respir Crit Care Med 163:129–134.
46. Milross MA, Piper AJ, Norman M, et al. (2001) Predicting sleep-disordered breathing in patients with cystic fibrosis. Chest 120:1239–1248.
47. Frangolias MA, Wilcox PG (2001) Predictability of oxygen desaturation during sleep in patients with cystic fibrosis: clinical, spirometric, and exercise parameters. Chest 119:434–441.
48. Martin RJ (1992) Nocturnal asthma. Clin Chest Med 13:533–550.
49. Turner-Warwick M (1988) Epidemiology of nocturnal asthma. Am J Med 85(Suppl 118):6–8.
50. Calhoun WJ (2003) Nocturnal asthma. Chest 123:399S–405S.
51. Turner-Warwick M (1977) On observing patterns of airflow obstruction in chronic asthma. Br J Dis Chest 71:73–86.
52. Douglas NJ (1985) Asthma at night. Clin Chest Med 6:663–674.
53. Ryan G, Latimer KM, Dolovich J, et al. (1982) Bronchial responsiveness to histamine: relationship to diurnal variation of peak flow rate, improvement after bronchodilator, and airway caliber. Thorax 37:423–429.
54. Martin RJ, Cicutto LC, Ballard RD (1990) Factors related to the nocturnal worsening of asthma. Am Rev Respir Dis 141:33–38.
55. Sutherland ER, Martin RJ, Bowler RP, et al. (2004) Physiologic correlates of distal lung inflammation in asthma. J Allergy Clin Immunol 113:1046–1050.
56. Kraft M, Djukanovic R, Wilson S, et al. (1996) Alveolar tissue inflammation in asthma. Am J Respir Crit Care Med 154:1505–1509.
57. Kraft M, Martin RJ, Wilson S, et al. (1999) Lymphocyte and eosinophil influx into alveolar tissue in nocturnal asthma. Am J Respir Crit Care Med 129:228–234.
58. Kraft M, Pak J, Martin RJ (2001) Distal lung dysfunction at night in nocturnal asthma. Am J Respir Crit Care Med 163:1551–1556.
59. Kraft M, Striz I, Georges G, et al. (1998) Expression of epithelial markers in nocturnal asthma. J Allergy Clin Immunol 102:376–381.
60. Platts-Mills TAE, Mitchell BB, Nock P, et al. (1982) Reduction of bronchial reactivity during prolonged allergen avoidance. Lancet 2:675–677.
61. Turki J, Pak J, Green SA, et al. (1995) Genetic polymorphisms of the beta 2-adrenergic receptor in nocturnal and non-nocturnal asthma: evidence that the Gly-16 correlates with the nocturnal phenotype. J Clin Invest 95:1635–1641.
62. Sutherland ER, Kraft M, Rex MD, et al. (2003) Hypothalamic pituitary-adrenal axis dysfunction during sleep in nocturnal asthma. Chest 123:405S.
63. Sutherland ER, Ellison MC, Kraft M, et al. (2003) Altered pituitary adrenal interaction in nocturnal asthma. J Allergy Clin Immunol 112:52–57.

64. Kraft M, Vianna E , Martin RJ, et al. (1999) Nocturnal asthma is associated with reduced glucocorticoid receptor binding affinity. J Allergy Clin Immunol 103:66–71.
65. Sutherland ER, Ellison MC, Kraft M, et al. (2003) Elevated serum melatonin is associated with the nocturnal worsening of asthma. J Allergy Clin Immunol 112:513–517.
66. Morrison JF, Pearson SB, Dean HG (1988) Parasympathetic nervous system in nocturnal asthma. BMJ 296:1427–1429.
67. Mackay TW, Hulks G, Douglas NJ (1998) Non-adrenergic, non-cholinergic function in the human airway. Respir Med 92:461–466.
68. Chen WY, Chai H (1982) Airway cooling and nocturnal asthma. Chest 81:675–680.
69. Catterall JR, Rhind GB, Stewart IC, et al. (1986) Effects of sleep deprivation on overnight bronchoconstriction in nocturnal asthma. Thorax 41:676–680.
70. Kales A, Beall GN, Bajor GF, et al. (1968) Sleep studies in asthmatic adults: relationship of attacks to sleep stage and time of night. J Allergy 41:164–173.
71. Ballard RD, Irvin CG, Martin RJ, et al. (1990) Influences of sleep on lung volume in asthmatic patients and normal subjects. J Appl Physiol 68:2034–2041.
72. Irvin CG, Pak J, Martin RJ (2000) Nocturnal asthma. Airway-parenchyma uncoupling in nocturnal asthma. Am J Respir Crit Care Med 161:50–56.
73. Fitzpatrick MF, Engleman H, Whyte KF, et al. (1991) Morbidity in nocturnal asthma: sleep quality and daytime cognitive performance. Thorax 46:569–657.
74. Weersink EJ, van Zomren EH, Köeter GH, et al. (1997) Treatment of nocturnal airway obstruction improves daytime cognitive performance in asthmatics. Am J Respir Crit Care Med 156:1144–1150.
75. Qureshi A, Ballard RD (2003) Obstructive sleep apnea. J Allergy Clin Immunol 112:613–651.
76. Ciftci TV, Ciftci B, Guren SF, et al. (2005) Effect of nasal continuous positive airway pressure in uncontrolled nocturnal asthmatic treatment with obstructive sleep apnea studies. Respir Med 99:529–534.
77. Chan CS, Woolcock AJ, Sullivan CE (1988) Nocturnal asthma: role of snoring and obstructive sleep apnea. Am Rev Respir Dis 137:1502–1504.
78. Martin RJ, Pak J (1991) Nasal CPAP in non-apneic nocturnal asthma. Chest 100:1024–1027.
79. Harding SM (1999) Nocturnal asthma: role of nocturnal gastroesophageal reflux. Chronobiol Intl 16:641–662.
80. Harding SM (1999) Gastroesophageal reflux and asthma: insight into the association. J Allergy Clin Immunol 105:251–259.
81. Davis RS, Larsen GL, Grunstein MM (1983) Respiratory response to intraesophageal acid infusion in asthmatic children during sleep. J Allergy Clin Immunol 72:393–399.
82. Martin ME, Grunstein MM, Larsen GL (1982) The relationship of gastroesophageal reflux to nocturnal wheezing in children with asthma. Ann Allergy 49:318–322.
83. Cuttita G, Cibella F, Visconti A, et al. (2000) Spontaneous gastroesophageal reflux and airway patency during the night in adult asthmatics. Am J Respir Crit Care Med 161:177–181.
84. Harding SM, Richter JE, Guzzo MR, et al. (1996) Asthma and gastroesophageal reflux: acid suppressive therapy improves asthma outcome. Am J Med 100:395–405.
85. National Institutes of Health. National asthma education and prevention program expert panel report 2: guidelines for the diagnosis and management of asthma. 1997; publication No 97-4051A, 1-80. Available at: www.nhlbi.nih.gov/guidelines/asthma/asthgdln.pdf. Accessed Oct. 2006.
86. Harding SM, Guzzo MR, Richter JE (2000) The prevalence of gastroesophageal reflux in asthma patients without reflux symptoms. Am J Respir Crit Care Med 162:34–39.
87. Hakala K, Stenius-Aanius-Aarnislaee B, Sovigarvi A (2000) Effects of weight loss on peak flow variability, airways obstruction, and lung volumes in obese patients with asthma. Chest 118:1315–1321.
88. Fitzpatrick MF, Mackay T, Driver H, et al. (1990) Salmeterol in nocturnal asthma: a double-blind, placebo-controlled trial of a long-acting inhaled beta-2 agonist. BMJ 301:1365–1368.
89. Lockey RF, DuBuske LM, Friedman B, et al. (1999) Nocturnal asthma: effect of salmeterol on quality of life and clinical outcomes. Chest 115:666–673.
90. Kraft M, Wenzel SE, Bettinger GM, et al. (1997) The effect of salmeterol on nocturnal symptoms, airway function, and inflammation in asthma. Chest 111:1249–1254.
91. Martin RJ, Kraft M, Beaucher WN, et al. (1999) A comparative study of extended release albuterol sulfate and long-acting inhaled salmeterol xinafoate in the treatment of nocturnal asthma. Ann Allergy Asthma Immunol 83:121–126.
92. Bogin RM, Ballard RD (1992) Treatment of nocturnal asthma with pulse-release albuterol. Chest 102:362–366.

93. Pincus PJ, Szefler SJ, Ackerson CM, et al. (1995) Chronotherapy of asthma with inhaled steroids: the effect of dosage timing on drug efficacy. J Allergy Clin Immunol 95:1172–1178.
94. Weersink EJ, Douma RR, Postma DS, et al. (1997) Flulticasone propionate, salmeterol xinafoate, and their combination in the treatment of nocturnal asthma. Am J Respir Crit Care Med 155: 1241–1246.
95. Beam RW, Weiner DE, Martin RJ, et al. (1992) Timing of prednisone and alterations of airways inflammation in nocturnal asthma. Am Rev Respir Dis 146:1524–1530.
96. Reiss TF, Chervinsky P, Dockhorn RJ, et al. (1998) Montelukast, a once-daily leukotriene receptor antagonist, in the treatment of chronic asthma: a multicenter, randomized, double-blind trial. Arch Intern Med 158:1213–1230.
97. Ilowite J, Webb R, Friedman B, et al. (2004) Addition of montelukast or salmeterol to fluticasone for protection against asthma attacks: a randomized, double-blind, multicenter study. Ann Allergy Asthma Immunol 92:641–648.
98. Bjermen L, Bisgaaard H, Bousquet J, et al. (2003) Montelukast and fluticasone compared with salmeterol and fluticasone in protecting against asthma exacerbation in adults: one year, double blind, randomized comparative trial. BMJ 327:871–897.
99. Kraft M, Torvik JA, Trudeau JB, et al. (1996) Theophylline: potential anti-inflammatory effects in nocturnal asthma. J Allergy Clin Immunol 97:1242–1246.
100. Selby C, Engleman HM, Fitzpatrick MF, et al. (1997) Inhaled salmeterol or oral theophylline in nocturnal asthma? Am J Respir Crit Care Med 155:104–108.
101. Westby M, Benson M, Gibson P (2004) Anticholinergic agents for chronic asthma in adults. Cochrane Database Syst Rev 3:CD.
102. Skloot GS (2002) Nocturnal asthma: mechanisms and management. Mt Sinai J Med 69:140–147.
103. McNicholas WT, Coffey M, Fitzgerald MX (1986) Ventilation and gas exchange during sleep in patients with interstitial lung disease. Thorax 41:777–782.
104. Perez-Padilla R, West P, Lertzman M, et al. (1985) Breathing during sleep in patients with interstitial lung disease Am Rev Respir Dis 132:224–229.
105. Clark M, Cooper B, Singh S, et al. (2001) A survey of nocturnal hypoxaemia and health-related quality of life in patients with cryptogenic fibrosing alveolitis. Thorax 56:482–486.
106. Turner GA, Lower EE, Corser BC, et al. (1997) Sleep apnea in sarcoidosis. Sarcoidosis Vasc Diffuse Lung Dis 14:61–64.
107. Krachman SL, Criner CJ, Chatila W (2003) Cor pulmonale and sleep-disordered breathing in patients with restrictive lung disease and neuromuscular disease. Semin Respir Crit Care Med 24:297–306.
108. González MM, Parreira VF, Rodenstein DO (2002) Non-invasive ventilation and sleep. Sleep Med Revie 6:29–44.

17 Pediatric Sleep I

Normal Sleep and Nonrespiratory Sleep Complaints—Infancy Through Adolescence

David M. Hiestand, MD, PhD

CONTENTS

INTRODUCTION

Sleep in children is a subject of tremendous anxiety for most parents. In fact, there are few issues in early childhood development that stimulate more conversation and debate. The timing and duration of "normal" sleep can be the source of many questions and concerns. Most sleep issues in early childhood are seen and treated by the general pediatrician or primary care doctor.

Sleep concerns change throughout childhood. Early issues relate to poor sleep and fragmentation of sleep. Commonly, caregiver lack of sleep becomes a significant clinical problem because of its impact on mood, behavior, and cognition. As children approach 1 year of age, bedtime resistance and movement disorders become significant concerns. Movement disorders such as head banging and body rocking are quite disconcerting to some parents, occasionally raising concern about possible autism and other developmental abnormalities. In toddlerhood, bedtime resistance persists and some children develop nonrapid eye movement (NREM) sleep parasomnias. Snoring frequently begins in toddlerhood and extends into the preschool years. As children reach early school years, nocturnal enuresis may become a focal issue. In adolescence, poor sleep hygiene becomes prevalent, leading to excessive daytime sleepiness. Sleep phase delay also occurs during this time, leading to excessive daytime sleepiness when schedules prevent later morning rising times.

In 2002, the American Academy of Pediatrics published guidelines related to pediatric sleep-disordered breathing *(1)*. These guidelines have not only led to heightened

From: *Current Clinical Practice: Primary Care Sleep Medicine: A Practical Guide*
Edited by: J. F. Pagel and S. R. Pandi-Perumal © Humana Press Inc., Totowa, NJ

awareness of sleep-disordered breathing, but also stimulated discussion about general sleep concerns, increasing referrals to sleep specialists. The majority of sleep specialists, however, have little pediatric training. Of approx 3000 individuals certified in sleep medicine by The American Board of Sleep Medicine, only about 100 have post-graduate pediatric training.

Nonrespiratory sleep disorders are fairly common in children. Night wakings can affect 50% of children in early childhood. Nocturnal parasamonias affect up to 5% throughout childhood. Insufficient sleep may affect one-third of children, and prevalence appears to be increasing. Delayed sleep phase may affect 10% of adolescents. Restless legs syndrome (RLS) and periodic leg movements (PLMs) appear to have a prevalence similar to that in adults (up to 15%). Narcolepsy affects 1 in 2000 and symptoms can often develop during late childhood and adolescence. Sleep specialists, therefore, need focused training on common sleep problems of childhood and on the pediatric presentation of those disorders also seen in adults.

NORMAL SLEEP STRUCTURE AND TIME ACROSS CHILDHOOD

One of the challenges in pediatric sleep medicine is the significant change in sleep architecture that occurs through early childhood. Although changes occur across the entire life-span, the most significant changes occur within the first few years. Total sleep time (TST) gradually decreases throughout childhood. The normal newborn sleeps 16–20 hours per day. Sleep generally occurs in 1–4-hour periods, followed by 1–2-hour wake periods. There is little distinction between day and night time sleep. Classic electroencephalography patterns are not present in the first months of life, and sleep staging is divided into active sleep (the forerunner to rapid eye movement [REM] sleep) and quiet sleep (the forerunner to NREM sleep). In the first few months of life, the amount of active and passive sleep is divided approximately equally and sleep is entered through the active stage. By 3–6 months of age, NREM stages 1–4 can be identified, and sleep is entered through one of these stages. The proportion of REM sleep begins to decline around 3 months of age.

Throughout the first 12 months of life, TST decreases to about 14 hours per day. Sleep consolidation into a 6- to 8-hour nighttime period occurs in about 75% by age of 9 months and in nearly all children by 12 months. Naps persist about twice a day in 2- to 4-hour blocks. In the toddler years (age 1–3 years), TST decreases to about 12 hours per day. Toddlers continue to take about one nap per day, but the duration of the single nap decreases to 1–3 hours. In the preschool years (age 3–6 years), TST may decrease slightly and generally is 11–12 hours per day. Most children stop taking naps by age 5, corresponding to the age of school attendance.

In middle childhood years (age 6–12 years), children still obtain 10–11 hours of sleep and a regular routine develops as a result of school schedules. Daytime sleepiness is classically considered rare. In adolescent years, sleep requirements continue to be 8–9 hours, but sleep attainment is usually variable and less than desired. Phase delay develops during these years.

NORMAL SLEEP DIFFICULTIES IN YOUNG CHILDREN

In the first 12 months of life, few true sleep problems occur. Parents must adjust to the sleep–wake cycle of the infant; therefore, questions posed to physicians generally regard the fragmentation of sleep. Reassurance that this pattern is normal is appropriate, along with insight into coping mechanisms. This is a time of intense focus on the activities and behaviors of the child, particularly first children. Much attention may be directed toward the sleeping child. Hypnic jerks may be noted and misinterpreted as abnormal behavior. Perhaps the most significant medical concern relates to respiratory patterns in the infant. In all infants, especially premature infants, ventilatory control centers are immature. Apneas can occur in central, obstructive, or mixed form. Mixed apneas are most common in infants. In premature infants, the prevalence of apnea is inversely proportional to gestational age at birth. Premature infants also manifest periodic breathing, cycles of regular breathing with 3- to 10-second pauses. Reassurance regarding periodic breathing is often resisted, particularly if the caregiver has any knowledge about sudden infant death syndrome (SIDS).

The *apparent life-threatening event* is a loosely defined term describing an acute, unexpected respiratory event that was frightening to the observer. It typically includes a combination of apnea, color change, tone change (predominantly limpness), and choking or gagging *(2)*. These episodes are exceptionally disconcerting for the caregiver and require careful evaluation. A comprehensive review of apparent life-threatening events has been recently published *(3)*. Caregivers frequently request home monitoring as a means to identify early events and prevent SIDS. Standards for home monitoring have been published; monitoring should not be routinely prescribed to prevent SIDS, as it has not been proved to do such. It may be warranted in at-risk premature infants and infants with tracheotomy, noninvasive ventilation, and congenital or acquired respiratory disorders *(4)*. The most important intervention that prevents SIDS is placing the infant on the back for sleep. Although this intervention has correlated with a significant decline in the prevalence of SIDS, there is still resistance to this in some cultures.

By age 9–12 months, children have more interaction with caregivers and the ability to sleep through the night. At this point and through the remainder of childhood, behavioral insomnias of childhood may occur. These include difficulty falling asleep, staying asleep, or both in association with a behavioral etiology. The most representative of these is limit-setting disorder. This disorder results from insufficient caregiver limit-setting and results in bedtime noncompliance, resistance, and "curtain calls." The behavioral insomnias can have night waking with associated fearful or resistive behaviors. They must be differentiated from medical or psychiatric illness. Associated night waking episodes must be differentiated from NREM parasomnias and nightmares. The distinguishing feature of the behavioral insomnias is consistency and lack of symptoms in nonroutine environments.

Night wakings are actually the norm in early childhood. They occur in association with the normal sleep cycle, so that brief awakenings occur every 90–120 minutes. The response to this waking, however, is variable. Children who are able to go back to sleep without parental intervention are referred to as *self-soothers*. Children who alert their parents with crying or getting out of bed are referred to as *signalers*. These signalers typically develop the pattern as a result of reinforcement by the caregiver (feeding, other soothing). Self-soothers, on the other hand, have typically been put to bed sleep but awake and tend to develop associations with sleep onset that do not involve interaction with the caregiver. Good sleep hygiene is key in promotion of self-soothing. This typically involves a regular sleep schedule with a consistent bedtime routine and use of transitional objects. Several methods have been used to treat signalers. Positive rewards for sleeping through the night should be used when possible. Either complete or graduated extinction may be utilized when reinforcement is not possible or practical.

Some night wakings are associated with clearly stated fears. This is most common in preschool- and school-aged children. In the preschool age, fears are commonly associated with darkness, monsters, and storms. In the school-aged group, fears center on threats (both physical and psychological) and disasters. A recent study of children aged 4–12 years revealed a prevalence of 73%. Another interesting finding from this study was the discordance of parental perception of both prevalence and content *(5)*. Treatment of night time fears centers on reassurance and development of coping skills. Although night time fears are quite common, it is important to assess the child for anxiety disorders and child abuse, as these have obvious long-term consequences.

PARASOMNIAS

Parasomnias are fairly common in children, and perhaps more common in children than adults. Disorders of arousal (the typical NREM parasomnias) include confusional arousals, sleepwalking, and sleep terrors. Parasomnias associated with REM sleep include REM behavior disorder, sleep paralysis, and nightmare disorder. Finally, another parasomnia nearly exclusive to children is sleep enuresis.

The NREM parasomnias are fairly common in children, occurring sporadically in up to 40%. Recurrent sleepwalking and sleep terrors occur in about 3–4%. These events occur in the first third of the night when slow-wave sleep pressure is the highest. All of the NREM parasomnias involve transition from slow-wave sleep to another stage. These partial arousals occur as a result of inability to shift to a different stage or awaken. Individuals tend to have a genetic predisposition that is stimulated by poor sleep hygiene, sleep deprivation, or psychological factors. Other precipitating factors that can induce partial arousals include sleep-disordered breathing, gastroesophageal reflux, RLS, seizures, and intercurrent illness.

Confusional arousals are seen earliest in childhood and are defined as awakenings with signaling, but without interaction. Reassurance and comforting is not helpful and the child cannot be awakened. Sleepwalking is also seen in early-middle childhood. It is identified by stereotypical behavior that can be appropriate or inappropriate. Sleep terrors can be seen in young children, but are more common in adolescence. Treatment is generally limited to reassurance. When indicated, treatment of underlying causes is usually effective. In individuals at risk of injury to self or others, effective treatment has been delivered with benzodiazepines, tricyclic antidepressants, and selective serotonin reuptake inhibitors *(6)*.

Of the REM-related parasomnias, nightmares are the most common in children. Nightmares are common in children, occurring sporadically in 75%. These events more commonly lead to early morning arousals because of the higher REM pressure in the second half of the night. In younger children who are unable to distinguish fantasy from reality, refusal to go back to sleep may occur. Treatment is typically limited to reassurance. REM behavior disorder and sleep paralysis can also be seen in children, although the prevalence is not well-defined.

Sleep (or nocturnal) enuresis is common in children. It is defined as enuresis in a child meeting the following criteria:

1. A chronological age of at least 5 years with a mental age of 4 years.
2. Two or more incontinent events in a month between age 5 and 6 years; or one or more events after age 6 years.
3. Absence of a physical disorder associated with incontinence such as diabetes, urinary tract infection, or seizure disorder.

Sleep enuresis is *primary* if a child has never had a period of prolonged nocturnal continence and *secondary* if wetting recurs after 1 year of continence. Sleep enuresis is quite common, affecting up to 25% of boys and 15% of girls at age 6. There is a natural regression of the disorder, and prevalence at the age of 12 is 8% in boys and 4% in girls. Enuresis typically occurs in NREM sleep and is uncommon in REM sleep. There is generally a family history of sleep enuresis. Sleep-disordered breathing has been identified as a potential cause of sleep enuresis.

Routine evaluation should include a comprehensive history with an evaluation for emotional or psychological abnormalities. Examination should focus on identification of masses in the abdomen and motor/sensory disturbances that can be associated with spina bifida. Limited testing is needed, although most individuals would recommend urinalysis for assessment of infection, proteinuria, and glucosuria.

Treatment should be directed at underlying disorders first, then at development of skills and behaviors to promote dryness. These include alarms, retention-control training, waking, and responsibility training. Drug treatment does not have long-term effectiveness. Therapy such as tricyclic antidepressants and antidiuretics can be used for short-term management. The most common agents used are imipramine at a dose of 25–75 mg at bedtime and desmopressin acetate (Aventis Pharmaceuticals Inc; Bridgewater, NJ) at a dose of 20–40 μg (1–2 sprays in each nostril).

SLEEP-RELATED MOVEMENT DISORDERS

Head banging and body rocking are very common in late infancy and early toddlerhood. This behavior is seen in about 67% of 9-month-olds, declining to 50% of 18-month-olds, and about 10% of 4-year-olds. It is commonly believed to be a means of soothing in the transition to sleep. There is little need for intervention, as behaviors do not cause harm to the infant. In some instances, the behavior is used for getting attention, and in these circumstances extinction is appropriate.

Bruxism is another movement disorder that can occur in children, though the prevalence is not well-defined. Treatment is usually not indicated, as the disorder is self-limited. In adolescents with dental damage or persistent head or jaw pain, consideration of an oral appliance may be indicated. RLS and PLMs also occur in children. Prevalence is not well-defined, particularly in younger children in whom communication limitations preclude accurate assessment of the historical features. The same essential criteria apply as in adult RLS:

1. Urge to move or unpleasant sensation of the legs.
2. Sensation worse with inactivity.
3. Sensation improved with activity.
4. Sensation occurs predominantly at night.

Commonly, diagnosis requires parental observation of leg movements or associated conditions. Current diagnostic guidelines for definite RLS in children are as follows *(7)*:

1. The child meets all four essential adult criteria and the child relates a description in his or her own words that is consistent with leg discomfort; or
2. The child meets all four essential adult criteria and two of the three following supportive criteria are present:
   a. Sleep disturbance for age.
   b. A biological parent or sibling has definite RLS.

c. The child has a polysomnographically documented periodic limb movements in sleep index of more than 5 per hour of sleep.

Recent studies have correlated RLS or periodic limb movements in sleep with conduct and behavior problems *(8,9)*. PLMs have been correlated and associated with "growing pains" in recent studies. And two recent studies have identified RLS symptoms or PLMs in newly diagnosed, drug-naive patients with attention-deficit/hyperactivity disorder *(10,11)*. Whether RLS is a cause or effect of attention-deficit/ hyperactivity disorder remains to be determined.

EXCESSIVE DAYTIME SLEEPINESS

Excessive daytime sleepiness is generally considered uncommon in early and middle childhood. Its prevalence in adolescence, however, compares with or exceeds the adult prevalence. By far the most common cause of excessive daytime sleepiness is inadequate sleep. Sleep need is on the order of 8–9 hours for most adolescents. Actual sleep time, however, is less than 7 hours for a significant number of adolescents. Frequently cited reasons for restricted sleep are evening activity levels (sports, homework, television viewing, and so on) and early school start times. Delayed sleep phase syndrome is common in children, and may result in daytime sleepiness when school start times lead to reduced total hours of sleep. Insomnia in children is not uncommon, but can only be diagnosed after an appropriate sleep schedule with adequate sleep has been attempted. Other common causes of sleepiness in children include sleep-disordered breathing and RLS. Uncommon causes that must be considered after appropriate sleep time and other secondary causes have been ruled out are narcolepsy, idiopathic hypersomnolence, and Kleine-Levin syndrome.

Although the diagnosis of narcolepsy typically occurs after puberty, at least half of patients report symptoms before the age of 15 years. This disorder should be considered early on in those individuals with a family history of narcolepsy and in those individuals presenting with sleepiness and cataplexy. Standard diagnostic multiple sleep latency criteria apply, although a high index of suspicion must be maintained for those individuals with borderline studies. Treatment can be challenging. Pharmacotherapy is similar to that used in adults; stimulants such as methylphenidate and dextroamphetamine have been used extensively in children. Modafinil has been used in children. Control of sleep hygiene is much more challenging. Children must comply with a strict sleep–wake cycle. Napping can be beneficial, but is seldom done by active adolescents.

Kleine-Levin syndrome is commonly reported as a cause of episodic hypersomnolence. It is associated with other behaviors such as overeating and sexual disinhibition. It is distinguished from narcolepsy and idiopathic hypersomnolence by these features. In summary, sleep medicine in the pediatric population can be challenging because of the dynamic nature of sleep architecture and sleep complaints. A thorough understanding of childhood development helps in categorizing sleep problems. Sleep disorders in children have some similar features to those seen in adults, but the manifestations and relative prevalence of the disorders may be different. Evaluation of the child with sleep problems requires a history from all caregivers as well as the child when possible.

REFERENCES

1. American Academy of Pediatrics (2002) Clinical practice guideline: diagnosis and management of childhood obstructive sleep apnea syndrome. Pediatrics 109:704–712.
2. National Institutes of Health Consensus Development Conference on Infantile Apnea and Home Monitoring, Sept 29 to Oct 1, 1986. (1987) Pediatrics 79:292–299.
3. Dewolfe CC (2005) Apparent life-threatening event: a review. Pediatr Clin North Am 52:1127–1146, ix.
4. American Academy of Pediatrics (2003) Apnea, sudden infant death syndrome, and home monitoring. Pediatrics 111:914–917.
5. Muris P, Merckelbach H, Ollendick TH, et al. (2001) Children's nighttime fears: parent-child ratings of frequency, content, origins, coping behaviors and severity. Behav Res Ther 39:13–28.
6. Remulla A, Guilleminault C (2004) Somnambulism (sleepwalking). Expert Opin Pharmacother 5:2069–2074.
7. American Academy of Sleep Medicine (2005) *The International Classification of Sleep Disorders Diagnostic and Coding Manual, ICSD-2*. 2nd ed. American Academy of Sleep Medicine, Westchester, IL.
8. Chervin RD, Archbold KH, Dillon JE, et al. (2002) Associations between symptoms of inattention, hyperactivity, restless legs, and periodic leg movements. Sleep 25:213–218.
9. Chervin RD, Dillon JE, Archbold KH, et al. (2003) Conduct problems and symptoms of sleep disorders in children. J Am Acad Child Adolesc Psychiatry 42:201–208.
10. Picchietti DL, Underwood DJ, Farris WA, et al. (1999) Further studies on periodic limb movement disorder and restless legs syndrome in children with attention-deficit hyperactivity disorder. Mov Disord 14:1000–1007.
11. Rajaram SS, Walters AS, England SJ, et al. (2004) Some children with growing pains may actually have restless legs syndrome. Sleep 27:767–773.

18 Pediatric Sleep II

Pediatric Sleep-Disordered Breathing

David M. Hiestand, MD, PhD

CONTENTS

INTRODUCTION

Sleep-disordered breathing (SDB) in children encompasses a continuum of upper airway obstruction during sleep. Intermittent snoring represents the mildest form of this disorder and appears to have few significant clinical consequences. Obstructive sleep apnea (OSA), on the other hand, represents the other extreme, with gas exchange abnormalities and sleep disruption. With the American Academy of Pediatrics Clinical Practice Guideline (published in April 2002) *(1)*, the primary care physician gained further awareness of the need to screen for SDB, leading to increased referrals to otolaryngology and sleep specialists. The American Academy of Pediatrics guideline recommends the following:

1. All children should be screened for snoring.
2. Complex, high-risk patients should be referred to a specialist.
3. Patients with cardiorespiratory failure cannot await elective evaluation.
4. Diagnostic evaluation is useful in discriminating between primary snoring (PS) and OSA syndrome; the gold standard is polysomnography (PSG).
5. Adenotonsillectomy is the first line of treatment for most children, and continuous positive airway pressure (CPAP) is an option for those who are not candidates for surgery or do not respond to surgery.
6. High-risk patients should be monitored as inpatients postoperatively.
7. Patients should be reevaluated postoperatively to determine whether additional treatment is required.

From: *Current Clinical Practice: Primary Care Sleep Medicine: A Practical Guide*
Edited by: J. F. Pagel and S. R. Pandi-Perumal © Humana Press Inc., Totowa, NJ

Although there is increased awareness of the possible detrimental effect of SDB, it is only beginning to understand the full characteristics and consequences of this disorder in children. It is clearly not the adult form of the disease in younger patients, and the clinical characteristics are somewhat different depending on the age and associated medical conditions of the child.

The prevalence of primary habitual snoring among all children (age 1–18) is probably between 8 and 12%. This estimate is the product of several studies of varied design and composition. OSA has traditionally been considered to have a prevalence of 1–3%, though more recent studies including older, more obese children indicate a prevalence as high as 5%. Epidemiological studies indicate several factors that influence the development of SDB in children. A clear racial predilection has been noted, with higher prevalence among African-American and Asian children than among Caucasians. Although many children with SDB are not obese, the presence of obesity does increase the risk of SDB. Gender appears to play no significant role in pediatric SDB. A family history of SDB (among parents or siblings) is common among children with SDB. Studies of specific populations with underlying genetic or developmental disorders have demonstrated that those disorders associated with upper airway obstruction (from any anatomical abnormality) or neuromuscular weakness can predispose to SDB.

A key question regarding pediatric SDB is the exact definition of clinically significant disease. Although the traditional teaching has identified PS as a benign disorder not associated with disturbed sleep or daytime executive function, data discovered during the last decade has demonstrated that even PS may have detrimental effects. O'Brien and colleagues *(2)* recently published a study demonstrating adverse neurobehavioral consequences of habitual snoring. In this study, PS was defined as habitual snoring with an apnea–hypopnea index of less than 5 and no gas exchange abnormalities. PS was associated with significant alterations in respiratory arousal and rapid eye movement percentages, compared with controls. Children with PS were more likely to have problems with attention, anxious/depressive symptoms, and social problems. Finally, children with PS had deficits in language and visuospacial ability, in addition to overall cognitive ability. Gottlieb and colleagues *(3)* demonstrated that 5-year olds with habitual snoring scored significantly lower than those without habitual snoring on tests of executive function, memory, and general intellectual ability. Chervin and colleagues *(4)* published a study of 2- to 14-year olds in whom a positive, pediatric, sleep-disordered questionnaire correlated with conduct problems.

These studies demonstrate that a relatively mild form of SDB can have clinical consequences. The optimal form of treatment for PS, however, remains to be defined. So, while a child with significant adenotonsillar hypertrophy, an apnea-hypopnea index of 10 with desaturations less than 92%, and behavioral and cognitive symptoms clearly should be considered for adenotonsillectomy, what should be recommended for the child with modest adenotonsillar hypertrophy, habitual snoring, and behavioral problems? These questions remain to be answered.

ETIOLOGY AND PATHOGENESIS

As noted above, a number of risk factors for pediatric SDB have been identified. Adenotonsillar hypertrophy is the predominant underlying mechanism in nonadolescent children. Adenotonsillar hypertrophy is the most prominent in children up to about age 6–8, when natural regression of this tissue begins to occur. Adenotonsillar hypertrophy results from multiple etiologies; the most common are recurrent upper respiratory infection and allergic irritants. Other causes of upper airway obstruction include chronic nasal obstruction from allergies and pharyngeal edema from gastroesophageal reflux disease (GERD).

In addition to anatomic obstruction, upper airway size and muscle tone also contribute to the etiology and pathogenesis of pediatric SDB. Obesity is the most common contributor to decreased airway size in adults, and, with the increasing prevalence of obesity in children, it will likely play a larger role in SDB in children. Airway size is also decreased in many syndromes such as Prader-Willi, achondroplasia, mucopolysaccharidoses, Pierre Robin, Treacher Collins, Apert, and many others. Decreased upper airway tone results from brainstem lesions (such as tumors and malformations) and diseases affecting overall neuromuscular tone.

Down syndrome is perhaps the most prevalent of the pediatric conditions leading to risk for SDB. Children with Down syndrome may have any or all of the predisposing factors for SDB, including macroglossia, midface hypoplasia, micrognathia, and muscular hypotonia. Other genetic syndromes are relatively uncommon but may be encountered by the sleep specialist. An excellent and valuable resource for such disorders is *Smith's Recognizable Patterns of Human Malformation (5).*

CLINICAL MANIFESTATIONS

The clinical manifestations of SDB in children are fairly broad. Within the broad category of SDB, the classic presentation of OSA in children involves obstructive hypoventilation without marked daytime somnolence. This presentation is somewhat different from that seen in the classic adult form of the disease. A comparison of the clinical features of these classic forms of the disease is provided in Table 1.

In reality, however, pediatric SDB exists as a continuum under which individuals can be categorized in one of four clinical variants or phenotypes. This continuum progresses in severity from an anatomic and physiological perspective, and it is inferred that this continuum translates into increase clinical severity. These include the following:

1. Chronic, habitual snoring that results in sleep disruption without associated blood-gas abnormalities.
2. Upper airways resistance similar to that seen in adults, including snoring without identifiable airflow obstruction and increasingly negative esophageal pressure swings and arousals.
3. Obstructive hypoventilation, which consists of long periods of persistent, partial, upper airway obstruction associated with hypercarbia with or without arterial oxygen desaturation (*classic* pattern).
4. Cyclic episodes of obstructive apnea, similar to that of adults with OSA.

The relative prevalence of each of these patterns is not well-studied. Empirically, habitual snoring would seem to be more common than cyclic obstructive events, and this is generally supported by the literature. A broader, population-based analysis across the full pediatric age range needs to be conducted to determine the true prevalence of these phenotypes and further assess the clinical consequences of each.

Among all variants, the most commonly encountered presenting symptom is snoring. Some parents report the child has difficulty breathing during sleep. Snoring is usually loud and may have associated breathing pauses and gaps, with movements. Some patients, particularly infants and those who are weak, may not snore. Patients with obstructive

Table 1
Comparison of Pediatric and Adult OSA

	Children	*Adults*
Demographics		
Estimated prevalence	Variable depending on phenotype; 1–3% in young children	Up to 5% in most populations
Peak age	2–6 years for classic phenotype	30–60 years
Gender	M = F	M > F
Weight	Commonly normal, but can be underweight or overweight	Majority overweight or obese until advanced age
Snoring	Often continuous	Usually alternating, with pauses
Excessive daytime sleepiness	Uncommon (?)	Very common
Major cause	Adenotonsillar hypertrophy	Obesity

hypoventilation often have continuous snoring without pauses or arousals. Sweating during sleep, restless sleep, nocturnal enuresis, and sleeping with a hyperextended neck are common, but do occur in the absence of SDB. In one study, sweating during sleep occurred in 36% of never snorers, and restless sleep occurred in 24% of never snorers *(6)*, making these symptoms very nonspecific markers of SDB. Witnessed apnea requiring parental intervention (such as shaking to reinitiate breathing) is probably the most specific symptom, although it is relatively uncommon among all children with SDB.

Daytime symptoms are frequently encountered in children. Excessive daytime sleepiness has traditionally been considered a rare feature in pediatric SDB. This concept is being challenged by numerous studies that identify a correlation between sleepiness, behavioral and cognitive dysfunction, and SDB symptoms *(3,7)*. The more typical presentation, however, is that of alteration in daytime function such as hyperactivity, inattentiveness, or other cognitive/behavioral abnormalities. It is likely that these symptoms represent a spectrum of interpretation of behaviors among children and that behavioral problems are a manifestation of sleepiness. Other daytime symptoms may include mouth breathing, difficulty swallowing, morning headaches, and poor appetite.

COMPLICATIONS

Complications arising as a consequence of SDB can be difficult to ascertain. It is often unclear whether the complication is a caused by SDB or an effect of SDB. Obesity, for instance, is often considered an associated feature in older children. But persistent behavioral sleep deprivation may result in weight gain, leading to decreased airway size, which predisposes to SDB. Additionally, many complications are theoretical with little data to identify the true prevalence of the complication and even less data to correlate the complication with the severity of SDB.

The most severe potential complications of SDB include death, growth failure, and cardiac, gastrointestinal, or pulmonary system disorders. More common, however, are the cognitive and behavioral complications of SDB. The incidence of death as a result of SDB is unknown. There is an association of OSA in patients with a family history of sudden infant death syndrome (SIDS) *(8)*. Although it is unlikely that SIDS represents a pure form OSA, some characteristics of this disorder may lead to death in these infants. On the whole, however, death as a complication of SDB is likely limited to the extremes of OSA when it is associated with other medical or surgical conditions.

Cardiovascular complications typically attributed to OSA include cor pulmonale, pulmonary hypertension, polycythemia, chronic respiratory acidosis, and hypertension. Although all must be considered, they generally occur at the extremes of OSA, in association with other disorders. OSA has been established as a clear cause of secondary hypertension in adults. There are limited data, however, on the association of pediatric SDB to hypertension. One recent study of 60 children demonstrated that children with OSA had significantly higher mean blood pressure (BP) variability during wakefulness and sleep, higher night-to-day systolic BP, and smaller nocturnal dipping of mean BP *(9)*. A smaller study of 23 patients also demonstrated that BP positively correlated with the degree of SDB *(10)*. What remains to be demonstrated is whether BP elevation related to childhood SDB contributes to adulthood hypertension and its consequences.

Gastrointestinal complications attributed to OSA include feeding difficulties and GERD. Feeding difficulties can be broadly ascribed to poor sleep and, possibly, to aversion associated with GERD. The mechanism of GERD relates to increased intra-abdominal pressures and more negative intrathoracic pressures during apneas and hypopneas, which favors movement of gastric contents into the esophagus. GERD has been clearly associated with OSA in adults, and there is one small study in children *(11)*. Pulmonary complications can include chronic aspiration, pulmonary edema, and development of a pectus excavatum. Chronic aspiration may result from repeated gastroesophageal reflux. Pulmonary edema, a rare complication is described following severe upper airway obstructive events. Development of a pectus excavatum occurs when the developing chest wall is subjected the effects of nightly, severe, upper airway resistance and the pressure required to overcome this resistance. Behavioral and cognitive consequences of OSA have been well-described. As noted above, these consequences are being attributed to milder forms of SDB, including PS. Further study is needed to determine what treatment is optimal for milder forms of SDB.

DIAGNOSIS AND ASSESSMENT

Because of the broad range of clinical symptoms and the incremental nature of severity in SDB, clinical evaluation of the child with suspected SDB can be challenging. Currently, a clinical evaluation should be considered in any child with frequent snoring who also has cognitive or behavioral problems, enuresis, hypertension, or significant parental concern. In addition to these commonly encountered symptoms, individuals with Down syndrome, anatomic abnormalities of the face, and neuromuscular weakness should undergo evaluation because of the high likelihood of SDB in these populations. Finally, children with signs of pulmonary hypertension, right ventricular failure, or growth delay may benefit from a clinical evaluation for SDB.

As noted above, questions related to the severity and frequency of snoring are imperative. Snoring is usually loud and may have associated breathing pauses and gaps, with movements. Important exceptions to this rule are infants and children with underlying neuromuscular weakness. Patients with obstructive hypoventilation often have continuous snoring without pauses or arousals. A parental description consistent with paradoxical breathing is a prominent physical sign in young children. Further history should include an assessment of overall sleep duration and quality, including timing of bedtime/wake time, duration of sleep, night awakenings, arousal parasomnias, enuresis, and body position. For infants, an apparent life-threatening event (ALTE) may be a presenting complaint. In these circumstances, a full history of the event is warranted (a comprehensive review of ALTE is included in the ref. *12*). A comprehensive past medical history should be conducted and include pregnancy and perinatal history; medical conditions such as sinus problems, asthma, chronic cough, and GERD; behavior issues such as hyperactivity or inattentiveness; and surgery involving the upper airway. Family history should include information about other family members with suspected or confirmed SDB, ALTEs, or SIDS, and congenital syndromes.

Physical examination should include a careful inspection of the upper airway. An assessment of the patency of the nose should be made, including position of the septum and size of the turbinates. The oropharynx should be inspected for tongue size, uvula size, and tonsil size. A standardized scale is published and utilized by pediatricians and otolaryngologists. Further inspection of the oropharynx should include assessment of the hard palate, mandible, and maxilla. Other examination should include an assessment of body fat and its distribution as well as evaluation for the presence of a pectus excavatum. Objective confirmation of SDB requires some form of testing. Debate continues regarding the efficacy of home monitoring. Portable, multichannel, unattended monitoring has been utilized successfully in research studies *(13)*. However, other studies comparing unattended portable monitoring to standard PSG have demonstrated that home monitoring in pediatric SDB is presently not a reliable substitute for standard PSG *(14)*. Furthermore, portable monitoring based only on oximetry does not appear to be adequate for identification of OSA in otherwise healthy children *(15)*.

In the laboratory, overnight PSG is considered the gold standard and the only means of excluding the diagnosis of SDB. PSG is not, however, universally standardized in configuration. PSG studies in children generally include the standard adult-montage, with added channels in some laboratories. This typically includes measurement with 4-channel electroencephalogram, left and right electrooculogram, submental electromyogram, leg electromyogram, chest and abdomen movement (by various means), oronasal thermistor, oximetry, and electrocardiogram. Other commonly added channels include infrared video and end-tidal or transcutaneous CO_2 assessment. Some laboratories substitute a nasal pressure transducer, which is likely more sensitive in assessing upper airways resistance *(16)*.

PSG normative values, however, have not been definitively established for children. Two recent studies have been published supporting common empiric norms for apneas and desaturation in normal children *(17,18)*. In these studies, obstructive apnea was defined as absence of airflow for ≥2 respiratory cycles, with paradoxical movement of the chest and abdomen. Hypopnea was defined as a 50% decrease in flow associated with arousal or SpO_2 fall of ≥3%. Central apnea was defined as absence of flow and effort not immediately preceded by an arousal or awakening and lasting ≥20 seconds or any associated with an SpO_2 fall of ≥3%. These studies support the following normal values in children:

1. Central apneas lasting for more than 20 seconds *without*
   a. SpO_2 drop of less than 89%; or
   b. SpO_2 drop of more than 4% from baseline.

2. A central apnea index of less than 1.
3. An obstructive apnea index of less than 1.
4. SpO_2 nadir of more than 92%.
5. Partial pressure of CO_2 level more than 45 mmHg for less than 10% of total sleep time.

There are no standard criteria for defining severity of SDB, and most clinicians grade the disease based on clinical judgment. Typically, severe disease is defined as a respitory disturbance index (RDI) of ≥10 or any RDI with a desaturation nadir less than 92; moderate disease is defined as an RDI of 5–10 without desaturation; and mild disease is defined as an RDI of 1–5. In light of mounting evidence that habitual snoring has detrimental behavioral and cognitive consequences, it seems reasonable to consider treatment for even mild SDB when these features are present. The complete diagnostic criteria, as defined by the *International Classification of Sleep Disorders*, is provided in Table 2 *(19)*.

TREATMENT

Treatment of SDB in children may encompass the spectrum of therapy from surgery, to medical therapy, to device therapy. Because adenotonsillar hypertrophy is the most common condition associated with pediatric OSA, adenotonsillectomy provides definitive therapy in the majority of patients. Certain patients may not derive full benefit from adenotonsillectomy. In a recent, population-based study of children from 1 to 18, 6% of children postadenoidectomy with or without tonsillectomy snored nightly *(20)*. Guilleminault and colleagues *(21)* recently published a prospective study of surgical outcomes. Children were evaluated by a multidisciplinary team, and recommendations were made for surgical therapy. Eleven children were treated by the multidisciplinary team, and 10 had complete resolution of symptoms. A total of 45 children were treated by other specialists. Only one of these children had the procedure recommended by the multidisciplinary team. Children with residual symptoms after the procedure totaled 58%, and 27% had residual PSG abnormalities. A full 29% underwent a second surgical procedure.

Conclusions to be drawn from these two studies are that all children who undergo adenoidectomy and/or tonsillectomy should undergo at least a repeat clinical evaluation to assure resolution of symptoms. This examination should take place at least 6–8 weeks after the procedure to allow for adequate healing time. Furthermore, more research and teaching is needed for individuals performing pediatric adenotonsillectomy to determine what procedures are the most important for SDB. Medical management can encompass pharmacotherapy and positive airway pressure. Both have been demonstrated in several small studies to provide some improvement in symptoms. Other treatments such as weight management, avoidance of passive and active smoke, and oral appliances may also play a role in selected populations.

Nasal CPAP, the standard of care in adults with OSA is effective in children. There have been at least eight studies of nasal CPAP in children, validating its effectiveness in children aged 6 weeks through adolescence, and several of these have been recently reviewed and summarized *(22)*. Because CPAP requires both a motivated patient *and* family, it is usually reserved for children in whom adenotonsillectomy has failed or is not possible. Because CPAP is not a Food and Drug Administration-approved device in children, mask manufacturers cannot provide masks designed for pediatric patients. The

Table 2
Diagnostic Criteria for Pediatric OSA

Caregiver reports snoring, labored or obstructed breathing, or both snoring and labored or obstructed breathing during sleep
Caregiver reports observing at least one of the following:
Paradoxical, inward, rib cage motion during inspiration
Movement arousals
Diaphoresis
Neck hyperextension during sleep
Excessive daytime sleepiness, hyperactivity, or aggressive behavior
Slow rate of growth
Morning headaches
Secondary enuresis
PSG recording demonstrates one or more scoreable respiratory events per hour (i.e., apnea or hypopnea of at least two respiratory cycles in duration)
Very few normative data are available for hypopneas, and the data that are available have been obtained using a variety of methodologies. These criteria may be modified in the future, once more comprehensive data become available
PSG recording demonstrates either 1 or 2 (next)

1. At least one of the following is observed:
   Frequent arousals from sleep associated with increased respiratory effort
   Arterial oxygen desaturation in association with the apneic episodes
   Hypercapnia during sleep
   Markedly negative esophageal pressure swings
2. Periods of hypercapnia, desaturation, or hypercapnia and desaturation during sleep, associated with snoring; paradoxical, inward, rib-cage motion during inspiration; and at least one of the following:
   Frequent arousals from sleep
   Markedly negative esophageal pressure swings

The disorder is not better explained by another current sleep disorder, medical or neurological disorder, medication use, or substance use disorder

Adapted from ref. *19*.

use of this therapy, however, is clearly efficacious, and families should be well-informed about the potential risks and benefits. CPAP requires frequent follow-up to assure appropriate mask fit and pressure titration.

The routine use of autotitrating CPAP would seem an ideal therapeutic option for children, particularly those with rapid growth or increasing weight. One study has demonstrated efficacy of automated CPAP in a group of 14 children, aged 8 months–12 years. Although this treatment was effective in most children, the authors conclude that larger studies are needed and routine follow-up is still necessary *(23)*. The common practice in adult patients of initiating auto-CPAP without in-laboratory assessment of tolerance is probably not appropriate for the pediatric population.

Medical therapy for SDB has been limited to those agents that reduce upper airway tissue burden. Two studies have demonstrated efficacy of nasal steroids in pediatric SBD *(24,25)*. One preliminary study has shown effectiveness of the leukotriene modifying agent, montelukast, in mild SDB *(26)*. Other agents such as nasal decongestants, may be helpful for intermittent snoring associated with intercurrent illness, but these agents should not be considered for long-term management. In obese patients, weight management is likely to be of benefit. Weight management in children should include comprehensive nutritional, exercise, and behavioral counseling for both the patient and the family. When appropriate, smoking cessation counseling should be offered to parents and caregivers. Finally, oral appliances may be utilized in adolescents when growth is completed.

CONCLUSIONS

Pediatric SDB is a dynamic and variable disease with significant physical and neurobehavioral consequences. Diagnoses and management requires full consideration of concurrent illnesses and complications. Much more research is needed to identify the long-term consequences of the spectrum of SDB. At present, it appears appropriate to offer treatment options to all children with any form of SDB in which behavioral or cognitive deficits are noted.

REFERENCES

1. American Academy of Pediatrics (2002) Clinical practice guideline: diagnosis and management of childhood obstructive sleep apnea syndrome. Pediatrics 109:704–712.
2. O'Brien LM, Mervis CB, Holbrook CR, et al. (2004) Neurobehavioral implications of habitual snoring in children. Pediatrics 114:44–49.
3. Gottlieb DJ, Chase C, Vezina RM, et al. (2004) Sleep-disordered breathing symptoms are associated with poorer cognitive function in 5-year-old children. J Pediatr 145:458–464.
4. Chervin RD, Dillon JE, Archbold KH, et al. (2003) Conduct problems and symptoms of sleep disorders in children. J Am Acad Child Adolesc Psychiatry 42:201–208.
5. Jones KL, Smith DW (2006) *Smith's Recognizable Patterns of Human Malformation*. 6th ed. Elsevier Saunders, Philadelphia, PA.
6. Ersu R, Arman AR, Save D, et al. (2004) Prevalence of snoring and symptoms of sleep-disordered breathing in primary school children in Istanbul. Chest 126:19–24.
7. Chervin RD, Archbold KH, Dillon JE, et al. (2002) Inattention, hyperactivity, and symptoms of sleep-disordered breathing. Pediatrics 109:449–456.
8. Tishler PV, Redline S, Ferrette V, et al. (1996) The association of sudden unexpected infant death with obstructive sleep apnea. Am J Respir Crit Care Med 153(6 Pt 1):1857–1863.
9. Amin RS, Carroll JL, Jeffries JL, et al. (2004) Twenty-four-hour ambulatory blood pressure in children with sleep-disordered breathing. Am J Respir Crit Care Med 169:950–956.
10. Kohyama J, Ohinata JS, Hasegawa T (2003) Blood pressure in sleep disordered breathing. Arch Dis Child 88:139–142.
11. Wasilewska J, Kaczmarski M (2004) Sleep-related breathing disorders in small children with nocturnal acid gastro-oesophageal reflux. Rocz Akad Med Bialymst 49:98–102.
12. Dewolfe CC (2005) Apparent life-threatening event: a review. Pediatr Clin North Am 52:1127–1146.
13. Goodwin JL, Enright PL, Kaemingk KL, et al. (2001) Feasibility of using unattended polysomnography in children for research: report of the Tucson Children's Assessment of Sleep Apnea study (TuCASA). Sleep 24:937–944.
14. Zucconi M, Calori G, Castronovo V, et al. (2003) Respiratory monitoring by means of an unattended device in children with suspected uncomplicated obstructive sleep apnea: a validation study. Chest 124:602–607.
15. Kirk VG, Bohn SG, Flemons WW, et al. (2003) Comparison of home oximetry monitoring with laboratory polysomnography in children. Chest 124:1702–1708.
16. Epstein MD, Chicoine SA, Hanumara RC (2000) Detection of upper airway resistance syndrome using a nasal cannula/pressure transducer. Chest 117:1073–1077.
17. Uliel S, Tauman R, Greenfeld M, et al. (2004) Normal polysomnographic respiratory values in children and adolescents. Chest 125:872–878.
18. Traeger N, Schultz B, Pollock AN, et al. (2005) Polysomnographic values in children 2–9 years old: additional data and review of the literature. Pediatr Pulmonol 40:22–30.

19. American Academy of Sleep Medicine (2005) *The International Classification of Sleep Disorders Diagnostic and Coding Manual.* 2nd ed. American Academy of Sleep Medicine, Westchester, IL.
20. Kaditis AG, Finder J, Alexopoulos EI, et al. (2004) Sleep-disordered breathing in 3,680 Greek children. Pediatr Pulmonol 37:499–509.
21. Guilleminault C, Li K, Quo S, et al. (2004) A prospective study on the surgical outcomes of children with sleep-disordered breathing. Sleep 27:95–100.
22. Guilleminault C, Lee JH, Chan A (2005) Pediatric obstructive sleep apnea syndrome. Arch Pediatr Adolesc Med 159:775–785.
23. Palombini L, Pelayo R, Guilleminault C (2004) Efficacy of automated continuous positive airway pressure in children with sleep-related breathing disorders in an attended setting. Pediatrics 113:e412-e417.
24. Alexopoulos EI, Kaditis AG, Kalampouka E, et al. (2004) Nasal corticosteroids for children with snoring. Pediatr Pulmonol 38:161–167.
25. Brouillette RT, Manoukian JJ, Ducharme FM, et al. (2001) Efficacy of fluticasone nasal spray for pediatric obstructive sleep apnea. J Pediatr 138:838–844.
26. Goldbart AD, Goldman JL, Veling MC, et al. (2005) Leukotriene modifier therapy for mild sleep-disordered breathing in children. Am J Respir Crit Care Med 172:364–370.

19 Sleep and Sleep Disorders in Women

Fiona C. Baker, PhD, Kathryn A. Lee, PhD, and R. Manber, RN, PhD, FAAN

CONTENTS

THE NORMAL MENSTRUAL CYCLE, ORAL CONTRACEPTIVES, AND MENSTRUAL-ASSOCIATED DISORDERS

The ovulatory menstrual cycle is characterized by a regulated variation in reproductive hormones across a 25- to 35-day period (Fig. 1). Coordinated through the central nervous system, pulsatile release of gonadotropin-releasing hormone from the hypothalamus, regulates the release of the hypothalamic hormones, luteinizing hormone, and follicle-stimulating hormone that in turn regulate the secretion of estrogen. Day 1 is identified as the first day of bleeding (menses) and ovulation occurs around day 14, dividing the cycle into two phases: a preovulatory follicular phase and a postovulatory luteal phase. In the luteal phase, progesterone dominates, being released from the corpus luteum, together with estradiol. Approximately 14 days after ovulation, if there is no implantation of a fertilized ovum, hormone levels rapidly drop and menses begin. During the late luteal phase (when hormone levels are declining) and the first day of menstruation, women experience the most negative symptoms.

Sleep Across the Normal Menstrual Cycle

Surveys and studies based on subjective reports have found that women across a wide age range (aged 18–50 years) report more sleep disturbances during the premenstrual week and during the first few days of menstruation than at other times *(1–3)*. The Study of Women's Health Across the Nation (SWAN), which included 630 women in their late reproductive stage or entering the menopausal transition, also showed that trouble sleeping varied with cycle phase, being more likely to occur during the early

From: *Current Clinical Practice: Primary Care Sleep Medicine, A Practical Guide*
Edited by: J. F. Pagel and S. R. Pandi-Perumal © Humana Press Inc., Totowa, NJ

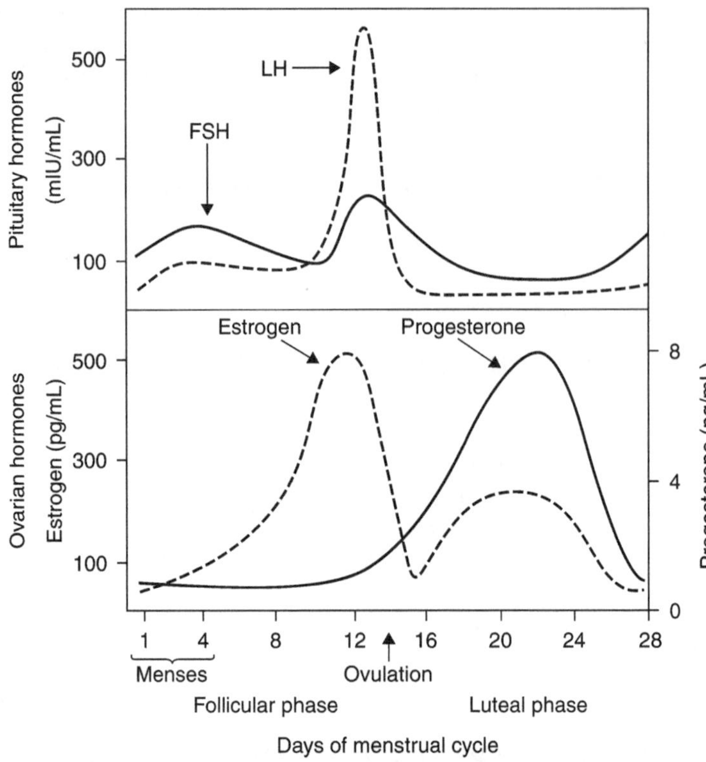

Fig. 1. Schematic representation of the reproductive hormone variations across a typical 28-day menstrual cycle. Day 1 is identified as the first day of bleeding (menses). Ovulation occurs just after the surge in luteinizing hormone.

follicular and late luteal phases of the menstrual cycle *(4)*. Therefore, there is strong evidence that women perceive the quality of their sleep as poorer around the time of menstruation.

Most polysomnographic (PSG) studies have found that sleep continuity and sleep efficiency remain stable at different phases of the ovulatory menstrual cycle in young, healthy women (*see* refs. *5,6* for review). Percentages of slow-wave sleep (SWS) and slow wave activity in nonrapid eye movement sleep also are unchanged *(7,8)*, suggesting that sleep homeostasis is maintained across the menstrual cycle. Rapid eye movement (REM) sleep may be influenced by menstrual phase to a limited extent: some studies have found that REM sleep has an earlier onset *(9)* and the percentage of REM sleep tends to decrease *(7,10–14)* in association with raised body temperature in the luteal phase.

Although there are not large changes in visually-scored sleep structure, the sleep electroencephalography is influenced by the hormonal variations of the menstrual cycle. Specifically, electroencephalography activity in the frequency range of sleep spindles is significantly increased *(7,8)* during the luteal phase compared with other phases of the menstrual cycle, hypothesized to represent an interaction between endogenous progesterone metabolites and $GABA_A$, membrane receptors *(7)*.

To summarize, with the exception of REM sleep and spindle activity, sleep-stage distribution is stable across the normal menstrual cycle despite substantial changes in the hormonal milieu. The subjective worsening of sleep quality around the time of menstruation in women may be because of increased physical discomfort such as bloating or cramps, impacting perceived sleep quality without affecting PSG-defined wake time. Women who suffer from menstrual-related disorders are more likely to have substantial disturbances in sleep, as discussed later.

The Effect of Oral Contraceptives on Sleep

Oral contraceptives suppress endogenous reproductive hormones and therefore prevent ovulation, so the women taking them do not have normal menstrual cycles. Oral contraceptives do not appear to influence subjective sleep quality *(15)*, but do alter sleep architecture. Women taking oral contraceptives have less SWS *(12,15–17)*, associated with more Stage 2 sleep *(15)*, and have also been found to have a shorter REM onset latency and more REM sleep *(16)*, compared with women with natural menstrual cycles. Exogenous steroid hormones therefore have a more pronounced effect on sleep architecture than do endogenous progesterone and estrogen during the natural luteal phase. The consequences of these changes in sleep structure, if any, are unknown.

Menstrual Cycle-Associated Sleep Disorders

Two sleep disorders that are temporally related to the menses have been proposed in the International Classification of Sleep Disorders—premenstrual insomnia and premenstrual hypersomnia *(18)*. Reports of the sleep characteristics of these disorders are rare and their underlying causes are unclear *(18)*. Women with premenstrual insomnia complain of difficulty in falling asleep or remaining asleep only during the premenstrual phase of the menstrual cycle. The insomnia occurs on a recurrent basis for at least three consecutive months *(18)*. There is some evidence from a case study that desynchronization of temperature and sleep–wake rhythms in the luteal phase could be a contributing factor to this disorder *(19)*. Premenstrual hypersomnia is characterized by excessive sleepiness that typically begins a few days before menstruation onset and ends a few days after *(18)*. Few cases have been published, and most of the patients have had unremarkable hormonal changes accompanying their symptoms *(20,21)*. Oral contraceptives have been successfully used to treat this condition *(21,22)*.

Premenstrual Syndrome and Premenstrual Dysphoric Disorder

Up to 17% of women have severe premenstrual syndrome (PMS) that significantly impacts their function and 3–8% report disabling premenstrual symptoms such as depressed mood, irritability, and anxiety that qualify them for a diagnosis of premenstrual dysphoric disorder (PMDD) *(23,24)*. Sleep disturbance (hypersomnia or insomnia) is included as one of 11 symptoms for a diagnosis of PMDD in the American Psychiatric Association's DSM-IV *(23)*. Women with severe PMS typically report sleep-related complaints such as hypersomnia, insomnia, fatigue, sleep perturbation by body movements and awakenings, and disturbing dreams associated with their PMS symptoms *(25)*. However, PSG studies have not found any evidence of increased sleep disturbance in the symptomatic luteal phase compared with the asymptomatic follicular phase in women with PMDD or severe PMS *(9,14,25–27)*. Possibly there is variation within the population of women with PMDD, such that sleep disturbances are only apparent in some women. Women with severe PMS should be encouraged to monitor their premenstrual symptoms, including sleep disturbances, in a daily diary so that appropriate treatment can be provided for severe symptoms.

Interestingly, total and partial sleep deprivation improve mood in women with PMDD *(14,28)*, although positive effects are more evident after recovery sleep than immediately following sleep deprivation, which differs from findings in patients with major depressive disorder. The mechanisms underlying the effects of sleep deprivation in women with PMDD remain to be determined. Appropriately timed light therapy has also shown some promise as a treatment strategy for PMDD, possibly by altering nocturnal melatonin secretion *(29)* but larger trials are needed to define what role bright light therapy has in treatment of PMDD *(30)*.

Dysmenorrhea

Dysmenorrhea refers to painful uterine cramps during menstruation and is the most common gynecological condition in women *(31)*. Primary dysmenorrhea is menstrual pain without organic disease and secondary dysmenorrhea is menstrual pain associated with conditions such as endometriosis and pelvic inflammatory disease *(31)*. The painful menstrual cramps experienced by these women every month significantly impact productivity and quality of life and are associated with a restriction of activity and absenteeism from work and school *(31,32)*. A PSG study of women with primary dysmenorrhea found that the painful menstrual cramps were associated with disturbed sleep (poorer subjective sleep quality; lower sleep efficiency, increased time spent awake, moving, and in Stage 1, light sleep and less REM sleep) compared with pain-free phases of the menstrual cycle, and compared with women who do not suffer menstrual pain *(11)*. Disturbed sleep, in turn, may exacerbate pain, as sleep deprivation is associated with a decreased pain threshold *(33)*. Treatment of nocturnal pain with analgesics should alleviate painful cramps and consequently improve sleep quality in women with primary dysmenorrhea.

Polycystic Ovarian Syndrome

Polycystic ovarian syndrome (PCOS) affects 4–12% of women of reproductive age *(34)*. Women with PCOS typically present with irregular or absent cycles, androgen excess (evident as hirsutism), and bilateral polycystic ovaries *(35)*. Insulin resistance is also an important component of PCOS *(35)* and obesity occurs in approx 50% of cases *(36)*. The combination of obesity, excess androgen production, and insulin resistance places women with PCOS at an increased risk for sleep disordered breathing (SDB). The prevalence of SDB in women with PCOS is 30–40 times that observed in age- and weight-matched controls *(37–39)*. Women with PCOS should be evaluated for SDB and treated appropriately, not only to improve alertness but also to address potential insulin resistance, which is common in both disorders *(38)*. Indeed, glucose tolerance and SDB may be influenced by a common mechanism in PCOS *(38)*.

PREGNANCY

Sleep patterns vary across trimesters as hormonal and physical changes take place. Both hormonal (prolactin and progesterone) and physical changes associated with pregnancy contribute to poor sleep (*see* refs. *40,41* for thorough reviews). Pregnant women commonly report sleep disruption because of nausea, backache, frequent urination, heartburn, leg cramps, and shortness of breath, especially in the third trimester *(42–45)*. Both longitudinal and cross-sectional PSG studies have also indicated an increase in wake after sleep onset in pregnant women, particularly in the third trimester *(13,42–45)*. Findings regarding changes in total sleep time and amounts of REM sleep and SWS are mixed, although most studies have found less REM sleep and SWS *(13,44)*, more α–δ sleep *(43)*, and more time in Stage 1 light sleep *(42)* in the third trimester. Despite the ubiquitous nature of frequent night waking during the third trimester, less than 20% view their awakenings as problematic *(13)*. The impact of poor sleep during pregnancy on labor and delivery is not clear. Although Evans *(46)* found no significant correlations between the length of labor and self-reported sleep quality during the day or the week preceding labor, another group found that women who slept less than 6 hours at night, or who were awake more than 15% of the night (by actigraphy recording) during the ninth month of pregnancy had longer labors and more incidence of cesarean deliveries *(47)*.

Sleep Disorders During Pregnancy

Data on the prevalence of sleep disorders during pregnancy are lacking. Pregnancy is associated with an increased risk for two sleep disorders, SDB and restless legs syndrome (RLS). The incidence of snoring is higher for pregnant women during the second half of pregnancy (12–23%) than for age-matched nonpregnant controls (~4%). Symptoms of SDB, including snoring, choking, and apneic events, increase as pregnancy progresses *(48–51)*. Women with pre-existing SDB, and those at high risk for SDB because of obesity should be carefully monitored during pregnancy as SDB may be associated with pre-eclampsia and neonatal complications *(52–54)*.

The incidence of RLS during pregnancy is 2–3 times higher than in the general population *(55)*, most likely because of iron deficiency and folate deficiency associated with pregnancy. Women with restless legs during pregnancy, compared with those without, have low serum ferritin and folate levels at preconception *(56)*, but whether iron and folate supplements before conception reduce the incidence of RLS during pregnancy, remains to be determined. Prospective studies find the incidence of RLS increases as pregnancy progresses, to about 20% before delivery *(55,56)*. For most women, RLS remits following delivery *(55)*. Rather than taking a dopaminergic medication for RLS during pregnancy, most women would favor nonpharmacological therapy to alleviate severity of symptoms such as warm baths and massage. Reduction in caffeine intake is also helpful to promote iron and folate absorption *(41)*.

POSTPARTUM

The first 6 months postpartum are associated with a substantial increase in time awake after sleep onset and a decrease in sleep efficiency relative to the last trimester of pregnancy *(57–60)*. However, this period is also associated with increases in SWS and REM pressure *(13)*, as evidenced by earlier REM onset that normalizes by 3 months postpartum *(13,42,57)*. The increase in slow wave sleep and early REM onset are likely to be a result of the chronic partial sleep deprivation that many mothers experience early in the postpartum period, as both are commonly found following sleep deprivation. Maternal sleep gradually improves during postpartum recovery *(61)*, but remains closely tied to the infant's sleep patterns and mode of feeding. Compared with nonlactating mothers, breastfeeding mothers report more night awakenings when first establishing feedings with their infants *(61)*, but report similar amounts of sleep time *(62)*. New mothers who are breastfeeding have been noted to have more SWS than nonlactating mothers in controlled laboratory studies *(63)*. Breastfeeding is closely tied to cosleeping

Table 1
Bed-Sharing Safety Measures for Parents and Infants

Never leave an infant alone on an adult bed
Infants should be placed on their backs for sleep
Infants should always sleep on a firm mattress without pillows or soft bed covers
Infants should not sleep on sofas or waterbeds
There should be no narrow spaces between the infant's sleep surface and the wall or other furniture
It is best for your infant's sleep, and for a parent's sleep, to place the infant in his or her own crib or bassinet, whether it is located in the parent's bedroom or elsewhere
An infant should not sleep in the same bed (cosleep) with a sibling
If an infant is going to sleep in the same bed with parents, the parents should not be under the influence of any sleep medication or alcohol, the infant should be placed in the center of the bed inside a contained structure with a firm surface to prevent accidental falls or suffocation

Adapted from ref. *139*.

behavior, where the infant shares the same bed with the mother. Although few (7%) women having their first baby indicate that they plan to bed-share or cosleep with their infant, bed-sharing occurs in a majority (60%) of cases, particularly during the first 1–2 months postpartum *(64)*. Reasons for initiating bed-sharing are unrelated to socioeconomic status, household space or cultural expectations, but rather are related to the attempt to feel emotionally and physically closer to the infant, and to get more sleep *(64)*. Even though parents may not be planning to bed-share with their infant when specifically asked, safety measures suggested by the American Academy of Pediatrics *(65)* are detailed in Table 1 and should be provided to all expectant parents.

As would be expected, maternal sleep fragmentation leads to increased self-reported daytime sleepiness, fatigue, and negative affect, and may contribute to the development of postpartum depression *(66,67)*. With the similarities in clinical presentation, it may be especially difficult for family members or clinicians to distinguish postpartum depression from chronic sleep deprivation. With chronic sleep loss, most new mothers report no difficulty falling asleep at night after their infant has fallen asleep. With depression, however, a new mother is still likely to report more difficulty with falling asleep at night *(68)*. As with other types of major depressive episodes, antidepressant medication and supportive counseling are the treatment options of choice. As breastfeeding mothers are often reluctant to take antidepressant medications, researchers have explored other options such as bright light therapy *(69)* and REM sleep deprivation *(70)*; however, both require further research and empirical testing.

MENOPAUSE TRANSITION (PERIMENOPAUSE)

The menopausal transition refers to the period of time between the first onset of menstrual irregularity, or skipped menses, and the final menstrual period *(71)*. The median age of onset of perimenopause is 47 years *(71)*. The median age at final menstrual period, marking the end of the perimenopausal period, is 51.4 years. This transition period is marked by wide fluctuations in reproductive hormones and is accompanied by changes in other aspects of a woman's life, including sleep.

Ample data show that sleep difficulties increase as women enter the menopausal transition *(4,72–80)*. This increase is observed even after adjustment for age and ethnicity *(4)*. A longitudinal study, conducted during 10 years, reported that problems with sleeping, and secondarily, vasomotor symptoms were the most bothersome symptoms associated with the transition to menopause *(81)*.

The SWAN, a multi-ethnic, community-based cohort study of 3302 women found that the odds of reporting difficulty sleeping were more for women who were in early or late menopausal transition compared with premenopausal women *(4,73)*. A recent epidemiological study further illuminates the prevalence of symptoms of insomnia as well as clinically significant chronic insomnia (more than 6 months of nocturnal symptoms associated with daytime distress or impairment) in peri- and postmenopausal women *(80)*. Similar to others, this study found that the most common persistent nocturnal symptom during the perimenopause is difficulty maintaining sleep, present in 50% of women; an increase from 30% in premenopausal women *(80)*. In contrast, sleep-onset difficulty and nonrestorative sleep were reported by approx 16 and 20% of perimenopausal women, respectively *(80)*. To the best of the knowledge, Ohayon's epidemiological study is the first to provide estimates as to the prevalence of chronic insomnia as a disorder (using DSM-IV criteria), which was estimated as 26% in perimenopausal women-double the prevalence in premenopausal women in the same study.

Whereas studies that rely on subjective methodology clearly document increases in self-reported sleep difficulties, studies that have measured sleep objectively have not found strong evidence for alteration in measures of sleep continuity in association with the transition to menopause *(79,82)*. The Wisconsin Sleep Cohort Study, the largest study measuring sleep objectively in perimenopausal women *(79)* found that although menopausal status was associated with self-reported sleep dissatisfaction, it was not associated with objectively measured sleep quality, total sleep time, or the percent of time spent in slow wave (stages 3 and 4) sleep *(79)*.

An increase in self-reported sleep difficulties during perimenopause has been associated with vasomotor symptoms such as hot flashes *(73)*, hormone levels *(4)*, and psychological factors or mood *(4,75,83)*. The direction of causality for some of these factors such as whether or not the mood changes experienced by perimenopausal women predict sleep disturbance, or are a consequence of sleep disturbance *(75)*, still needs to be determined. A possible link between the hormonal changes of the menopausal transition and self-reported sleep difficulties emerges from a study conducted by Kravitz et al. *(4)* who found that pregnanediol glucuronide, a progesterone metabolite was significantly associated with increased trouble sleeping across the menstrual cycle in perimenopausal women, but not in premenopausal women. The link between poor sleep and nocturnal vasomotor events has received much attention and is discussed later in this chapter.

POSTMENOPAUSE

Postmenopause begins at the time of the last menstrual period, although it is not recognized until after 12 months of amenorrhea *(84)*. Population-based surveys find evidence for a link between postmenopause and self-reported sleep difficulties even after controlling for age and depression scores *(79)*. Odds ratios for comparisons of sleep difficulties between pre- and postmenopausal women range between 1.3 and 3.4 *(73,74,79)*. The increase in sleep difficulty and dissatisfaction with sleep in postmenopausal women appears to be primarily because of difficulty maintaining sleep, reported by 35–60% of postmenopausal women *(80,84)*. In contrast, the prevalence of persistent (at least 6 months) self-reported sleep-onset difficulties, nonrestorative sleep, and a diagnosis of DSM-IV defined insomnia, are similar in pre- and postmenopausal women *(80)*.

Most PSG studies have not found evidence of disturbed sleep in postmenopausal women compared with premenopausal women *(78,79)*. In fact, in the large, population-based Wisconsin Cohort study, postmenopausal women had significantly better objectively defined sleep quality (3.4% more time spent in SWS, 13.4 minutes more total sleep time, and a lower proportion of time spent a wake) than premenopausal women. A smaller study of women without sleep complaints also found no evidence for poorer sleep quality in post compared with premenopausal women *(85)*. Recovery from sleep deprivation is also relatively well-preserved in postmenopausal women when compared with very young women, despite poorer sleep at baseline *(86)*.

Taken together, the data from studies that have compared sleep during the pre-, peri-, and postmenopausal periods suggest an increase in insomnia symptoms from pre- to perimenopause and, although there is some improvement in sleep maintenance during postmenopause, the postmenopausal period is associated with more self-reported sleep maintenance problems than the premenopausal period. Several factors have been evaluated for their potential contribution to observed increases in subjective insomnia symptoms in postmenopausal women relative to premenopausal women, of which vasomotor symptoms are most commonly cited.

Relation of Sleep Continuity Disturbance to Hot Flashes

Some studies have shown that the presence of vasomotor symptoms is associated with subjective and objective sleep disturbance *(87–89)*. Moreover, the prevalence of subjectively defined poor sleep and a diagnosis of chronic insomnia seem to increase with the severity of hot flashes *(80)*. However, not all studies that examined this relationship found a strong association between the experience of vasomotor symptoms and sleep disturbance. For example, the Wisconsin Cohort Study found that objectively defined sleep quality did not differ between women who did or did not report hot flashes *(78,79)*. Prospective outcome studies evaluating efficacy of interventions that target hot flashes, do not always find an association between reductions in nocturnal hot flash severity and clinically meaningful improvements in sleep (e.g., *see* refs. *90,91*). The Women's Health Initiative study, which found a statistically significant improvement in self-reported sleep quality after one year of hormone replacement therapy (HRT), considered the difference small and clinically insignificant. Moreover, the difference was not present at the 3-year follow-up *(90)*.

Studies that have tried to ascertain what proportion of awakenings result from nocturnal hot flashes, compared with the proportion that occur when flashes are absent, have also yielded inconsistent results. Because the ability to perceive and report phenomena that occur during sleep is limited, the most reliable data to answer this question come from studies that use objective measures of sleep and hot flashes. Using such measures, Freedman and Roehrs *(92)* concluded that the link between hot flashes and awakenings is not as strong as was previously believed. This study of postmenopausal women found that "of awakenings occurring within 2 minutes of a hot flash, 55.2% occurred before, 40% after, and 5% simultaneously" *(92)*. In other words, a similar proportion of arousals and awakenings occur shortly after a hot flash, and therefore presumably were "caused" by a hot flash, as those that occur before a hot flash. A study of sleep in breast cancer survivors that also used objective measures of sleep and hot flashes found that the 10-minute periods around hot flashes included significantly more wake time and more stage changes to lighter sleep than other 10-minute periods during the night *(93)*. The difference in the populations sampled in these two studies might explain the apparent discrepancy in their findings as hot flashes that occur in the context of natural menopause might differ from those that occur in breast cancer patients. It is possible that the association between nocturnal hot flashes and awakenings might be mediated by another, yet unidentified, common pathway.

Other Factors Potentially Impacting Sleep of Postmenopausal Women

Factors other than unstable hormone levels and vasomotor symptoms may contribute to the disruption of sleep or to the perceived poor sleep quality in postmenopausal women. These include adjustment to role transition as children leave the home or aging parents require caregiving *(94)*, changes in health, and age-related alteration in the sleep regulation systems (such as impaired photic input) *(95)*. The relative contributions of the different factors have not been systematically investigated.

It is also not known what proportion of postmenopausal women, whose sleep continuity disturbance was triggered during the transition to menopause, develop chronic insomnia that persists even after other menopausal symptoms abate. For example, with time, the negative association between the bed and the unpleasant experience of tossing and turning in bed when unable to return to sleep could lead to increased sleep effort and hyper arousal. Both might render the bed a cue for sleep-related arousal that can serve to prolong insomnia.

Little is known about the treatment of peri- and postmenopausal insomnia. A randomized, controlled treatment study, which included 141 women with perimenopausal and postmenopausal insomnia, concluded that zolpidem 10 mg daily was well-tolerated and effective *(96)*. Preliminary results from a study that included 410 women with insomnia associated with the menopause transition, showed that subjects receiving eszopiclone reported significantly more improvements in sleep, compared with those subjects taking placebo *(97)*. Whereas brief cognitive behavioral therapy for insomnia is effective for the treatment of primary insomnia and its effects last long after the termination of treatment *(98–101)*, it is not known if it is equally effective for menopausal emergent insomnias.

SDB During Menopause

The prevalence of SDB increases with menopause, even after controlling for age and body mass index *(78,102,103)*. It is, therefore, important to assess SDB in postmenopausal women with complaints of snoring, daytime sleepiness, or unsatisfactory sleep *(104)*. A recent small study also underscores the importance of ruling out SDB in postmenopausal women with insomnia. This study found that 50% of postmenopausal women with insomnia had obstructive sleep apnea (OSA) *(105)*. Although the severity of SDB in postmenopausal women is not related to the severity of vasomotor symptoms or to circulating estradiol levels *(106)*, the incidence of SDB is lower in women on HRT *(78,103,107)* and estrogen therapy can reduce respiratory disturbance in postmenopausal women *(108)*.

The increased incidence of SDB in postmenopausal women is thought to be related to an increase in abdominal fat distribution *(109)* and a decline in estrogens and progestins *(110)*. The relevance of hormones to the presentation of SDB in postmenopausal women is evident from several lines of research. For example, the prevalence of SDB in postmenopausal women on HRT is similar to that found in premenopausal women *(102,107)*. Studies that experimentally induced hypocapnia found that the change in the end-tidal CO_2 at the apnea threshold was the highest in premenopausal women, with no difference between postmenopausal women and men *(111)*. Using a similar methodology, Rowley and colleagues *(111)* found that HRT increased the change in end-tidal CO_2 at the apnea threshold *(111)* lending further support for the role of progesterone in the regulation of breathing during sleep. Progesterone is also known to increase the ventilatory response to hypercapnia and hypoxia *(112–115)* and may increase activity of the upper-airway dilator muscles *(116)*. Although HRT might reduce SDB severity in postmenopausal women, continuous positive airway pressure remains the most effective treatment of SDB in both men and women.

SEX DIFFERENCES IN SLEEP AND SLEEP DISORDERS*

As described earlier, different stages of the reproductive cycle in women are associated with an increased prevalence and/or severity of self-reported sleep difficulty, insomnia, SDB, and RLS. Sex is also a relevant factor in the study of sleep and sleep disorders. Women have a more need for sleep, spend more time in bed, and have a longer sleep duration than men *(117,118)*. However, women report more sleep problems and poorer sleep quality than do men *(119,120)*. Women have an increased risk of suffering insomnia (risk ratio 1.41) across different age groups, which is the most pronounced among the elderly *(121)*. Women also are more likely than are men to be diagnosed with insomnia by a physician and to receive a prescription for a hypnotic *(119)*. Paradoxically, PSG recordings indicate that men have a more disturbed, lighter sleep *(122–124)*, and show a faster age-related decline in SWS than is seen in women *(123,125)*, although not all studies have found sex differences in sleep architecture *(126,127)*.

The sex difference in the prevalence of insomnia may be explained by several factors, including comorbid psychiatric illness and social factors. Women have an increased risk for psychiatric disorders that are associated with sleep disturbances such as depression. However, sex differences in sleep quality persist even after adjusting for comorbid psychiatric disorders in adults and in adolescents *(118,128)*. Even within depressed populations there is a sex difference in sleep architecture changes; depressed men are more likely to have deficiencies in SWS whereas depressed women are more likely to show ultradian rhythm abnormalities (low degree of synchronization between 90 minutes sleep EEG rhythms) compared with healthy controls *(129,130)*. Social role factors also cannot entirely explain the sex difference in insomnia *(131)*. It is likely that inherent biological differences contribute significantly to the sex difference in sleep quality and incidence of insomnia.

---

*The term *sex* is commonly used as a biological category of male or female and the term *gender* is most often used in reference to social or cultural categories (The American Heritage® book of English usage [digital]: a practical and authoritative guide to contemporary English. 1996; Available from: Bartleby.com).

As is the case for insomnia, the prevalence of RLS is approximately twice as high in women as in men *(132,133)*; however, there are few sex differences in the clinical presentation of RLS, based on self-reports *(134)*. In contrast, recent data suggest sex differences in some physiological markers of RLS such as changes in heart rate following a leg movement in periodic limb movement disorder *(135)* and in levels of cerebrospinal fluid ferritin *(136)*.

OSA is more common in men, with a male-to-female ratio of between 2:1 and 4:1 *(102,104,110,137,138)*. Biological sex differences in OSA can be explained by several mechanisms, including obesity pattern and fat distribution, upper airway anatomy and function, the control of breathing, and hormone status *(110)*.

CONCLUSIONS

Women's sleep is influenced by unique reproductive events such as the menstrual cycle, pregnancy, and menopause. At these different stages of the reproductive cycle, sleep quality as well as the incidence and presentation of sleep disorders varies and may also differ from that of men. The treatment of sleep disorders in women, therefore, should be considered in the context of their reproductive cycle.

REFERENCES

1. Baker FC, Driver HS (2004) Self-reported sleep across the menstrual cycle in young, healthy women. J Psychosom Res 56:239–243.
2. Manber R, Bootzin RR (1997) Sleep and the menstrual cycle. Health Psychol 16:209–214.
3. National Science Foundation NSF. *Women and Sleep Poll* 1998 [cited 2006 March 13]; Available from: http://web.archive.org/web/20040608054453/www.sleepfoundation.org/publications/1998womenpoll.cfm. Accessed Dec. 2006.
4. Kravitz HM, Janssen I, Santoro N, et al. (2005) Relationship of day-to-day reproductive hormone levels to sleep in midlife women. Arch Intern Med 165:2370–2376.
5. Dzaja A, Arber S, Hislop J, et al. (2005) Women's sleep in health and disease. J Psychiatr Res 39:55–76.
6. Moline ML, Broch L, Zak R, Gross V (2003) Sleep in women across the life cycle from adulthood through menopause. Sleep Med Rev 7:155–177.
7. Driver HS, Dijk DJ, Werth E, Biedermann K, Borbely AA (1996) Sleep and the sleep electroencephalogram across the menstrual cycle in young healthy women. J Clin Endocrinol Metab 81:728–735.
8. Ishizuka Y, Pollak CP, Shirakawa S, et al. (1994) Sleep spindle frequency changes during the menstrual cycle. J Sleep Res 3:26–29.
9. Lee KA, Shaver JF, Giblin EC, Woods NF (1990) Sleep patterns related to menstrual cycle phase and premenstrual affective symptoms. Sleep 13:403–409.
10. Baker FC, Driver HS, Paiker J, Rogers GG, Mitchell D (2002) Acetaminophen does not affect 24-h body temperature or sleep in the luteal phase of the menstrual cycle. J Appl Physiol 92:1684–1691.
11. Baker FC, Driver HS, Rogers GG, Paiker J, Mitchell D (1999) High nocturnal body temperatures and disturbed sleep in women with primary dysmenorrhea. Am J Physiol 277:E1013–E1021.
12. Baker FC, Waner JI, Vieira EF, Taylor SR, Driver HS, Mitchell D (2001) Sleep and 24 hour body temperatures: a comparison in young men, naturally cycling women and women taking hormonal contraceptives. J Physiol 530:565–574.
13. Lee KA, McEnany G, Zaffke ME (2000) REM sleep and mood state in childbearing women: sleepy or weepy? Sleep 23:877–885.
14. Parry BL, Mostofi N, LeVeau B, et al. (1999) Sleep EEG studies during early and late partial sleep deprivation in premenstrual dysphoric disorder and normal control subjects. Psychiatry Res 85:127–143.
15. Baker FC, Mitchell D, Driver HS (2001) Oral contraceptives alter sleep and raise body temperature in young women. Pflugers Arch 442:729–737.
16. Burdick RS, Hoffmann R, Armitage R (2002) Short note: oral contraceptives and sleep in depressed and healthy women. Sleep 25:347–349.

17. Henderson A, Nemes G, Gordon NB, Roos L (1970) Sleep of regularly menstruating women and of women taking an oral contraceptive. Psychophysiology 7:337.
18. American Academy of Sleep Medicine AAoSM, International classification of sleep disorders, revised: Diagnostic and coding manual. American Academy of Sleep Medicine, Chicago, 2001.
19. Suzuki H, Uchiyama M, Shibui K, Kim K, Tagaya H, Shinohara K (2002) Long-term rectal temperature measurements in a patient with menstrual-associated sleep disorder. Psychiatry Clin Neurosci 56:475–478.
20. Billiard M, Guilleminault C, Dement WC (1975) A menstruation-linked periodic hypersomnia. Kleine-Levin syndrome or new clinical entity? Neurology 25:436–443.
21. Sachs C, Persson HE, Hagenfeldt K (1982) Menstruation-related periodic hypersomnia: a case study with successful treatment. Neurology 32:1376–1379.
22. Papy JJ, Conte-Devolx B, Sormani J, Porto R, Guillaume V (1982) [The periodic hypersomnia and megaphagia syndrome in a young female, correlated with menstrual cycle (author's transl)]. Rev Electroencephalogr Neurophysiol Clin 12:54–61.
23. *American Psychiatric Association, Diagnostic and Statistical Manual of Mental Disorders (DSM-IV)*. 4th ed. American Psychiatric Association, Washington, DC, 1994.
24. Halbreich U (2004) The diagnosis of premenstrual syndromes and premenstrual dysphoric disorder—clinical procedures and research perspectives. Gynecol Endocrinol 19:320–334.
25. Mauri M (1990) Sleep and the reproductive cycle: a review. Health Care Women Int 11:409–421.
26. Chuong CJ, Kim SR, Taskin O, Karacan I (1997) Sleep pattern changes in menstrual cycles of women with premenstrual syndrome: a preliminary study. Am J Obstet Gynecol 177:554–558.
27. Parry B, Mendelson W, Duncan W, Sack D, Wher T (1989) Longitudinal sleep EEG, temperature, and activity measurements across the menstrual cycle in patients with premenstrual depression and age matched controls. Psychiatry Res 30:285–303.
28. Parry BL, Wehr TA (1987) Therapeutic effect of sleep deprivation in patients with premenstrual syndrome. Am J Psychiatry 144:808–810.
29. Parry BL, Udell C, Elliott JA, et al. (1997) Blunted phase-shift responses to morning bright light in premenstrual dysphoric disorder. J Biol Rhythms 12:443–456.
30. Krasnik C, Montori VM, Guyatt GH, Heels-Ansdell D, Busse JW (2005) The effect of bright light therapy on depression associated with premenstrual dysphoric disorder. Am J Obstet Gynecol 193:658–661.
31. Proctor M, Farquhar C (2006) Diagnosis and management of dysmenorrhoea. BMJ 332:1134–1138.
32. Dawood MY (1990) Dysmenorrhea. Clin Obstet Gynecol 33:168–178.
33. Kundermann B, Krieg J, Schreiber W (2004) The effect of deprivation on pain. Pain Res Manag 9:25–32.
34. Sheehan MT (2004) Polycystic ovarian syndrome: diagnosis and management. Clin Med Res 2:13–27.
35. Sartor BM, Dickey RP (2005) Polycystic ovarian syndrome and the metabolic syndrome. Am J Med Sci 330:336–342.
36. Dunaif A (1997) Insulin resistance and the polycystic ovary syndrome: mechanism and implications for pathogenesis. Endocr Rev 18:774–800.
37. Fogel RB, Malhotra A, Pillar G, Pittman SD, Dunaif A, White DP (2001) Increased prevalence of obstructive sleep apnea syndrome in obese women with polycystic ovary syndrome. J Clin Endocrinol Metab 86:1175–1180.
38. Tasali E, Van Cauter E, Ehrmann DA (2006) Relationships between sleep disordered breathing and glucose metabolism in polycystic ovary syndrome. J Clin Endocrinol Metab 91:36–42.
39. Vgontzas AN, Legro RS, Bixler EO, Grayev A, Kales A, Chrousos GP (2001) Polycystic ovary syndrome is associated with obstructive sleep apnea and daytime sleepiness: role of insulin resistance. J Clin Endocrinol Metab 86:517–520.
40. Gaylor E, Manber R (2005) Pregnancy and Postpartum. In: *Sleep Deprivation: Clinical Issues, Pharmacology, and Sleep Loss Effects*, (Kushida C, ed.); Marcel Dekker Inc, New York, pp. 177–194.
41. Lee KA, Caughey AB (2006) Evaluating insomnia during pregnancy and postpartum. In: *Sleep Disorders in Women: A Guide to Practical Management*, (Attarian HP, ed.) Humana Press, New Jersey, pp. 185–198.
42. Lee KA, Zaffke ME, McEnany G (2000) Parity and sleep patterns during and after pregnancy. Obstet Gynecol 95:14–18.
43. Schorr SJ, Chawla A, Devidas M, Sullivan CA, Naef RW 3rd, Morrison JC (1998) Sleep patterns in pregnancy: a longitudinal study of polysomnography recordings during pregnancy. J Perinatol 18:427–430.

44. Wolfson A, Crowley SJ, Anwer U, Bassett JL (2003) Changes in sleep patterns and depressive symptoms in first-time mothers: Last trimester to 1-year postpartum. Beh Sleep Med 1:54–67.
45. Baratte-Beebe KR, Lee K (1999) Sources of midsleep awakenings in childbearing women. Clin Nurs Res 8:386–397.
46. Evans ML, Dick MJ, Clark AS (1995) Sleep during the week before labor: relationships to labor outcomes. Clin Nurs Res 4:238–249, discussion 250–252.
47. Lee KA, Gay CL (2004) Sleep in late pregnancy predicts length of labor and type of delivery. Am J Obstet Gynecol 191:2041–2046.
48. Edwards N, Blyton DM, Hennessy A, Sullivan CE (2005) Severity of sleep-disordered breathing improves following parturition. Sleep 28:737–741.
49. Guilleminault C, Querra-Salva M, Chowdhuri S, Poyares D (2000) Normal pregnancy, daytime sleeping, snoring and blood pressure. Sleep Med 1:289–297.
50. Izci B, Vennelle M, Liston WA, Dundas KC, Calder AA, Douglas NJ (2006) Sleep-disordered breathing and upper airway size in pregnancy and post-partum. Eur Respir J 27:321–327.
51. Pien GW, Fife D, Pack AI, Nkwuo JE, Schwab RJ (2005) Changes in symptoms of sleep-disordered breathing during pregnancy. Sleep 28:1299–1305.
52. Connolly G, Razak AR, Hayanga A, Russell A, McKenna P, McNicholas WT (2001) Inspiratory flow limitation during sleep in pre-eclampsia: comparison with normal pregnant and nonpregnant women. Eur Respir J 18:672–676.
53. Edwards N, Blyton CM, Kesby GJ, Wilcox I, Sullivan CE (2000) Pre-eclampsia is associated with marked alterations in sleep architecture. Sleep 23:619–625.
54. Franklin KA, Holmgren PA, Jonsson F, Poromaa N, Stenlund H, Svanborg E (2000) Snoring, pregnancy-induced hypertension, and growth retardation of the fetus. Chest 117:137–141.
55. Manconi M, Govoni V, De Vito A, et al. (2004) Pregnancy as a risk factor for restless legs syndrome. Sleep Med 5:305–308.
56. Lee KA, Zaffke ME, Baratte-Beebe K (2001) Restless legs syndrome and sleep disturbance during pregnancy: the role of folate and iron. J Womens Health Gend Based Med 10:335–341.
57. Coble P, Reynolds CF, Kupfer DJ, Houck PR, Day NL, Giles DE (1994) Childbearing in women with and without a history of affective disorder. II. Electroencephalographic sleep. Compr Psychiatry 35:215–224.
58. Kang MJ, Matsumoto K, Shinkoda H, Mishima M, Seo YJ (2002) Longitudinal study for sleep-wake behaviours of mothers from pre-partum to post-partum using actigraph and sleep logs. Psychiatry Clin Neurosci 56:251–252.
59. Nishihara K, Horiuchi, S (1998) Changes in sleep patterns of young women from late pregnancy to postpartum: Relationships to their infants' movements. Percept Mot Skills 87:1043–1056.
60. Shinkoda H, Matsumoto K, Park YM (1999) Changes in sleep-wake cycle during the period from late pregnancy to puerperium identified through the wrist actigraph and sleep logs. Psychiatry Clin Neurosci 53:133–135.
61. Mosko S, Richard C, McKenna J (1997) Maternal sleep and arousals during bedsharing with infants. Sleep 20:142–150.
62. Quillin SI, Glenn LL (2004) Interaction between feeding method and co-sleeping on maternal-newborn sleep. J Obstet Gynecol Neonatal Nurs 33:580–588.
63. Blyton DM, Sullivan CE, Edwards N (2002) Lactation is associated with an increase in slow-wave sleep in women. J Sleep Res 11:297–303.
64. Gardiner A, Gay CL, Lee KA (2005) Sleep and fatigue in bed-sharing and room-sharing parents. 289(Abstract suppl): A76.
65. American Academy of Pediatrics Task Force on Sudden Infant Death Syndrome. (2005) The changing concept of sudden infant death syndrome: diagnostic coding shifts, controversies regarding the sleeping environment, and new variables to consider in reducing risk. Pediatrics 116:1245–1255.
66. Hiscock H, Wake M (2001) Infant sleep problems and postnatal depression: a community-based study. Pediatrics 107:1317–1322.
67. Hiscock H, Wake M (2002) Randomised controlled trial of behavioural infant sleep intervention to improve infant sleep and maternal mood. BMJ 324:1062–1065.
68. Kennedy HP, Beck CT, Driscoll JW (2002) A light in the fog: caring for women with postpartum depression. J Midwifery Womens Health 47:318–330.
69. Corral M, Kuan A, Kostaras D (2000) Bright light therapy's effect on postpartum depression. Am J Psychiatry 157:303–304.
70. Parry BL, Curran ML, Stuenkel CA, et al. (2000) Can critically timed sleep deprivation be useful in pregnancy and postpartum depressions? J Affect Disord 60:201–212.

71. Santoro N (2005) The menopausal transition. Am J Med 118:8–13.
72. Owens JF, Matthews KA (1998) Sleep disturbance in healthy middle-aged women. Maturitas, 30:41–50.
73. Kravitz HM, Ganz PA, Bromberger J, Powell LH, Sutton-Tyrrell K, Meyer PM (2003) Sleep difficulty in women at midlife: a community survey of sleep and the menopausal transition. Menopause 10:19–28.
74. Kuh DL, Wadsworth M, Hardy R (1997) Women's health in midlife: the influence of the menopause, social factors and health in earlier life. Br J Obstet Gynaecol 104:923–933.
75. Baker A, Simpson S, Dawson D (1997) Sleep disruption and mood changes associated with menopause. J Psychosom Res 43:359–369.
76. Woods NF, Mitchell ES (2005) Symptoms during the perimenopause: prevalence, severity, trajectory, and significance in women's lives. Am J Med 118:14–24.
77. Shin C, Lee S, Lee T, et al. (2005) Prevalence of insomnia and its relationship to menopausal status in middle-aged Korean women. Psychiatry Clin Neurosci 59:395–402.
78. Young T, Finn L, Austin D, Peterson A (2003) Menopausal status and sleep-disordered breathing in the Wisconsin Sleep Cohort Study. Am J Respir Crit Care Med 167:1181–1185.
79. Young T, Rabago D, Zgierska A, Austin D, Laurel F (2003) Objective and subjective sleep quality in premenopausal, perimenopausal, and postmenopausal women in the Wisconsin Sleep Cohort Study. Sleep 26:667–672.
80. Ohayon MM (2006) Severe hot flashes are associated with chronic insomnia. Arch Intern Med, 166:1262–1268.
81. Ford K, Sowers M, Crutchfield M, Wilson A, Jannausch M (2005) A longitudinal study of the predictors of prevalence and severity of symptoms commonly associated with menopause. Menopause 12:308–317.
82. Shaver J, Giblin E, Lentz M, Lee K (1988) Sleep patterns and stability in perimenopausal women. Sleep 11:556–561.
83. Kloss JD, Tweedy K, Gilrain K (2004) Psychological factors associated with sleep disturbance among perimenopausal women. Behav Sleep Med 2:177–190.
84. National Institutes of Health State-of-the-Science Conference statement: management of menopause-related symptoms. (2005) Ann Intern Med 142:1003–1013.
85. Sharkey KM, Bearpark HM, Acebo C, Millman RP, Cavallo A, Carskadon MA (2003) Effects of menopausal status on sleep in midlife women. Behav Sleep Med 1:69–80.
86. Kalleinen N, Polo O, Himanen SL, Joutsen A, Urrila AS, Polo-Kantola P (2006) Sleep deprivation and hormone therapy in postmenopausal women. Sleep Med 7:436–447.
87. Polo-Kantola P, Erkkola R, Irjala K, Helenius H, Pullinen S, Polo O (1999) Climacteric symptoms and sleep quality. Obstet Gynecol 94:219–224.
88. Woodward S, Freedman RR (1994) The thermoregulatory effects of menopausal hot flashes on sleep. Sleep 17:497–501.
89. Erlik Y, Tataryn IV, Meldrum DR, Lomax P, Bajorek JG, Judd HL (1981) Association of waking episodes with menopausal hot flushes. JAMA 245:1741–1744.
90. Hays J, Hunt JR, Hubbell FA, et al. (2003) The Women's Health Initiative recruitment methods and results. Ann Epidemiol 13:S18–S77.
91. Huang MI, Nir Y, Chen B, Schnyer R, Manber R (2006) A randomized controlled pilot study of acupuncture for postmenopausal hot flashes: effect on nocturnal hot flashes and sleep quality. Fertil Steril 86:700–710.
92. Freedman RR, Roehrs TA (2004) Lack of sleep disturbance from menopausal hot flashes. Fertil Steril 82:138–144.
93. Savard J, Davidson JR, Ivers H, et al. (2004) The association between nocturnal hot flashes and sleep in breast cancer survivors. J Pain Symptom Manage 27:513–522.
94. Hislop J, Arber S (2003) Sleep as a social act: a window on gender roles and relationships. In: *Gender and Ageing: Changing Roles and Relationships*, (Arber S, Davidson K, Ginn J, eds.) Open University Press, Maidenhead, pp. 186–205.
95. Herljevic M, Middleton B, Thapan K, Skene DJ (2005) Light-induced melatonin suppression: age-related reduction in response to short wavelength light. Exp Gerontol 40:237–242.
96. Dorsey CM, Lee KA, Scharf MB (2004) Effect of zolpidem on sleep in women with perimenopausal and postmenopausal insomnia: a 4-week, randomized, multicenter, double-blind, placebo-controlled study. Clin Ther 26:1578–1586.
97. Soares CN, Joffe H, Rubens R, Amato D, Roach J, Caron J (2006) Eszopiclone treatment during menopausal transition: sleep effects, impact on menopausal symptoms and mood. In: *American Psychiatric Association 159th Annual Meeting*. Toronto, Ontario, Canada, Abstract NR857.

98. Morin CM, Colecchi C, Stone J, Sood R, Brink D (1999) Behavioral and pharmacological therapies for late-life insomnia: a randomized controlled trial. JAMA 281:991–999.
99. Sivertsen B, Omvik S, Pallesen S, et al. (2006) Cognitive behavioral therapy vs zopiclone for treatment of chronic primary insomnia in older adults: a randomized controlled trial. JAMA 295:2851–2858.
100. Edinger JD, Wohlgemuth WK, Radtke RA, Marsh GR, Quillian RE (2001) Cognitive behavioral therapy for treatment of chronic primary insomnia: a randomized controlled trial. JAMA 285: 1856–1864.
101. Jacobs GD, Pace-Schott EF, Stickgold R, Otto MW (2004) Cognitive behavior therapy and pharmacotherapy for insomnia: a randomized controlled trial and direct comparison. Arch Intern Med 164: 1888–1896.
102. Bixler EO, Vgontzas AN, Lin HM, et al. (2001) Prevalence of sleep-disordered breathing in women: effects of gender. Am J Respir Crit Care Med 163:608–613.
103. Polo-Kantola P, Erkkola R, Helenius H, Irjala K, Polo O (1998) When does estrogen replacement therapy improve sleep quality? Am J Obstet Gynecol 178:1002–1009.
104. Kripke DF, Ancoli-Israel S, Klauber MR, Wingard DL, Mason WJ, Mullaney DJ (1997) Prevalence of sleep-disordered breathing in ages 40-64 years: a population-based survey. Sleep 20:65–76.
105. Hachul de Campos H, Brandao LC, D'Almeida V, et al. (2006) Sleep disturbances, oxidative stress and cardiovascular risk parameters in postmenopausal women complaining of insomnia. Climacteric 9:312–319.
106. Polo-Kantola P, Saaresranta T, Polo O (2001) Aetiology and treatment of sleep disturbances during perimenopause and postmenopause. CNS Drugs 15:445–452.
107. Shahar E, Redline S, Young T, et al. (2003) Hormone replacement therapy and sleep-disordered breathing. Am J Respir Crit Care Med 167:1186–1192.
108. Manber R, Kuo TF, Cataldo N, Colrain IM (2003) The effects of hormone replacement therapy on sleep-disordered breathing in postmenopausal women: a pilot study. Sleep 26:163–168.
109. Young T (1993) Analytic epidemiology studies of sleep disordered breathing—what explains the gender difference in sleep disordered breathing? Sleep 16:S1–S2.
110. Kapsimalis F, Kryger MH (2002) Gender and obstructive sleep apnea syndrome, part 2: mechanisms. Sleep 25:499–506.
111. Rowley JA, Zhou XS, Diamond MP, Badr MS (2006) The determinants of the apnea threshold during NREM sleep in normal subjects. Sleep 29:95–103.
112. Hannhart B, Pickett CK, Moore LG (1990) Effects of estrogen and progesterone on carotid body neural output responsiveness to hypoxia. J Appl Physiol 68:1909–1916.
113. Regensteiner JG, Woodard WD, Hagerman DD, et al. (1989) Combined effects of female hormones and metabolic rate on ventilatory drives in women. J Appl Physiol 66:808–813.
114. Zwillich CW, Natalino MR, Sutton FD, Weil JV (1978) Effects of progesterone on chemosensitivity in normal men. J Lab Clin Med 92:262–269.
115. Edwards N, Wilcox I, Polo OJ, Sullivan CE (1996) Hypercapnic blood pressure response is greater during the luteal phase of the menstrual cycle. J Appl Physiol 81:2142–2146.
116. Popovic RM, White DP (1998) Upper airway muscle activity in normal women: influence of hormonal status. J Appl Physiol 84:1055–1062.
117. Ferrara M, De Gennaro L (2001) How much sleep do we need? Sleep Med Rev 5:155–179.
118. Lindberg E, Janson C, Gislason T, Bjornsson E, Hetta J, Boman G (1997) Sleep disturbances in a young adult population: can gender differences be explained by differences in psychological status? Sleep 20:381–387.
119. Collop NA, Adkins D, Phillips BA (2004) Gender differences in sleep and sleep-disordered breathing. Clin Chest Med 25:257–268.
120. Reyner LA, Horne JA, Reyner A (1995) Gender- and age-related differences in sleep determined by home-recorded sleep logs and actimetry from 400 adults. Sleep 18:127–134.
121. Zhang B, Wing YK (2006) Sex differences in insomnia: a meta-analysis. Sleep 29:85–93.
122. Bixler EO, Kales A, Jacoby JA, Soldatos CR, Vela-Bueno A (1984) Nocturnal sleep and wakefulness: effects of age and sex in normal sleepers. Int J Neurosci 23:33–42.
123. Hume KI, Van F, Watson A (1998) A field study of age and gender differences in habitual adult sleep. J Sleep Res 7:85–094.
124. Williams RL, Karacan I, Hursch CJ (1974) *Electroencephalography (EEG) of Human Sleep: Clinical Applications*. John Wiley, New York.
125. Ehlers CL, Kupfer DJ (1997) Slow-wave sleep: do young adult men and women age differently? J Sleep Res 6:211–215.

126. Carrier J, Land S, Buysse DJ, Kupfer DJ, Monk TH (2001) The effects of age and gender on sleep EEG power spectral density in the middle years of life (ages 20-60 years old). Psychophysiology 38:232–242.
127. Voderholzer U, Al-Shajlawi A, Weske G, Feige B, Riemann D (2003) Are there gender differences in objective and subjective sleep measures? A study of insomniacs and healthy controls. Depress Anxiety 17:162–172.
128. Johnson EO, Roth T, Schultz L, Breslau N (2006) Epidemiology of DSM-IV insomnia in adolescence: lifetime prevalence, chronicity, and an emergent gender difference. Pediatrics 117:e247–e256.
129. Armitage R, Hoffmann R, Fitch T, Trivedi M, Rush AJ (2000) Temporal characteristics of delta activity during NREM sleep in depressed outpatients and healthy adults: group and sex effects. Sleep 23:607–617.
130. Armitage R, Hoffmann R, Trivedi M, Rush AJ (2000) Slow-wave activity in NREM sleep: sex and age effects in depressed outpatients and healthy controls. Psychiatry Res 95:201–213.
131. Chen WC, Lim PS, Wu WC, et al. (2006) Sleep behavior disorders in a large cohort of chinese (Taiwanese) patients maintained by long-term hemodialysis. Am J Kidney Dis 48:277–284.
132. Hogl B, Kiechl S, Willeit J, et al. (2005) Restless legs syndrome: a community-based study of prevalence, severity, and risk factors. Neurology 64:1920–1924.
133. Tison F, Crochard A, Leger D, Bouee S, Lainey E, El Hasnaoui A (2005) Epidemiology of restless legs syndrome in French adults: a nationwide survey: the INSTANT Study. Neurology 65:239–246.
134. Bentley AJ, Rosman KD, Mitchell D (2006) Gender differences in the presentation of subjects with restless legs syndrome. Sleep Med 7:37–41.
135. Gosselin N, Lanfranchi P, Michaud M, et al. (2003) Age and gender effects on heart rate activation associated with periodic leg movements in patients with restless legs syndrome. Clin Neurophysiol 114:2188–2195.
136. Earley CJ, Connor JR, Beard JL, Clardy SL, Allen RP (2005) Ferritin levels in the cerebrospinal fluid and restless legs syndrome: effects of different clinical phenotypes. Sleep 28:1069–1075.
137. Redline S, Kump K, Tishler PV, Browner I, Ferrette V (1994) Gender differences in sleep disordered breathing in a community-based sample. Am J Respir Crit Care Med 149:722–726.
138. Young T, Palta M, Dempsey J, Skatrud J, Weber S, Badr S (1993) The occurrence of sleep-disordered breathing among middle-aged adults. N Engl J Med 328:1230–1235.

20 Parasomnias in Adults

Ruth M. Benca, MD, PhD

CONTENTS

INTRODUCTION

The term parasomnia, meaning "around sleep," refers to a group of disorders that are characterized by "unpleasant or undesirable behavioral or experiential phenomena that occur predominantly or exclusively during the sleep period" *(1)*. Parasomnias have been categorized by the sleep state from which they arise, for example, nonrapid eye movement (NREM) sleep, rapid eye movement (REM) sleep, or those that are not specific to sleep state. They can also be categorized based on whether they are primary disorders of the sleep state from which they arise (e.g., sleepwalking) or are secondary to other medical or psychiatric disorders (e.g., nocturnal panic attacks). REM sleep behavior disorder and childhood parasomnias are covered elsewhere.

NREM PARASOMNIAS

Disorders of arousal during NREM sleep include *sleepwalking*, *night terrors*, and *confusional arousals*. These disorders are thought to occur as a result of sleep-state instability during NREM slow-wave sleep. Sleepwalking (somnambulism) may occur in up to 4% of adults, and behavior ranges from calm to agitated, as in children *(2)*. Night terrors or sleep terrors (pavor nocturnus) also occur in up to 4% of adults *(3)*; they are paroxysmal events that usually begin with a loud scream and are characterized by extreme fear, sometimes accompanied by violent behavior and/or running out of bed, which can result in injury. The term *confusional arousals* is used to describe partial arousals characterized by confusion, usually when subjects are aroused from slow-wave sleep during the early part of the night. Confusional arousals are seen in about 4% of adults *(2)*. *Sleep drunkenness* has also been used to describe the confusion, disorientation, impaired cognition, and behavioral disturbance that occurs following arousal of individuals with this disorder.

From: *Current Clinical Practice: Primary Care Sleep Medicine: A Practical Guide*
Edited by: J. F. Pagel and S. R. Pandi-Perumal © Humana Press Inc., Totowa, NJ

Although these disorders typically arise in childhood, they are also found in adults. They typically arise during slow-wave sleep and are therefore most common during the first one-third of the night, although they can also arise from other NREM stages and/or later in the night (e.g., sleep drunkenness upon arising in the morning). There may be a familial predisposition, and sleepwalking has been associated with the *HLA-DQB1* gene *(4)*. Subjects may have little or no recollection of the events, and are usually difficult to awaken fully in the midst of an episode, despite the fact that they may appear highly aroused or agitated.

Other factors that may precipitate or exacerbate these parasomnias in adults include alcohol and a variety of drugs such as sedative/hypnotics, benzodiazepines, antihistamines, lithium, and others that may increase arousal threshold *(5)*. Anxiety, sleep deprivation, fever, and endocrine factors (such as pregnancy) can also increase the frequency of episodes *(6)*. In adults, other primary sleep disorders such as apnea or periodic limb movements can trigger episodes as well. Parasomnias in adults are not generally associated with psychopathology *(7,8)*.

Related disorders include sleep-related eating disorder and sleep sex. In sleep-related eating disorder *(9–13)*, individuals may have episodes of eating at night, sometimes eating large amounts of high-calorie foods, typically, or even inappropriate or odd foods such as frozen or uncooked food, animal food, or kitchen cleaning compounds. Unlike the parasomnias above, these episodes can occur at any time in the sleep cycle and may occur multiple times per night. The prevalence is about 4% in adults, but may be as high as 8–17% in patients with eating disorders; the disorder occurs predominantly in women (75% of cases). The predisposing and exacerbating factors for sleep-related eating disorder are similar to those for the parasomnias above (e.g., primary sleep disorders, medications, and so on). *Sleep sex* describes sexual activity that occurs during sleep, without conscious awareness. It can be exacerbated by alcohol or sedative/hypnotic use as well.

Diagnosis of parasomnias is usually made by clinical history, but cases that are potentially dangerous to the patient or bed partner, are disruptive to the patient or family members, lead to excessive daytime sleepiness or other significant sequelae, or are associated with other medical/psychiatric/sleep disorders generally require further evaluation, including sleep laboratory studies. If nocturnal seizures are considered, an extended electroencephalography montage may be needed. Sleep laboratory evaluation of parasomnias must also include video monitoring. In some cases, more than one night of recording may be required. The differential diagnosis of the parasomnias described above includes nocturnal seizures, obstructive sleep apnea, nocturnal panic attacks, and REM sleep behavior disorder. Psychiatric disorders such as dissociative states or malingering may also present with similar features.

Treatment includes attention to good sleep hygiene and avoidance of sleep deprivation, alcohol, and drug use. The sleep environment should be assessed to avoid conditions that might lead to injury. In mild cases, reassurance may be adequate, but more severe or frequent episodes can be treated with medication. Benzodiazepines, tricyclic antidepressants, trazodone, and paroxetine have all been reported to be effective in some cases. Cognitive behavior therapy may also be helpful.

REM SLEEP PARASOMNIAS

Nightmares, frightening dreams that cause awakenings are the most common REM sleep-related parasomnia. Although they typically are characterized by fear and anxiety, they may also elicit feelings of intense sadness, anger, or disgust. Nightmares occur throughout the life-span and are more prevalent in childhood *(14,15)*; virtually everyone has had experienced at least one nightmare at some point in his or her lifetime. Frequent nightmares occur in less than 5% of young adults and in 1–2% of adults *(16)*. After childhood, women report nightmares more frequently than men *(17)*. A variety of psychiatric disorders are associated with complaints of nightmares, including depression, anxiety disorders (particularly post-traumatic stress disorder, generalized anxiety disorder, and panic disorder), and substance abuse disorders. It is not clear if psychiatric patients actually have more nightmares or simply report them more; subjects without psychiatric disorders are known to underreport the frequency of nightmares *(18,19)*. Women are more frequently affected than men, possibly related to their increased tendency for depression and anxiety disorders. There also appears to be a genetic component for nightmares, based on a twin cohort study *(20)*.

Increased rates of nightmares have been reported in association with a number of medications, particularly those that affect monoaminergic systems (e.g., amphetamines, antidepressants, β-blockers, catecholamines, and antiparkinsonian agents) *(21,22)*. Sedative/hypnotics and barbiturates may also lead to nightmares as well as withdrawal from barbiturates and alcohol. REM sleep behavior disorder is covered elsewhere.

OTHER PARASOMNIAS

A variety of other parasomnias, many of which are related to medical or psychiatric disorders, have been described. There are also several sleep-related behaviors that are not considered to be pathologic. Sleeptalking (somniloquy) is common, occurs in all sleep stages and is not considered as a disorder. Hypnic jerks or sleep starts typically occur during the transition from waking to sleep and are also quite common in the general population. Typically, they are characterized by a sudden jerk, often accompanied by the sense of falling. In more complicated cases, they may also include visual hallucinations, or auditory experiences (sudden loud noise), or other sensory phenomena. In some cases, they can be repetitive. They may be exacerbated by sleep deprivation. Exploding head syndrome likely is a variation of sleep starts; it is an abrupt arousal accompanied by hearing a loud noise, sometimes described as an exploding sound in the head. Given the benign nature of these conditions, they usually do not require treatment.

Bruxism, or teeth grinding, occurs in up to 20% of children and decreases with age *(23)*. It can occur in any stage of sleep, although may be more common in stages 1 and 2 as well as in supine sleep *(24–26)*. Nocturnal bruxism may cause jaw pain and tooth sensitivity during waking. Factors that contribute to bruxism include genetic/familial predisposition and medications (e.g., serotonin reuptake inhibitors, amphetamines, antipsychotics) *(27)*. Bruxism may lead to excessive wear or damage to teeth, and is often treated with splints. A variety of other treatments are in widespread use, but without clear evidence regarding efficacy; these include cognitive behavior therapy, antidepressants, benzodiazepines, nonsteroidal antiinflammatory drugs, dopaminergic agents, and propranolol.

Catathrenia or sleep-related expiratory groaning *(28)* can be particularly disturbing to bed partners or family members. It occurs in NREM or REM sleep, and consists of a loud and prolonged groan with exhaling. It is not known to be associated with any significant medical or psychiatric illnesses and does not respond to treatments for other sleep disorders, including medications or continuous positive airway pressure. A variety of medical conditions can become exacerbated during sleep and lead to arousals, including sleep-related headaches, cardiac arrhythmias, angina pectoris, asthma, gastroesophageal reflux, tinnitus, muscle cramps, pruritis related to dermatological conditions, and sweating (night sweats).

FORENSIC ISSUES

Because of the nature of some parasomnias, there is potential for patients to engage in violent or injurious behavior while not fully conscious. The criteria for evaluating sleep-related violence, as developed by Mahowald and colleagues *(29)*, include the following:

1. Reason from individual's history to suspect a sleep disorder, based on similar episodes in the past.
2. Duration of the activity is brief (minutes, not hours).
3. The behavior is abrupt, impulsive, and senseless (i.e., without apparent motivation).
4. The victim is someone who happened to be nearby.
5. After fully awakening, the individual is horrified and does not attempt to conceal the action.
6. Some degree of amnesia may persist.
7. If a slow-wave sleep parasomnia, the action may have occurred at least 1 hour after sleep onset or on attempts to awaken the subject, and/or it may have been potentiated by alcohol, drugs, or sleep deprivation.

REFERENCES

1. Mahowald MW, Cramer Bornemann MA (2005) NREM sleep-arousal parasomnias. In: *Principles and Practice of Sleep Medicine*. 4th ed. (Kryger MH, Roth T, Dement WC, eds.) Elsevier Saunders, Philadelphia, PA, pp. 889–896.
2. Ohayon MM, Guilleminault C, Priest RG (1999) Night terrors, sleepwalking, and confusional arousals in the general population: their frequency and relationship to other sleep and mental disorders. J Clin Psychiatry 60:268–276.
3. Crisp AH (1996) The sleepwalking/night terrors syndrome in adults. Postgrad Med J 72:599–604.
4. Lecendreux M, Bassetti C, Dauvilliers Y, et al. (2003) HLA and genetic susceptibility to sleepwalking. Mol Psychiatry 8:114–117.
5. Mendelson WB (1994) Sleepwalking associated with zolpidem. J Clin Psychopharmacol 14:150.
6. Mahowald MW, Schenck CH (2005) Non-rapid eye movement sleep parasomnias. Neurol Clin 23:1077–1106, vii.
7. Schenck CH, Milner DM, Hurwitz TD, et al. (1989) A polysomnographic and clinical report on sleep-related injury in 100 adult patients. Am J Psychiatry 146:1166–1173.
8. Llorente MD, Currier MB, Norman SE, et al. (1992) Night terrors in adults: phenomenology and relationship to psychopathology. J Clin Psychiatry 53:392–394.
9. Benca RM, Schenck CH (2005) Sleep and eating disorders. In: *Principles and Practice of Sleep Medicine*. 4th ed. (Kryger MH, Roth T, Dement WC, eds.) Elsevier Saunders, Philadelphia, PA, pp. 1337–1344.
10. Schenck CH, Hurwitz TD, Bundlie SR, et al. (1991) Sleep-related eating disorders: polysomnographic correlates of a heterogeneous syndrome distinct from daytime eating disorders. Sleep 14:419–431.
11. Schenck CH, Hurwitz TD, O'Connor KA, et al. (1993) Additional categories of sleep-related eating disorders and the current status of treatment. Sleep 16:457–466.
12. Schenck CH, Mahowald MW (1994) Review of nocturnal sleep-related eating disorders. Int J Eat Disord 15:343–356.
13. Winkelman JW (1998) Clinical and polysomnographic features of sleep-related eating disorder. J Clin Psychiatry 59:14–19.
14. Salzarulo P, Chevalier A (1983) Sleep problems in children and their relationship with early disturbances of the waking-sleeping rhythms. Sleep 6:47–51.

15. Fisher BE, Pauley C, McGuire K (1989) Children's sleep behavior scale: normative data on 870 children in grades 1 to 6. Percept Mot Skills 68:227–236.
16. Partinen M (1994) Epidemiology of sleep disorders. In: *Principles and Practice of Sleep Medicine.* 2nd ed. (Kryger MH, Roth T, Dement WC, eds.) Elsevier Saunders, Philadelphia, PA, pp. 437–452.
17. Coren S (1994) The prevalence of self-reported sleep disturbances in young adults. Int J Neurosci 79:67–73.
18. Zadra A, Donderi DC (2000) Nightmares and bad dreams: their prevalence and relationship to well-being. J Abnorm Psychol 109:273–281.
19. Wood JM, Bootzin RR (1990) The prevalence of nightmares and their independence from anxiety. J Abnorm Psychol 99:64–68.
20. Hublin C, Kaprio J, Partinen M, et al. (1999) Nightmares: familial aggregation and association with psychiatric disorders in a nationwide twin cohort. Am J Med Genet 88:329–336.
21. Thompson DF, Pierce DR (1999) Drug-induced nightmares. Ann Pharmacother 33:93–98.
22. Pagel JF, Helfter P (2003) Drug induced nightmares: an etiology based review. Hum Psychopharmacol 18:59–67.
23. Montplaisir J, Allen RP, Walters AS, et al. (2005) Restless legs syndrome and periodic limb movements during sleep. In: *Principles and Practice of Sleep Medicine*. 4th ed. (Kryger MH, Roth T, Dement WC, eds.) Elsevier Saunders, Phildelphia, PA, pp. 839–852.
24. Lavigne GJ, Rompre PH, Montplaisir JY (1996) Sleep bruxism: validity of clinical research diagnostic criteria in a controlled polysomnographic study. J Dent Res 75:546–552.
25. Macaluso GM, Guerra P, Di Giovanni G, et al. (1998) Sleep bruxism is a disorder related to periodic arousals during sleep. J Dent Res 77:565–573.
26. Miyawaki S, Lavigne GJ, Pierre M, et al. (2003) Association between sleep bruxism, swallowing-related laryngeal movement, and sleep positions. Sleep 26:461–465.
27. Lavigne GJ, Manzini C, Kato T (2005) Sleep bruxism. In: *Principles and Practice of Sleep Medicine.* 4th ed. (Kryger MH, Roth T, Dement WC, eds.) Elsevier Saunders, Philadelphia, PA, pp. 946–959.
28. Vetrugno R, Provini F, Plazzi G, et al. (2001) Catathrenia (nocturnal groaning): a new type of parasomnia. Neurology 56:681–683.
29. Mahowald MW, Bundlie SR, Hurwitz TD, et al. (1990) Sleep violence—forensic science implications: polygraphic and video documentation. J Forensic Sci 35:413–432.

21 Clinical Features, Diagnosis, and Treatment of Narcolepsy

Lois E. Krahn, MD

CONTENTS

INTRODUCTION

Narcolepsy, a chronic sleep disorder that typically begins at a young age, has the potential to greatly disrupt social, educational, and vocational development. Because of the nature of its symptoms (e.g., excessive daytime sleepiness and cataplexy, in particular), narcolepsy provides insights to mechanisms regarding human sleep regulation. Its universal symptom of inappropriate daytime sleepiness probably contributes most substantially to the resulting impaired quality of life that has been documented *(1)*. A specific and intriguing sign of narcolepsy, experienced by 60% of patients, is cataplexy, or transient muscle weakness triggered by emotions. Other classic, but less specific symptoms include sleep paralysis and hypnagogic hallucinations. Disturbed nocturnal sleep is the most recent addition to the constellation of symptoms.

Narcolepsy is an uncommon but not rare sleep disorder that occurs in 0.05% of the population *(2)*. In contrast to most other sleep disorders, it begins at a younger age, generally in the second decade of life and is a chronic process. Narcolepsy is difficult to diagnose; the typical patient is symptomatic for 10 years before the diagnosis is established *(3)*. Multiple factors contribute to the challenges of diagnosing narcolepsy more promptly. These factors include the extensive differential diagnosis of excessive daytime sleepiness, which includes voluntary sleep restriction, obstructive sleep apnea, circadian rhythm disorders (such as delayed sleep phase disorder), chemical dependency, and mood disorder *(4)*. Another relevant factor is the cost and lack of access to very carefully conducted diagnostic sleep studies. For patients taking psychotropic medications, including psychostimulants or antidepressants prescribed for other indications,

From: *Current Clinical Practice: Primary Care Sleep Medicine: A Practical Guide*
Edited by: J. F. Pagel and S. R. Pandi-Perumal © Humana Press Inc., Totowa, NJ

an adequate washout must be obtained before sleep studies can proceed. Sometimes narcolepsy is suspected and diagnostic testing is undertaken without taking this step, yielding false-negative results that further delay the diagnosis of this condition.

CLINICAL FEATURES

In addition to the excessive daytime sleepiness associated with narcolepsy, cataplexy incurs in 60% of patients with this disorder; recognizing these symptoms is often problematic *(2)*. This is because cataplexy can be subtle enough to go unrecognized by patients and clinicians alike. The differential diagnosis of cataplexy includes complex partial seizures, syncope, and events related to psychological factors akin to a pseudoseizure *(5)*. The preserved consciousness, that is invariably associated with cataplexy, aids in discriminating these episodes from those with different pathophysiological mechanisms. Confirming the absence of deep tendon reflexes during the cataplectic episode can also be a useful physical examination procedure.

Classic cataplexy is a transient bilateral loss of muscle strength that is typically triggered by a positive emotion, such as laughter. The patient's symptoms can range from a slumping of the head and subtle weakness of the knees, to episodes where a patient gradually loses muscle strength throughout their body and collapses on the ground. The patient remains conscious and can recall events taking place during the episode. It is no longer believed that patients commonly transition from cataplexy into rapid eye movement (REM) sleep *(6)*. Patients generally are not injured by falls related to cataplexy, because the weakness develops progressively, allowing patients an opportunity to sit or lie down abruptly to break the fall *(7)*. The literature describes cataplexy as becoming a less common occurrence throughout the lifetime of the patient with narcolepsy and cataplexy. However, there are published cases of cataplexy starting well after the onset of excessive daytime sleepiness and persisting throughout the life-span of a patient.

Hypnagogic hallucinations may also occur with narcolepsy, and these are often upsetting for patients. On awakening, a patient may have difficulty determining whether such perceptions are real or part of a dream. Thus, there are published reports of patients with narcolepsy being misdiagnosed with schizophrenia *(8)*. As narcolepsy and schizophrenia both become better understood, little evidence has been found to support that the REM intrusion found in narcolepsy plays any role in schizophrenia. Nonetheless, the vivid, bizarre dreams of a patient with narcolepsy can be difficult to distinguish from chronic psychotic symptoms, based on clinical interview alone. These phenomena in narcolepsy are characterized by their primarily visual, and sometimes tactile nature, rather than an auditory form found in chronic psychotic disorders. These symptoms can also be distinguished from other clinical phenomena by their tendency to occur exclusively during the transition from sleeping to waking. Some patients find these dreams so distressing that they dread falling asleep and often awaken feeling emotionally distressed, which may contribute to their disturbed nocturnal sleep.

Sleep paralysis is another symptom experienced by many patients with narcolepsy and cataplexy. These episodes tend to be more prolonged than cataplexy but in many ways, are similar. Patients are unable to move voluntarily. Sleep paralysis occurs at the sleep–wake transition. As these episodes can be accompanied by hypnopompic or hypnagogic hallucinations, patients sometimes can have a frightening experience of feeling that they need to flee because of their frightening dream but are unable to move *(9)*. Difficulty with sleep maintenance was not included as part of the tetrad of narcolepsy symptoms first described in 1957 by Yoss and Daley *(10)*. Since then, investigators have become more aware of the relatively high prevalence of this symptom *(9)*. The causes of nocturnal awakenings are numerous (e.g., frightening dreams, coexisting obstructive sleep apnea, parasomnia, periodic limb movements, and the alerting affects of psychostimulant medications).

EVALUATION

When unequivocal cataplexy is present, many clinicians agree that narcolepsy can be diagnosed on the basis of the patient's clinical history alone *(11)*. Episodes of brief, reversible, bilateral muscle weakness provoked exclusively by laughter is the most specific symptom of narcolepsy, and essentially pathognomonic for this condition. However, cataplexy is often difficult to confirm. For patients who have narcolepsy without cataplexy, given the extensive differential diagnosis of excessive daytime sleepiness, laboratory sleep studies are necessary. Also, because the treatment of narcolepsy warrants the long-term use of many medications that are on the US Drug Enforcement Administration Schedule II or III, most practitioners prefer to base their diagnoses on laboratory testing. Clinicians must be alert to the possibility that a patient with drug dependence may simply be fabricating a history of sleep problems to obtain, in particular, psychostimulants. Human leukocyte antigen testing can support a diagnosis of narcolepsy, but it is certainly not conclusive. The *DQB1*0602* allele is found in 30% of the normal population, whereas it is lacking in some well-characterized patients who have narcolepsy with cataplexy *(12)*. This allele is found in 85% of patients with clear-cut cataplexy.

Sleep studies directed toward possible narcolepsy must be carefully planned and include more than polysomnography. Initial sleep testing is not always diagnostic and sometimes needs to be repeated at a later date. This is especially true because the symptoms of narcolepsy with or without cataplexy may develop over time. Also, medications that are sedating or alter REM sleep, in particular antidepressants, may interfere with testing. Optimal diagnostic testing includes a tool to characterize the patient's sleep–wake schedule over time. Having the patient keep a sleep diary for 1–2 weeks, ideally in conjunction with wrist actigraphy for more objective data, can be invaluable. The presence of an irregular sleep–wake cycle or circadian-rhythm issue, such as a delayed sleep phase, may invalidate subsequent testing. For example, a patient with a pronounced delayed sleep phase may have sleep-onset REM episodes occurring during a multiple sleep latency test (MSLT) that simply reflect delayed night time sleep, rather than daytime REM intrusion. An MSLT can be conducted in a manner that avoids this issue by coordinating the start time to match the patient's typical sleep–wake pattern. Assessment of the sleep–wake rhythm also can reveal that a patient has chronically insufficient sleep. Sleep deprivation can lead to a false-positive MSLT with REM sleep present, because the sleep depth increases REM pressure *(13)*. However, because disruptive night time sleep affects many patients with narcolepsy, it is sometimes not feasible to restrict an MSLT to patients who obtain ≥8 hours of sleep a day. The clinician must carefully review the patient's circumstances to determine if the patient has obtained adequate sleep to get a reliable MSLT. The standard of care to control sleep deprivation and to look for other explanations of excessive daytime sleepiness is to use a polysomnography before the MSLT to verify that the patient gets at least 6 hours of sleep at night. Ideally, the patient would get 7–8 hours of sleep the night before the MSLT.

The MSLT is the pivotal test for the diagnosis of narcolepsy. This daytime sleep study requires the patient to take four or five naps, during which the mean time to sleep onset and the presence of REM sleep are measured. The presence of REM sleep during two or more daytime naps is a currently accepted laboratory marker of narcolepsy. The mechanism behind this abnormally regulated REM sleep appears to be a dysfunctional switching mechanism that leads to the inappropriate intrusion of non-REM sleep or wakefulness during sleep *(14)*. To improve the validity of the MSLT, it should be interpreted within the context of the patient's clinical history. Cataplexy, sleep paralysis, and hypnagogic hallucinations may all be related to inappropriately regulated REM sleep or absent muscle tone, which is an isolated component of this sleep stage.

PATHOGENESIS

The exact mechanisms of these phenomena have not been conclusively demonstrated. Considerable evidence points to the deficiency of a recently described neuropeptide, known as hypocretin (also known as orexin) *(15)*. The neuropeptide can be reliably measured in human cerebrospinal fluid. At this time, the test has not yet become part of the standard diagnostic testing protocol for narcolepsy and cataplexy. The reasons are that there is no commercially available assay. The assays conducted in research settings have, until recently, been fraught with some quality assurance issues. At this point, other than cerebral spinal fluid, hypocretin deficiency cannot be documented in any other body fluid *(9)*. Attempts to develop a serum-based test have been unsuccessful, despite conflicting reports in the literature.

The International Classification of Sleep Disorders second edition modified the classification in use for narcolepsy subdividing this condition into the following four types:

1. Narcolepsy with cataplexy.
2. Narcolepsy without cataplexy.
3. Narcolepsy owing to medical condition.
4. Narcolepsy, unspecified.

The intent was to differentiate between narcolepsy with and without cataplexy on the basis that these conditions have different symptoms. These conditions do share the common abnormality of sleep architecture with REM sleep occurring abruptly during daytime naps. However the deficiency in the cerebro spinal fluid of the neuropeptide hypocretin applies only to narcolepsy with cataplexy. Nonetheless, in part to prevent potential disruption in access to treatment for many patients diagnosed with narcolepsy without cataplexy, these conditions were not separated in distinct diseases but renamed to be specific about the presence of cataplexy, as well as a relationship to a medical or neurological disorder. The medical disorders observed to cause narcolepsy with cataplexy include hypothalamic tumors or sarcoidosis, Niemann-Pick type C disease, and paraneoplastic syndrome with anti-Ma2 antibodies. For head trauma, multiple sclerosis, myotonic dystrophy, Prader-Willi syndrome, Parkinson's disease, and multiple system atrophy, rare cases have been associated with narcolepsy without cataplexy. In the most persuasive cases, the narcoleptic symptoms begin shortly after the onset of the other disease state.

TREATMENT

Because of the diverse symptomatology that can affect patients with narcolepsy, the treatment of this sleep disorder can be a complex process. Establishing the diagnosis is only the first phase of improving the quality of life of a patient with this chronic sleep disorder. Patient education is necessary to emphasize the importance of optimal sleep hygiene, as well as a consistent sleep–wake schedule to facilitate getting adequate sleep *(16)*. In addition to behavioral interventions, a simulating or alerting agent is typically used. Modafinil 200–400 mg/day is a Food and Drug Administration (FDA)-approved treatment for excessive daytime sleepiness associated with narcolepsy. It has been demonstrated to be effective to reduce the severity of mild-to-moderate sleepiness *(17)*. Modafinil is generally well tolerated but does have several side effects, of which headache is the most common. Unlike the psychostimulant medications, modafinil, although beneficial for excessive daytime sleepiness, does not appear to reduce cataplexy directly. The psychostimulants methylphenidate or amphetamine are often first-line choices for patients with severe, excessive daytime sleepiness *(4)*. Most of these agents have FDA indications for attention deficit hyperactivity disorder but have long been known to work for narcolepsy. The newer formulations that offer extended or continuous release are often especially valuable, because they have a longer duration of action. Many patients require treatment only with a stimulating agent. As daytime sleepiness is decreased, cataplectic episodes often become less frequent owing to an indirect effect. Generally, the higher the degree of sleepiness, the more likely it is for a patient to enter a cataplectic state.

For patients with cataplexy severe enough to warrant targeted treatment, antidepressant medications have been the mainstay of this treatment for years *(4)*. However, no antidepressant has a FDA indication for cataplexy. The more noradrenergic compounds, such as imipramine, venlafaxine, and duloxetine, are viewed as the most effective treatments for cataplexy. Side effects (e.g., constipation and cardiac conduction delay) may be limiting factors for some patients who use tricyclic agents. One published report of a small pilot study has indicated that selective noradrenergic reuptake inhibitor reboxetine is efficacious *(18)*. Selective serotonin reuptake inhibitors have also been prescribed for cataplexy. Although generally less effective, this class of antidepressant may be an appropriate choice because of its different profile of side effects.

Sodium oxybate received FDA approval in 2002 for its use in the treatment of cataplexy. This novel CNS depressant has an unknown mechanism of action but is believed to act through the mechanism of γ-aminobutyric acid. The main clinical effect is a pronounced increase in slow-wave sleep. γ-Aminobutyric acid appears to consolidate sleep and is associated with the reduction in cataplectic episodes *(19)*. To reduce the chance of injuries resulting from the rapid onset of sleepiness, this liquid medication is taken after the patient has gotten to bed. Patients may also experience enuresis, because they enter deep sleep and have a higher arousal threshold. In clinical trials, enuresis was reported in 9% of patients, but less than 1% discontinued the medication for this reason *(20)*. Sleepwalking has also been reported with prevalences ranging from 7 to 32%. Sleepwalking was identified as the reason for discontinuing sodium oxybate in 1% of patients. Because serious injury is possible during sleepwalking, patients should be advised to assess their sleeping environment carefully. Barriers should be placed to restrict access to potential hazards, such as staircases, windows, and balconies. The dose of sodium oxybate may need to be reduced, or even discontinued, in the rare cases that a patient appears to be at risk of serious injury because of a non-REM parasomnia. After trials with other medications, and despite the prospect of sleepwalking and enuresis, the benefits of sodium oxybate to treat daytime sleepiness can greatly outweigh the risks for patients with an unsatisfactory quality of life.

CONCLUSIONS

Narcolepsy with cataplexy remains difficult to detect and diagnose, even with the recent understanding of its association with hypocretin deficiency. Hopefully, new diagnostic tests will become available that utilize this finding. In the meantime, diagnostic testing must be conducted under rigorous conditions in order to prevent false-negative, as well as false-positive, diagnoses. The traditional treatment approach typically involves a set of diverse psychoactive medications that target the multiple symptoms of this fascinating sleep disorder.

REFERENCES

1. Broughton R, Guberman A, Roberts J (1984) Comparison of the psychosocial effects of epilepsy and narcolepsy/cataplexy: a controlled study. Epilepsia 25:423–433.
2. Silber M, Krahn L, Olson E, et al. (2002) The epidemiology of narcolepsy in Olmsted County, Minnesota: a population-based study. Sleep 25:197–202.
3. Aldrich M (1998) Diagnostic aspects of narcolepsy. Neurology 50(Suppl 1):S2–S7.
4. Krahn L, Black J, Silber M (2001) Narcolepsy: new understanding of irresistible sleep. Mayo Clin Proc 76:185–194.
5. Krahn L, Hansen M, Shepard J (2001) Pseudocataplexy. Psychosomatics 42:356–358.
6. Krahn L, Boeve B, Olson E, et al. (2000) A standardized test for cataplexy. Sleep Med 1:125–130.
7. Rubboli G, d'Orse G, Zaniboni A, et al. (2000) A video-polygraphic analysis of the cataplectic attack. Clin Neurophysiol 111(Suppl 2):S120–S128.
8. Shapiro B, Sptiz H (1976) Problems in the differential diagnosis of narcolepsy versus schizophrenia. Am J Psychiatry 133:1321–1323.
9. Overeem S, Mignot E, Gert van Dijk J, et al. (2001) Narcolepsy: clinical features, new pathophysiologic insights, and future perspectives. J Clin Neurophysiol 18:78–105.
10. Yoss R, Daly D (1957) Criteria for the diagnosis of the narcoleptic syndrome. Procedural Staff Meeting, Mayo Clinic vol. 32, pp. 320–328.
11. Parkes J, Fenton G, Struthers G, et al. (1974) Narcolepsy and cataplexy: clinical features, treatment and cerebrospinal fluid findings. Q J Med 43:525–536.
12. Mignot E, Hayduk R, Black J, et al. (1997) HLA DQB1*0602 is associated with cataplexy in 509 narcoleptic patients. Sleep 20:1012–1020.
13. Aldrich M, Chervin R, Malow B (1997) Value of the multiple sleep latency test (MSLT) for the diagnosis of narcolepsy. Sleep 20:620–629.
14. Scammell T (2003) The neurobiology, diagnosis and treatment of narcolepsy. Ann Neurol 53:154–166.
15. Mignot E, Lammers G, Ripley B, et al. (2002) The role of cerebrospinal fluid hypocretin measurement in the diagnosis of narcolepsy and other hypersomnias. Arch Neurol 59:1553–1562.
16. Garma L, Marchand F (1994) Non-pharmacological approaches to the treatment of narcolepsy. Sleep 17:S97–S102.
17. Mitler M, Harsh J, Hirshkowitz M, et al. (2000) Long-term efficacy and safety of modafinil (Provigil) for the treatment of excessive daily sleepiness associated with narcolepsy. Sleep Med 1:231–243.
18. Larrosa O, de la Llave Y, Bario S, et al. (2001) Stimulant and anticataplectic effects of reboxetine in patients with narcolepsy: a pilot study. Sleep 24:282–285.
19. Lammers G, Arends J, Declerck A, et al. (1993) Gamma-hydroxybutyrate and narcolepsy: a double blind placebo-controlled study. Sleep 16:216–220.
20. Reference PD (2004) *Xyrem Oral Solution*. Orphan Medical, Minnetonka, MN.

22 Mental Disorders Associated With Disturbed Sleep

Lois E. Krahn, MD

CONTENTS

INTRODUCTION

Clinicians are well aware that many psychiatric disorders are associated with disturbed sleep. As many as 3% of people in the community may have "insomnia related to mental disorders," a subtype of insomnia in the second edition of the *International Classification of Sleep Disorders (1)*. Insomnia is not the only sleep condition of interest when focusing on this population because excessive daytime sleepiness and rapid eye movement (REM) parasomnia can also be linked with psychiatric illness. Because of the variety of the conditions that can compromise sleep quality, identifying, and effectively managing sleep issues in the context of psychiatric disease requires knowledge of the pertinent psychiatric and sleep issues.

MOOD DISORDERS

Depressed patients often seek out medical care because of unsatisfactory or unrefreshing sleep. For decades psychiatrists and neuroscientists have examined the association between mood and sleep. The long-recognized relationship between sleep architecture, specifically reduced initial rapid eye movement (REM) latency and major depression, and has the potential to promote better understanding of the pathophysiological mechanisms of mood disorders.

According to the *Diagnostic and Statistical Manual of Mental Disorders*, Fourth Edition (DSM-IV) *(2)*, major depression involves a constellation of at least five symptoms, one of which is disturbed sleep. More than 90% of patients with major depression have sleep disturbances *(3)*. Insomnia, encompassing initial insomnia, sleep maintenance difficulties, and early morning awakenings, is the most common sleep symptom.

From: *Current Clinical Practice: Primary Care Sleep Medicine: A Practical Guide*
Edited by:J. F. Pagel and S. R. Pandi-Perumal © Humana Press Inc., Totowa, NJ

Major depression is a common medical problem with lifetime prevalence of 20% in the United States.

Twenty percent of patients with insomnia have major depression; women with depression are more likely to experience insomnia than men *(4)*. The presence of insomnia is risk factor for the development of major depression within the following year *(5)*. Because insomnia is a common symptom of major depression, controversy exists over whether insomnia is actually risk factor or rather a precursor symptom indicating an evolving depressive episode. Conceiving of insomnia as a precursor symptom is plausible because the two conditions have been theorized to have a similar mechanism of hyperarousal or an elevated level of alertness. In both conditions, increased cortisol or adrenocorticotropic hormone levels have been reported, suggesting an aberrant hypothalamic pituitary axis.

In addition to having delayed sleep onset, patients with major depression classically awaken 2–4 hours earlier than desired and are unable to fall back to sleep *(6)*. During the day, depressed patients report fatigue more likely than objective excessive daytime sleepiness. However, in atypical major depression, patients may have hypersomnia and increased appetite in place of insomnia and anorexia. Pharmacological treatment of depression can potentially exacerbate sleep difficulties. Selective serotonin reuptake inhibitors (SSRIs), the prototype of which is fluoxetine, and the newer selective serotonin norepinephrine reuptake inhibitors, the prototype is duloxetine, are known to sometimes cause insomnia in the first phase of treatment, generally resolving within a week. Over the course of the first month of therapy, as the depressive symptoms respond as a group, the insomnia has been expected to respond as well. Even a more stimulating antidepressant, as long as it modulates some of the underlying neurochemical abnormalities of major depression, should with time lead to remission. Nonetheless, there are indications that insomnia may be more refractory to treatment than other symptoms of depression *(7)*.

For several reasons it may be desirable to augment an antidepressant with a sedating agent. The justifications include more prompt improvement in sleep quality enhancing quality of life, as hypnotics generally have a quicker onset of action than antidepressants. Patients sometimes express having more confidence in medication therapy in general when they start to note clinical improvement quickly rather than waiting 3–4 weeks as with antidepressants. Based on the observations of Nierenberg et al. *(7)*, another possible rationale is that hypnotic augmentation may lead to more complete resolution of the depressive symptoms. Trazodone (25–100 mg) or, increasingly, nonbenzodiazepine hypnotics such as zolpidem (5–10 mg/day) or eszopiclone (2–3 mg) are prescribed concurrently to minimize SSRI-related insomnia.

Using polysomnography to confirm a suspected diagnosis of major depression is increasingly difficult. In current clinical practice, many patients are given medications relatively early in the course of their illness. Antidepressant medications alter sleep architecture, most typically by suppressing REM sleep. The opportunity to perform a polysomnographic study on an unmedicated depressed patient who also does not snore or have any sleep issue is increasingly rare. For this reason, polysomnography is not a part of standard clinical practice as a diagnostic test or outcome measure.

Nonetheless, polysomnography is of interest because research studies have consistently revealed decreased initial REM sleep latency. It is important to recognize that the shortened REM latency reported in depressive disorders is 45–60 min, markedly longer than the sleep-onset REM episodes that occur within minutes in narcolepsy. Reduced REM latency has also been reported in unaffected first-degree relatives of patients with major depression, raising the possibility that this is more of a trait rather than a state marker *(8)*. Reduced REM latency in major depression has been used as a predictor of response to antidepressant medications and psychotherapy *(9)*. Other abnormalities of REM sleep in major depression include a shortened initial REM period and increased REM density. Possible explanations are that REM sleep is phase advanced in major depression or associated with increased cholinergic activity relative to monoaminergic neurotransmission. Other nonspecific polysomnographic findings in major depression include increased awakenings and reduced slow-wave sleep.

Dysthymia is a milder but more chronic form of depression with two or more depressive symptoms lasting at least 2 years. Patients with dysthymia report significant fatigue in addition to their other depressive symptoms. A study of multiple sleep latency tests in apparently sleepy patients with dysthymia did not reveal any abnormal findings, suggesting the absence of actual sleepiness and rather the presence of fatigue or lethargy *(10)*.

Bipolar patients in the manic phase are in a markedly hyperaroused state presenting with pressured speech, elevated mood, distractibility, agitation, inflated self-esteem, and excessive involvement in pleasurable activities. They characteristically have a decreased need to sleep in spite of sustaining increased energy levels. Often patients have poor insight into their disorder and do not recognize the extent of their elevated mood state. Because of this poor insight, bipolar patients sometimes seek assistance specifically for their unsatisfying sleep without being aware that this is a component of an overarching mood disorder. By means of a history and a mental status examination, clinicians need to screen patients with insomnia for a possible evolving manic state. Patients with chronic bipolar disorder, who can experience mixed mood states with coexisting depressive and manic symptoms, can also present requesting intervention for their inability to sleep. Taking a careful history of past mood swings can aid in the identification of these patients. Appropriate treatment includes discontinuing antidepressant medications and starting mood stabilizers such as lithium, valproic acid, or other anticonvulsant agents like lamotrigine. In some cases, short-term use of benzodiazepines may be helpful for insomnia and daytime agitation.

A seasonal variant of major depression, commonly known as *seasonal affective disorder*, has a prevalence of up to 5% in North Americans *(11)*. This condition is more common in higher latitudes where there is less daylight during the winter months. Affected patients have a depressed mood that occurs exclusively during the winter months, and characteristically experience an increased need for sleep, increased appetite, and weight gain. This form of depression responds to antidepressant medications, particularly the SSRIs. Phototherapy in the morning has been demonstrated to be efficacious and leads support to the theory that this condition is linked to excessive production of melatonin. Bright light potentially improves the depression by suppressing melatonin secretion.

ANXIETY DISORDERS

Anxiety, defined as a subjective sense of unease, tension, or anticipation, often indicates a primary psychiatric disorder. Whether a symptom or a discrete disorder, anxiety is an important issue relative to sleep. Anxious patients typically do not enter the relaxed state necessary for sleep initiation. Insomnia, described in 38% of patients, is frequently a feature of anxiety disorders *(12)*. Anxiety disorders, the most prevalent psychiatric illnesses in the general community, are present in 15–20% of patients seeking health care.

It is important to recognize that anxiety can develop in the absence of a primary psychiatric disorder. For example, patients with respiratory diseases such as chronic obstructive pulmonary disease can experience fear if they are unable to readily breathe. In this situation, optimizing ventilation is the most immediate way to reduce the patient's anxiety. In another situation relevant to sleep medicine, some patients develop anxiety when initially using a nasal mask for continuous positive airway pressure because of unfamiliarity or a sensation of being smothered. Patient education with gradual and ongoing exposure is often sufficient to decrease this discomfort. If the problem persists, behavioral techniques and medications used for primary anxiety disorders may be required.

Generalized anxiety disorder, present in approx 4% of the US population *(13)*, is the presence of daily worrying or anxiety over a period of at least 6 months. The patients' worries are relentless and do not markedly fluctuate in intensity as seen in panic disorder. Experiencing stressful life events only complicates matters because susceptible individuals have more concerns to preoccupy them, thus perpetuating the anxiety. Patients often have increased tension in their muscles, which they are unable to consciously relax. Initial insomnia is common because patients lie awake at night in a stimulated or hyperaroused state. Additionally, patients with generalized anxiety disorder appear to have difficulty in accurately assessing their sleep. Overestimation of initial sleep latency and/or wakefulness time after sleep onset, now classified, as paradoxical insomnia rather than sleep state misperception, is common.

Many patients find psychotherapy, antidepressant medications, or a combination of the two modalities effective for generalized anxiety disorder. These treatment modalities are the standard of care for patients with and without prominent sleep complaints. Cognitive therapy that aims at the reduction of distorted perceptions (such as anticipating possible but improbable events like a natural disaster disrupting planned events), usually in conjunction with relaxation training, is a mainstay of treatment. Numerous studies have shown that essentially all antidepressants (tricyclic antidepressants, SSRIs, monoamine oxidase inhibitors, as well as most atypical agents) are useful treatments. The stimulating effects of bupropion make it a notable exception. Benzodiazepines are a less preferred therapeutic option than the antidepressants for long-term therapy because of the risk of daytime sedation, cognitive impairment, falls, and dependency issues.

Panic disorder, another common psychiatric disease with a prevalence rate of approx 3%, is more common in women than men *(14)*. This disorder is characterized by episodes of intense anxiety, which has two important components: (1) thoughts, for example, fear of injury or death, and (2) physical symptoms, including tachycardia, tachypnea, and diaphoresis. Many patients identify possible triggers—for example, feeling trapped and unable to get out of a public place—of these extremely unpleasant experiences and accordingly avoid these situations. When this avoidance causes them to steer clear of crowded spaces, as is often the case, the patient is said to experience agoraphobia.

Panic attacks that arise exclusively from sleep appear to be rare with relatively few reported cases in the literature *(15,16)*. Most panic attacks are not preceded by dreams and occur in NREM sleep at the transition from stage 2 to 3. In contrast to patients with sleep terrors who are not fully aware of their surroundings and return easily to sleep, nocturnal panic attack patients are awake and hyperalert, often for a considerable time. Insomnia is the most common sleep complaint reported by patients with panic disorder.

Treatment options include antidepressants, such as the SSRIs. For patients with predominantly nocturnal panic attacks, sedating antidepressants such as mirtazapine and nortriptyline may be particularly useful, despite not having specific Food and Drug Administration (FDA) approval for this condition. Benzodiazepines are useful in the acute management of severe panic disorder but are generally not preferred for the long-term, because of the same issues mentioned for generalized anxiety disorder. Behavioral therapy using exposure to anxiety-provoking situations as well as training in relaxation techniques has been repeatedly demonstrated to be effective for the motivated patient.

Post-traumatic stress disorder (PTSD) is characterized by chronic hyperarousal and anxiety. Patients recall and re-experience severely distressing life events like terrorist attacks, natural disasters, wartime incidents, and accidents. The most commonly reported sleep disturbances are insomnia and nightmares. Studies of PTSD using polysomnography show conflicting results, ranging from no objective abnormalities to increased wakefulness after sleep onset, frequent arousals, and occasional awakenings from NREM sleep. The nightmares occur primarily during REM sleep. Many studies have reported a high prevalence of other primary sleep disorders, especially sleep-disordered breathing *(17)*. Whether PTSD places a patient at increased risk for parasomnias remains controversial.

Treatment for PTSD includes careful use of exposure therapy to help patients reduce their arousal when confronted with circumstances that remind them of the original traumatic event. Individual and group supportive psychotherapy is often valuable. Valuable medications include the SSRIs, of which paroxetine and sertraline have received FDA approval for the treatment of PTSD. A recent study indicated that nightmares and insomnia substantially improved in chronic PTSD after a 20-week trial of the centrally acting α_1-adrenergic antagonist prazosin, which was added to patients' previous psychotropic medication or psychotherapy *(18)*.

PSYCHOTIC DISORDERS

Schizophrenia is a chronic disorder of thought and perception that affects 1% of the population. Schizophrenia is commonly associated with insomnia that may begin in the prodromal phase of the disorder before the first episode of psychotic symptoms. Polysomnography has shown an increase in sleep fragmentation, shortened REM latency, and a decrease in slow-wave sleep. In contrast with major depression, treatment with antipsychotic medication lengthens REM latency and thus its significance in the pathophysiology of the disorder is uncertain. Treatment also improves sleep continuity but is associated with a persistent reduction in slow-wave sleep *(19)*.

Treatment of schizophrenia consists primarily of antipsychotic medications. These reduce the positive symptoms of schizophrenia (auditory hallucinations, delusions, and unusual thought patterns) as well as negative symptoms (lack of motivation, inability to speak, and blunted affect). The primary mechanism of action of these newer medications is dopamine as well as serotonin antagonism; the latter factor is suspected to reduce the frequency of extrapyramidal side effects. Sedation is a feature of several of these newer medications, particularly quetiapine. This can be beneficial for insomnia, but at times the doses must be titrated downwards because of excessive daytime sleepiness. Many of the atypical antipsychotic medications approved in the mid-to-late 1990s are associated with weight gain, so the possibility of obstructive sleep apnea syndrome must be considered periodically in schizophrenic patients. Olanzapine, quetiapine, and clozapine have been reported to have the strongest association with weight gain, particularly in young adult patients.

CHEMICAL DEPENDENCY

Because of their effect on mood, alcohol and drugs are widely used. In typical Western communities, 90% of people consume alcohol at some point in their lives and 30% develop transient alcohol-related difficulties *(20)*. Alcohol and drugs have many possible effects on sleep, including insomnia, excessive daytime sleepiness, and parasomnias. When patients present with a sleep complaint, the clinical interview should always include questions about substance use.

Alcohol is often consumed with the intent of inducing relaxation and sleep. Acute alcohol use in a nonhabitual user typically leads to sedation. Alcohol intoxication has been linked to decreased REM sleep and increased stage shifting in NREM sleep, leading to sleep fragmentation. Alcohol is metabolized rapidly at a rate of 1 oz of hard alcohol per hour, resulting in the sedating effects being short-lived. Probably because of increased fragmentation of sleep, alcohol ingestion can induce NREM parasomnias primarily in adolescents and young adults. Within an hour or two of falling asleep, while in slow-wave sleep, affected patients can engage in inappropriate motor activities like sleepwalking. These behaviors must be differentiated from activities conducted when awake but intoxicated or in an alcohol-related blackout. Many patients consuming alcohol have coexisting sleep deprivation related to late-night partying, another well-established trigger for episodes of an NREM parasomnia. Because serious injury is possible, susceptible persons should be told to avoid both alcohol intoxication and an irregular sleep–wake schedule.

Alcohol is a potent muscle relaxant, decreasing the neural input to the upper airway muscles, and is a well-known precipitant of snoring and obstructive sleep apneas *(21)*. In persons who do not typically snore, consuming a small amount of alcohol can relax the muscles of the upper airway and lead to snoring, whereas patients with pre-existing snoring will be highly likely to experience obstructive breathing events. Similarly, patients with obstructive sleep apnea who consume intermittent or daily alcohol can experience aggravation of their sleep-disordered breathing.

Occasional alcohol use can evolve into alcohol abuse and dependence. Because alcohol leads to a positively reinforcing state of euphoria at lower levels of intoxication, people tend to continue drinking even in the face of adverse consequences. Daily alcohol use can lead to complex changes in the brain, mind, and body. Alcohol abuse is defined in DSM-IV as alcohol use leading to repeated undesirable consequences. Alcohol dependence by DSM-IV criteria is impairment in at least three areas of functioning, including occupational, academic, social, and recreational activities, for at least 12 months. The factors that make an individual vulnerable to alcohol dependence are unclear, but familial factors may play a significant contributing role. Physical dependence on alcohol can occur, with the presence of withdrawal symptoms when alcohol is abruptly discontinued.

Patients with alcohol abuse or dependence can have a wide variety of sleep complaints including insomnia, hypersomnia, and parasomnias. Sometimes the patients start using alcohol frequently because of a belief that an evening drink would enhance sleep. Acute alcohol intoxication causes sedation that starts 30 minutes after consumption, with the duration depending on the amount consumed. One study indicated that

61% of patients with alcohol dependence had insomnia before entering chemical dependency treatment *(22)*. Polysomnography in patients using alcohol on a habitual basis revealed shorter initial sleep latency, decreased wakefulness after sleep onset for the first half of the night, and decreased slow-wave sleep *(23)*. In the second half of the night, patients experience more indeterminate arousals, stage changes, and REM rebound, which may lead to nightmares.

Treatment typically includes advising the patients to reduce alcohol consumption. If they are unable to do so without assistance, referral to an outpatient or inpatient alcohol treatment program may be required. In these settings, patients are generally advised to abruptly discontinue alcohol use, and a benzodiazepine is given on a tapering schedule to prevent withdrawal symptoms. If a patient has entered alcohol withdrawal, delirium tremens, severe restlessness, visual hallucinations, seizures, and total absence of sleep can develop *(24)*. Polysomnography shows a marked reduction in slow-wave sleep, sleep fragmentation, and increased REM sleep with loss of muscle atonia. Slow-wave sleep may take months to years to recover. Aggressive treatment with benzodiazepines and possibly anticonvulsants is mandated by this condition associated with significant mortality.

If at all possible, other than benzodiazepines used for detoxification, behavioral measures should be used to address the insomnia that develops when an alcoholic patient starts abstaining from alcohol. Patient education should emphasize that sleep initiation and maintenance problems are a core component of the transition away from excessive drinking. Patients with persisting insomnia 5 months after stopping alcohol are at higher risk for relapse, likely because of a tendency to self-medicate the insomnia with alcohol *(22)*. Using a medication, especially a benzodiazepine but possibly nonbenzodiazepines like zolpidem, zaleplon, and eszopiclone, reinforces the patient's perspective that exogenous substances are necessary for satisfactory sleep. If a patient is in a rehabilitation setting, sedating antidepressants unknown to cause physical dependence such as trazodone are often preferred. Some patients experience distressing insomnia and daytime fatigue for up to 12 months after achieving sobriety *(22)*.

Polysomnography demonstrates reduced total sleep time and slow-wave sleep. The physician should consider whether a coexisting mood or anxiety disorder is contributing to the sleep disturbance that in general cannot be diagnosed for at least 4 weeks after alcohol cessation. However, clinicians treating a visibly symptomatic patient sometimes cannot adhere rigidly to this guideline. Sedating antidepressants and mood stabilizers are strongly preferred over benzodiazepines that may trigger craving for alcohol, as a result of crosstolerance. The potential exists for the nonbenzodiazepine receptor agonists to trigger a relapse with alcohol. Case reports indicate a risk of tolerance, dose escalation, and relapse with alcohol related to zolpidem in particular in this population of patients with demonstrated vulnerability to addiction *(24)*.

Disorders related to sedatives and anxiolytics are grouped together in the DSM-IV classification of chemical dependency-related sleep disorders. Because of related pharmacological actions and cross-tolerance, this cluster of sleep disorders is fairly similar to alcohol-induced sleep disorder. Benzodiazepines are commonly prescribed medications for insomnia and anxiety disorders. Although initially leading to desired sedation, over time they reduce the quality of sleep. Longer-acting agents (such as clonazepam or flurazepam) are prone to cause morning sedation with a hangover effect. Some patients might misinterpret this as a sign of inadequate sleep and lead to an increase in benzodiazepine dosage. Clinicians should intervene by designing a gradual taper of the benzodiazepine and re-evaluating sleep once this is complete. Withdrawal or abstinence from these agents, especially after years of usage, can contribute to insomnia similar to that seen after cessation of chronic alcohol use. When benzodiazepines are discontinued after long-term daily use, polysomnographic studies show a reduction in slow-wave sleep and increase in wakefulness after sleep onset.

The DSM-IV stimulant-dependent sleep disorder describes a reduction of sleep owing to either use of or abstinence from agents including cocaine, amphetamines, and methylphenidate. During binges of stimulant use, a user may not sleep for days, followed by marked hypersomnolence. These drugs reduce both total sleep time and REM sleep time. Stimulant abusers may also abuse sedatives in order to moderate the intensity of their intoxicated state or obtain sleep. Withdrawal from stimulants can cause excessive daytime sleepiness with coexisting depressed mood and increased appetite. During this phase, polysomnography shows an increase in total and REM sleep time that can result in sleep-onset REM periods on a multiple sleep latency test. Treatment depends on the stimulant abused. Users of potent medications like amphetamines and cocaine typically need medically supervised detoxification and rehabilitation. Caffeine users should gradually taper their usage over 1 week to reduce the likelihood of rebound headache.

REFERENCES

1. Campbell S, Murphy P (1998) Extraocular circadian phototransduction in humans. Science 279:396–399.
2. Czeisler C, Duffy J, Shanahan T, et al. (1999) Stability, precision, and near-24-hour period of the human circadian pacemaker. Science 284:2177–2181.
3. Naylor E, Bergmann B, Krauski K, et al. (2000) The circadian clock mutation alters sleep homeostasis in the mouse. J Neurosci 20:8138–8143.
4. Toh K, Jones C, He Y, et al. (2001) An hPer2 phosphorylation site mutation in familial advanced sleep phase syndrome. Science 291:1040–1043.
5. Hattar S, Lucas RJ, Mrosovsky N, et al. (2003) Melanopsin and rod-cone photoreceptive systems account for all major accessory visual functions in mice. Nature 424:75–81.
6. Schrader H, Bovim G, Sand T (1993) The prevalence of delayed and advanced sleep phase syndromes. J Sleep Res 2:51–55.
7. Cole R, Smith J, Alcala Y, et al. (2002) Bright-light mask treatment of delayed sleep phase syndrome. J Biol Rhythms 17:89–101.
8. Arendt J, Deacon S, English J, et al. (1995) Melatonin and adjustment to phase shift. J Sleep Res 4:74–79.
9. Kayumov L, Brown G, Jindal R, et al. (2001) A randomized, double-blind, placebo-controlled crossover study of the effect of exogenous melatonin on delayed sleep phase syndrome. Psychosom Med 63:40–48.
10. Nagtegaal JE, Kerkhof GA, Smits MG, et al. (1998) Delayed sleep phase syndrome: a placebo-controlled cross-over study on the effects of melatonin administered five hours before the individual dim light melatonin onset. J Sleep Res 7:135–143.
11. Campbell S, Dawson D, Anderson MW (1993) Alleviation of sleep maintenance insomnia with timed exposure to bright light. J Am Geriatr Soc 41:829–836.
12. Murphy P, Campbell S (1996) Enhanced performance in elderly subjects following bright light treatment of sleep maintenance insomnia. J Sleep Res 5:165–172.
13. Moldofsky H, Musisi S, Phillipson E (1986) Treatment of a case of advanced sleep phase syndrome by phase advance chronotherapy. Sleep 9:61–65.
14. De Leersnyder H, Bresson J, de Blois M, et al. (2003) Beta 1-adrenergic antagonists and melatonin reset the clock and restore sleep in a circadian disorder, Smith-Magenis syndrome. J Med Genet 40:74–78.

15. Leger D, Guilleminault C, Santos C, et al. (2002) Sleep/wake cycles in the dark: sleep recorded by polysomnography in 26 totally blind subjects compared to controls. Clin Neurophysiol 113:1607–1614.
16. Lewy AJ, Bauer VK, Hasler BP, et al. (2001) Capturing the circadian rhythms of free-running blind people with 0.5 mg melatonin. Brain Res 918:96–100.
17. Petrie K, Dawson AG, Thompson L, et al. (1993) A double-blind trial of melatonin as a treatment for jet lag in international cabin crew. Biol Psychiatry 33:526–530.
18. Spitzer RL, Terman M, Williams JB, et al. (1999) Jet lag: clinical features, validation of a new syndrome-specific scale, and lack of response to melatonin in a randomized, double-blind trial. Am J Psychiatry 156:1392–1396.
19. Wright S, Lawrence L, Wrenn K, et al. (1998) Randomized clinical trial of melatonin after night-shift work: efficacy and neuropsychologic effects. Ann Emerg Med 32:334–340.
20. Mohren DC, Jansen NW, Kant IJ, et al. (2002) Prevalence of common infections among employees in different work schedules. J Occup Environ Med 44:1003–1011.
21. Rosekind M, Smith R, Miller D, et al. (1995) Alertness management: strategic naps in operational settings. J Sleep Res 4:62–66.
22. Czeisler CA, Walsh JK, Roth T, et al. (2005) Modafinil for excessive sleepiness associated with shift-work sleep disorder. N Engl J Med 353:476–486.
23. Nickelsen T, Samel A, Vejvoda M, et al. (2002) Chronobiotic effects of the melatonin agonist LY 156735 following a simulated 9h time shift: results of a placebo-controlled trial. Chronobiol Int 19:915–936.
24. Hajak G, Muller W, Wittchen HU, Pittrow D, Kirch W (2003) Abuse and dependence potential for the non-benzodiazepine hypnotics zolpidem and zopiclone: a review of case reports and epidemiological data. Addiction 98: 1371–1378.

23 Sleep and the Esophagus

Susan M. Harding, MD, FCCP

CONTENTS

INTRODUCTION

Gastroesophageal reflux disease (GER) is very common in the adult population, with 7% of adults experiencing GER symptoms daily and 14% experiencing symptoms at least weekly *(1,2)*. Sleep-related GER is underappreciated and impacts sleep and daytime functioning. Potential extraesophageal manifestations of sleep-related GER include sleep-related asthma and sleep-related laryngospasm. There is also a common coexistence of obstructive sleep apnea (OSA) and GER *(3)*. This syllabus will review esophageal function during sleep and sleep-related GER.

ESOPHAGEAL FUNCTION DURING SLEEP

Esophageal functional anatomy, pathophysiological mechanisms of GER, sleep's influence on esophageal function, and esophageal acid clearance will be reviewed.

Esophageal Functional Anatomy

Esophageal functional anatomy is complex. At the cephalad (proximal) end is the upper esophageal sphincter (UES), a high-pressure zone that includes the cricopharyngeus muscle. The esophageal body is 18–22 cm in length and is made up of striated muscle in the proximal 4 cm, followed by a mixture of striated and smooth muscle (4–8 cm), followed exclusively by smooth muscle at the distal end. Diseases affecting striated muscle may also involve the upper third of the esophagus. Critical to the pathophysiology

From: *Current Clinical Practice: Primary Care Sleep Medicine: A Practical Guide*
Edited by: J. F. Pagel and S. R. Pandi-Perumal © Humana Press Inc., Totowa, NJ

of GER is the lower esophageal sphincter (LES) *(4)*. The LES is a 2–4 cm, dual-sphincter, high-pressure zone consisting of a muscular layer (intrinsic LES) and the diaphragmatic crura. The intrinsic LES has cholinergic innervation, and the crural diaphragm has bilateral phrenic nerve innervation. The intrinsic LES and the crural diaphragm are anchored to each other by the phreno-esophageal ligament. The intrinsic LES maintains a tonic contraction and relaxes with deglutination or esophageal distension. The diaphragmatic crura causes spike-like increases in LES pressure during inspiration and relaxes with vomiting and esophageal distension. The intrinsic LES and the diaphragmatic crura make up the two components of the LES antireflux barrier.

There are three types of esophageal contractions: primary, secondary, and nonperistaltic. Primary esophageal peristaltic contractions occur with swallowing, last 2–3 seconds, and have a propagation speed of approx 4 cm/second. The amplitude (or force of contraction) insures that there is adequate push of the solid or liquid bolus. Secondary peristaltic contractions are localized to the esophagus, not associated with a swallow or UES relaxation, and remove leftover residue. Nonperistaltic contractions, on the other hand, break up food in the esophagus. Esophageal manometry monitors esophageal contractions and measures UES and LES pressures.

Transient LES relaxations (TLESRs) occur without swallowing, are associated with belching, vomiting, rumination, and are vagally mediated *(5)*. During a TLESR, there is simultaneous relaxation of the LES and the crural diaphragm, with inhibition of esophageal body contractions. TLESRs are longer in duration than swallowing-induced LES relaxations. TLESRs are the major GER mechanism and are responsible for 63–74% of reflux episodes. Interestingly, sleep and the supine position increase the vagal threshold for triggering TLESRs. In general, TLESRs do not occur during stable sleep and are usually confined to arousals. Other TLESR triggers include gastric distension and pharyngeal intubation. Patients with GER have a higher frequency of TLESRs and a higher incidence of reflux episodes with TLESRs. Other GER-promoting factors include increased gastric acid production, delayed gastric emptying, and increased gastric pressure overcoming the LES barrier. In addition, large pleural-abdominal pressure gradients (as seen with OSA events), esophageal dysmotility, LES hypotension, and hiatal hernia also predispose to GER.

If a reflux episode occurs, esophageal acid clearance mechanisms, including volume clearance and acid neutralization, come into play *(6)*. Salivation stimulates swallowing, which triggers peristalsis. Most of the refluxate is cleared with the first two or three swallows. If an acid coating remains in the esophagus, subsequent swallows deliver saliva to the area, resulting in acid neutralization.

Sleep Influences on Gastric and Esophageal Function and Esophageal Acid Clearance

Sleep alters gastric physiology. The circadian rhythm for basal gastric acid secretion peaks between 8 PM and 1 AM *(7)*. Elsenbruch and colleagues *(8)* noted that sleep disrupts gastric myoelectric function, leading to delayed gastric emptying. Goo and colleagues *(9)* reported significantly delayed gastric emptying during the sleep period. Sleep also alters esophageal function. UES pressure drops from 44–10 mmHg with sleep onset, thus predisposing to aspiration if proximal migration of gastric contents occurs *(10)*. UES pressure does not significantly change with the various sleep stages. Esophageal acid clearance is markedly delayed because of multiple events that occur during sleep. First, swallowing is almost nonexistent during stable sleep and occurs primarily during brief arousals from sleep. The swallowing rate during wakefulness is 1.61/minute, compared with 0.06/minute during sleep stages 2, 3, 4, and REM *(11)*. Furthermore, salivary secretion is not measurable during stable sleep, hindering acid neutralization *(12)*.

Orr and colleagues *(11)* performed multiple experiments examining esophageal acid clearance during sleep utilizing esophageal acid infusions. For instance, 15 mL of 0.1 *N* HCl was cleared within 6 minutes during wakefulness, compared with 25 minutes during stable sleep. Esophageal acid clearance occurred primarily during brief arousals. Arousal responses and swallowing frequency were more prevalent with acid infusions, compared with water infusions. Furthermore, Orr and Johnson *(13)* noted that sleep prolonged the latency period between esophageal acid exposure and the first swallow. Orr and colleagues *(14)* also noted that sleep facilitated proximal acid migration if acid entered the distal esophagus. In 15 healthy adults, 1 mL of acid in the distal esophagus resulted in proximal migration 40% of the time during sleep, compared with less than 1% of the time during wakefulness. These physiological alterations can lead to the development of esophageal and extraesophageal GER manifestations during sleep.

Esophageal pH Testing

Sleep-related GER episodes can be monitored with esophageal pH testing that is optimally monitored over a 24-hour period to increase the test's sensitivity and specificity. Twenty-four-hour esophageal pH testing has a sensitivity and a specificity of approx 90% *(15)*. Esophageal pH testing can be integrated with polysomnography during the sleep time to correlate esophageal acid events with sleep events, including arousal, apnea, dyspnea, laryngospasm, and increased chin electromyelogram tone. Significant esophageal reflux events occur if the refluxate drops to pH less than 4.0. The distal pH probe is placed 5 cm above the LES. Manometric determination of the LES is the gold standard for determining pH probe placement *(16)*. Alternately, the LES locator can be used if esophageal manometry is not available. Many pH probes have two pH electrodes. The second pH electrode is often placed at the proximal esophagus, within 2 cm of the UES, or in the pharynx. A reference lead is placed on the anterior chest wall. The esophageal pH probe is connected to a portable data acquisition device that has an event marker to note when symptoms occur. Patients also record meal and sleep times *(16)*.

Esophageal pH can be integrated with polysomnographic monitoring. The esophageal pH probe and reference lead should be recorded through an electrical isolation box before connecting to the DC amplifier. The output needs to be in the range of 0–1 V. When examining reflux events with polysomnography, take note of which events occur on the time line axis when the esophageal pH drops to less than 4.0. Normal esophageal acid contact times for the distal (5 cm above the LES) and proximal probes (within 2 cm of the UES) are shown in Table 1 *(17)*. Note, supine, by definition, is the period of time the patient is in bed.

SLEEP-RELATED GER

Sleep-related GER is a primary sleep disorder *(18)*. Sleep-related GER is more injurious than diurnal GER and is associated with esophagitis, Barrett esophagitis, and adenocarcinoma of the esophagus *(19–21)*. Sleep-related GER may present with multiple awakenings, substernal burning, and/or chest discomfort, indigestion, or heartburn.

Table 1
Normal 24-Hour Esophageal pH Values[a]

Time (%) pH < 4.0	*Distal (%)[b]*	*Proximal (%)[c]*
Total	<5.8	<1.1
Upright	<8.2	<1.7
Supine	<3.5	<0.6

[a]University of Alabama at Birmingham *(17)*.
[b]Distal: pH probe placed 5 cm above LES.
[c]Proximal: pH probe placed 1–2 cm below UES.

Other symptoms may include a sour or bitter taste in the mouth, regurgitation, water brash, coughing, or choking. Some patients may not have esophageal symptoms and present with excessive daytime sleepiness without an obvious cause, so polysomnography with esophageal pH monitoring may be required to establish the diagnosis. Sleep-related GER can have a major impact on sleep and daytime functioning and cause excessive daytime sleepiness *(22,23)*.

To get a better understanding of the prevalence and impact of nocturnal heartburn, Shaker and colleagues *(3)* reported a national, population-based telephone survey conducted by the Gallup Organization of 1000 people who experienced heartburn at least once weekly. Night time heartburn was reported by 79% of respondents; among these, 75% reported that heartburn affected their sleep. Sixty-three percent believed that heartburn negatively affected their ability to sleep well, and 40% believed that nocturnal heartburn impaired their daytime functioning. Furthermore, of the 791 respondents with night time heartburn, 71% reported taking over-the-counter medications, but only 29% had adequate control of their GER symptoms. Also, of the 41% of respondents who were taking prescription medications, only 49% had adequate control of their GER symptoms. These investigators concluded that night time heartburn occurs quite frequently in the majority of adults with GER and causes sleep difficulties *(3)*.

Furthermore, Fass and colleagues *(24)* examined predictors of heartburn during sleep in 15,314 subjects of the Sleep Heart Health Study. Twenty-five percent (3806 subjects) reported having heartburn during sleep. In multivariant models, increased body mass index (BMI), carbonated drink consumption, snoring, sleepiness on Epworth Sleepiness Scale, insomnia, use of benzodiazepines, hypertension, and asthma were strong predictors of heartburn during sleep. This study also confirms that heartburn occurring once a week or more is common during sleep, and it is associated with daytime sleepiness and insomnia.

Chand and colleagues *(25)* examined consecutive patients with endoscopically proven erosive esophagitis who did not have a history of sleep disorders. Sleep was assessed with the Pittsburgh Sleep Quality Index (PSQI) and actigraphy. Eighteen subjects were treated with esomeprazole, 40 mg, 30 minutes before breakfast. At baseline, patients with erosive esophagitis had high values on the PSQI (8.5—a score of ≤5 indicates poor sleep) that improved with esomeprazole. Actigraphy did not change with GER treatment. Although not placebo-controlled, this study provides preliminary evidence that sleep disturbances are common in patients with erosive esophagitis and that sleep disturbance improves with GER therapy.

Johnson and colleagues *(26)* did perform a placebo-controlled trial utilizing esomeprazole, 40 mg, 20 mg, or placebo for 4 weeks in 750 adults with GER-associated sleep disturbance. The primary outcome was relief of night time heartburn and secondary outcomes, including resolution of the sleep disturbance, sleep quality as measured by the PSQI, and work productivity. More than 50% of the esomeprazole-treated subjects had resolution of their night time heartburn, compared with 13% of the placebo group. Furthermore, at baseline, 83% of subjects had poor sleep quality (global PSQI score >5). By 4 weeks, 73% of the esomeprazole-treated subjects had resolution of their GER-associated sleep disturbance. Work productivity also improved in the esomeprazole-treated groups. Both doses of esomeprazole improved sleep quality, reduced lost work hours, and increased work productivity.

When monitoring nocturnal acid reflux events during sleep, Freidin and colleagues *(27)* noted that reflux events and TLESRs occurred most commonly during brief arousals, rather than during stable sleep. Khoury and colleagues *(28)* observed that the right lateral decubitus position was associated with the highest esophageal acid contact times and the longest esophageal acid clearance times, even though GER episodes were noted more frequently while subjects were in the supine position. The left lateral decubitus position is the preferred sleep position in patients with GER, because reflux events are less likely to occur in this position.

Diagnostic criteria for sleep-related GER include recurrent awakenings from sleep with shortness of breath or heartburn, with either a sour bitter taste in the mouth upon awakening from sleep, sleep-related coughing, or choking, or awakening from sleep with heartburn. Polysomnography and esophageal pH monitoring demonstrate GER during sleep with associated arousal *(18)*.

EXTRAESOPHAGEAL MANIFESTATIONS OF SLEEP-RELATED GER IN ADULTS

Sleep-related GER may also trigger sleep-related asthma, cause sleep-related laryngospasm, and is often seen in patients with OSA *(29)*.

Sleep-Related Asthma

Nocturnal asthma is characterized by an exaggeration of the normal circadian variation in lung function, airway inflammation, and bronchial responsiveness *(30)*. Most asthma deaths occur between 6 PM and 3 AM. Gastroesophageal reflux is a potential trigger of asthma *(31)*. A cross-sectional epidemiological investigation, as part of the European Community Respiratory Health Survey of more than 2600 subjects, including more than 450 asthmatics, was recently reported by Gislason and colleagues *(32)*. Subjects with GER were more likely to have night time wheezing, breathlessness, and nocturnal cough, compared with subjects without GER. Asthma was more frequent in nocturnal subjects with GER, compared with those without nocturnal GER (9% vs 4%; $p < 0.005$). In the 5- to 10-year evaluation, 16,191 participants responded to a questionnaire to determine whether obesity, nocturnal GER, and snoring were independent risk factors for asthma development *(33)*. Again, nocturnal GER was independently related to asthma development. Obesity (BMI > 30 kg/m^2) was also independently related to asthma development *(26)*. Sontag and colleagues *(34)* examined 261 asthmatics and 218 controls and noted that twice as many asthmatics, compared with controls, had night time heartburn (98% vs 42%). Asthmatics were also more likely to eat before bedtime (60%), and these asthmatics were more likely to have severe night time GER.

Jack and colleagues *(35)* monitored both tracheal and esophageal pH in four nocturnal asthmatics with GER. There were 37 episodes of esophageal reflux, of which five episodes were associated with a fall in tracheal pH. Peak expiratory flow rates dropped 8 L/minute with esophageal acid, compared with 84 L/minute if there was also a fall in tracheal pH. Tracheal acid episodes were associated with prolonged reflux episodes, nocturnal awakenings, and bronchospasm during the night *(35)*.

In a different study design, Cuttitta and colleagues *(36)* evaluated spontaneous reflux episodes and airway patency during the night in seven asthmatics with GER. Multiple, step-wise, linear regression analysis revealed that the most important predictor of change in lower respiratory resistance was the duration of esophageal acid exposure. Both long and short GER episodes (those <5 minutes and those >5 minutes) were associated with higher respiratory resistance, compared with baseline. These data collectively suggest that esophageal acid is able to elicit nocturnal bronchoconstriction *(36)*.

Sleep-Related Laryngospasm

Sleep-related laryngospasm refers to episodic abrupt interruptions of sleep, accompanied by feelings of acute suffocation, followed by stridor. This condition is included in the diagnostic and coding manual of the American Academy of Sleep Medicine *(18)*. Differential diagnosis of sleep-related laryngospasm includes OSA, GER, epilepsy, panic disorder, sleep-choking syndrome, sleep terrors, vocal cord dysfunction, and other airway pathological processes. Evaluation of sleep-related laryngospasm may include an upper airway examination, polysomnography with esophageal pH monitoring, and seizure monitoring. Gastroesophageal reflux may precipitate sleep-related laryngospasm. Thurnheer and colleagues *(37)* reported a case series of 10 patients with sleep-related laryngospasm *(37)*. Patients had abrupt sleep interruption accompanied by feelings of acute suffocation associated with an apneic period lasting 5–45 seconds, followed by stridor. Nine of 10 patients had GER documented by esophageal pH testing, of which six responded to anti-reflux therapy. The presence of GER should be investigated in these patients *(37)*.

Sleep-Related GER and OSA

Sleep-related GER is common in patients with OSA. Janson and colleagues *(38)* examined more than 2200 young adults, 20–44 years old, as part of the European Community Respiratory Health Survey, finding that 5% of men and 2% of women snored nightly. Reflux symptoms were associated with disruptive breathing, with an odds ratio of 3.8 (95% confidence intervals 1.4–10). Using a similar database, Gislason and colleagues *(32)* noted that when comparing young adults with nocturnal GER symptoms with those without nocturnal GER symptoms, apnea was more likely to be present in the subjects with GER ($p < 0.01$). These epidemiological studies show that OSA symptoms are associated with nocturnal GER. More recently, Green and colleagues *(39)* prospectively examined 331 patients with OSA. Significant night time GER was found in 62% of subjects before OSA treatment. Patients compliant with continuous positive airway pressure (CPAP) had a 48% improvement in their nocturnal GER symptoms ($p < 0.001$). There was no change in night time reflux symptoms if patients did not use CPAP. Furthermore, there was a strong correlation between higher CPAP pressures and improvement in nocturnal GER symptom scores. This study shows that nocturnal reflux is common in patients with OSA and that nasal CPAP decreases the frequency of nocturnal GER symptoms by 48% *(39)*. Demeter and colleagues *(40)* performed endoscopy on 55 patients with OSA and GER. Esophagitis was present in 80%. Logistic regression analysis showed a positive correlation between severity of esophagitis and apnea hypopnea index ($p = 0.0167$). Ozturk and colleagues *(41)* examined potential variables affecting the occurrence of GER in patients with OSA, finding no differences in age, BMI, or OSA severity in patients with vs those without nocturnal GER.

To further evaluate the association between OSA and GER, Penzel and colleagues *(42)* monitored overnight polysomnography and esophageal pH in 15 patients with OSA or who are heavy snoring with GER, noting that 69 reflux events occurred with 68 arousals. Thirty-one reflux events occurred during wakefulness after sleep onset, and 37 reflux events occurred temporally with respiratory events. However, they cautioned that a temporal correlation between reflux events and respiratory events does not prove causality *(42)*. Furthermore, Graf and colleagues *(43)* examined 17 consecutive patients with OSA and divided them into two groups—those with a respiratory disturbance index (RDI) of 5–15, and those with an RDI of more than 15. Gastroesophageal reflux was present in both groups without a difference in distal and proximal esophageal acid contact times between groups. They also noticed that apneic episodes were not temporally related to reflux events *(43)*. Furthermore, Ing and colleagues *(44)* examined the relationship between OSA and GER in 63 patients with OSA (RDI >15), and in 41 age-, BMI-, FEV_1-, and alcohol-matched controls (RDI < 5). Forty-seven percent of reflux events had no temporal relationship with apneic events, whereas 11% of reflux events were preceded within 1 minute by apneic events; 30% were followed by apneic events; and 12% occurred simultaneously. Furthermore, 53% of respiratory events were unrelated to reflux events, and 56% of arousals were unrelated to reflux events. In conclusion, patients with OSA had more prolonged and more frequent reflux events, compared with control subjects, and acid reflux events were temporally related to 40–50% of arousals and apneas. However, the precise nature of the OSA-reflux relationship remains unclear *(44)*. Furthermore, Ing and colleagues *(44)* studied the effect of CPAP on reflux parameters in 14 patients with OSA and 8 controls, noting that CPAP decreased the number of reflux episodes and decreased esophageal acid contact times in the patients with OSA *(44)*. Twelve patients with OSA and GER were randomized to receive either 150 mg of nizatidine (H_2 blocker) or placebo. Nizatidine decreased the frequency of arousals and number of reflux events and improved esophageal acid contact times. Reflux may contribute to excessive sleepiness and arousals in patients with OSA and GER. Furthermore, Senior and colleagues *(45)* examined overnight polysomnography both before and after 30 days of omeprazole, 20 mg bid, in 10 men with OSA and GER, noting that the apnea index decreased from 45/hour to 31/hour, and the RDI decreased from 62/hour to 46/hour with proton pump inhibitor (PPI) therapy. More recently, Berg and colleagues *(46)* examined 14 consecutive men with suspected OSA, using polysomnography, esophageal pH, and esophageal pressure monitoring. Esophageal pH events were defined as a drop in esophageal pH by 1.0 U or more. There were many more respiratory events (AHI 33 ± 22) than esophageal pH events (7 ± 6) per hour of sleep. Eighty-one percent of all esophageal pH events occurred simultaneously with respiratory events. There was no relationship noted between esophageal pH events and esophageal pressure swings, or the AHI. The relationship between OSA and GER is more complex than might be expected from simple, passive, mechanical considerations, i.e., the transdiaphragmatic pressure gradient. This study supports the notion that GER is not caused by OSA, but may be facilitated by it *(46)*.

Another recent report by Morse and colleagues *(47)* explored the potential relationship between OSA and GERD. A total of 136 patients with suspected OSA underwent polysomnography (OSA defined as AHI >5), GERD symptoms checklist, and Sleep Health Heart Health Study Questionnaire. Seventy-four percent of subjects had OSA. Self-reported GER symptoms were unrelated to the severity of OSA, and OSA was not influenced by GER severity. In men, subjective sleep quality was affected by regurgitation. Kim and colleagues *(48)* also noted that there was no relationship between OSA and GER symptoms, nor the severity of OSA and the likelihood of GER symptoms. These data support the notion that OSA and GER are not causally linked *(49)*.

Data show that there is a coexistence of OSA and GER in many patients. With apnea, there is continued respiratory effort against a closed upper airway associated with marked intrathoracic pressure swings and increases in transdiaphragmatic pressures. Furthermore, OSA may cause arousals that trigger TLESRs and promote GER. The interactions between OSA and GER may be complex. The two are common disease states and share similar risk factors for development, including obesity. Both OSA and GER can disrupt subjective sleep findings and sleep architecture. Current data suggest that there is not a direct causal relationship between OSA and GER; however, further research will examine potential interactions.

MANAGEMENT OF SLEEP-RELATED GER

Management of sleep-related GER and its potential extraesophageal manifestations include conservative measures, medical therapy (acid secretion inhibitors and prokinetic agents), and surgical therapy. Nasal CPAP also improves esophageal acid contact times *(44)*. Surgical fundoplication may also have a role in controlling nocturnal symptoms in selected patients. There are many potential GER therapies that may provide even more optimal therapy *(50)*.

CONSERVATIVE MEASURES

It is extremely important to implement life style modifications for sleep-related GER. Patients should be instructed to sleep in the left lateral decubitus position, if possible *(28)*. Furthermore, sleeping on a wedge may decrease esophageal acid exposure by at least 30% *(51)*. This can be achieved by elevating the head of the bed by 6 in. or using a full-length wedge. Also, limit eating for at least 2 hours before bedtime. Patients should also abstain from foods that can worsen GER, including caffeine, chocolate, mints, alcohol (decreases LES pressure), and avoid high-fat foods (delays gastric emptying) *(52)*. Furthermore, tomato products and citric acid-containing products may worsen GER symptoms. Carbonated beverages have a pH of 1.0–2.0 and should be avoided. Medications that have the potential to worsen GER include calcium channel blockers, anticholinergics, theophylline (which can lower LES pressure and increase gastric acid secretion), prostaglandins, and alendronate. Smoking cessation is vital in controlling sleep-related GER, because smoking leads to marked lowering of the LES pressure. Antacids or alginic acid can be utilized to control acute GER symptoms *(53)*.

ACID SECRETION INHIBITORS

PPIs and H_2-receptor antagonists inhibit gastric acid secretion. H_2-receptor antagonists were introduced in the 1970s and are safe and well-tolerated *(52)*. Currently available H_2-receptor antagonists have equal efficacy and include cimetidine (up to 800 mg bid, or 400 mg qid), ranitidine (150 mg bid), nizatidine (150 mg bid), and famotidine (20 mg bid). H_2-receptor antagonists provide complete heartburn relief in approx 60% of patients.

PPIs provide superior gastric acid suppression and have excellent safety profiles. Patients have been on long-term omeprazole therapy for more than 15 years *(52)*. The PPIs have minimal, clinically relevant differences between them and include omeprazole (20 mg qd or 20 mg bid), lansoprazole (30 mg qd or bid), pantoprazole (40 mg qd), rabeprazole (20 mg qd), and esomeprazole (40 mg up to bid). Rabeprazole has a slightly quicker onset of action; omeprazole has the highest potential for drug interactions with warfarin, diazepam, and phenytoin; lansoprazole may alter theophylline levels. Pantoprazole has the lowest potential for drug interactions. None of the PPIs require dosing adjustments for hepatic or renal insufficiency. PPIs should be given before meals, because they require an active parietal cell for action. Recent data show that 40 mg of esompegrazole provides better control of night time GER symptoms than 20 mg of omeprazole or 30 mg lansoprazole. Faster relief of night time GER symptoms was obtained with 40 mg of pantoprazole, compared with 40 mg of esomeprazole *(54)*. In general, esomeprazole and pantoprazole appear to be equally effective in resolving night time GER symptoms; however, pantoprazole has a longer half-life than other PPIs *(54)*.

More recently, nocturnal gastric acid breakthrough was noted with PPIs. Omeprazole 40 mg with dinner or 20 mg in the morning and evening resulted in better gastric acid suppression than 40 mg before breakfast. Peghini and colleagues *(55)* noted that nocturnal gastric acid breakthrough occurred in 90% of normal control subjects using omeprazole 20 mg twice daily. Initial studies using ranitidine 150 mg before bedtime resulted in improvement in nocturnal gastric acid breakthrough. However, the effect was lost after 7 days *(56)*. This finding was verified by Orr and colleagues *(57)* who noted that 150 mg of ranitidine did not alter sleep-related GER in patients taking omeprazole twice daily.

Prokinetic Agents

GER is not an *acid* disease, but an esophageal *motility* disease. Prokinetic agents attempt to increase LES pressure, accelerate esophageal acid clearance mechanisms, and improve gastric emptying. Unfortunately, the only Food and Drug Administration-approved prokinetic agent in the United States is metoclopramide (10 mg qid). Central nervous system side effects, including drowsiness, irritability, and extrapyramidal effects, occur in 20–50% of patients. Prokinetic agents can be used in combination with acid suppressive agents.

Continuous Positive Airway Pressure

As previously noted, CPAP decreases esophageal acid contact times, decreases the number of reflux episodes, and improves night time esophageal symptoms in patients with OSA *(39,44)*. Although CPAP has been used rarely in patients with GER without OSA, further research is needed to examine CPAP utility and risks in these patients.

Surgical Fundoplication

Nissen fundoplication (open and laparoscopic techniques) provides symptom resolution in 80–90% of patients *(58)*. Surgical complications include dysphagia, chest herniation, slipped fundoplication, a wrap that is too tight, and vagal nerve injury. Interestingly, laparoscopic fundoplication is associated with a higher rate of dysphagia (8–12%), compared with open techniques. Long-term GER therapy outcomes were examined by Spechler and colleagues *(59)* who carried out a prospective randomized trial of medical vs surgical therapy in 160 patients with complicated GER, having a median follow-up of 10 years. Ninety-two percent of medically treated and 62% of surgically treated patients used antireflux medications regularly. Surgery often does not replace the need for antireflux medical therapy. A recent follow-up trial, examining 310 subjects randomized to receive either omeprazole or surgical fundoplication, showed that surgically treated patients had a higher GER remission rate, compared with those using omeprazole *(60)*. Surgical fundoplication can be considered in selected patients with GER, especially those with a low LES pressure, normal esophageal motility, and GER improvement with medical therapy.

POTENTIAL FUTURE THERAPIES

New potential GER therapies on the horizon include GABA β-agonists that inhibit TLESRs *(61)*. Currently, baclofen is available, but it has many side effects; however, newer agents are being developed with similar actions. Endoscopic LES therapies being investigated include endoscopic gastroplexy and the Stretta procedure, in which radio-frequency energy is transmitted to the lower esophagus; both are currently considered experimental *(62)*. Endoluminal therapies include the Enteryx® procedure (Enteric Medical Technologies, Inc., Foster City, CA), in which liquid copolymers are injected into the LES area, which then quickly solidify to bolster the LES. The Enteryx procedure was voluntarily withdrawn from the market on September 23, 2005, because of severe adverse events. Further research will examine these potential future therapies' efficacies.

In conclusion, esophageal function during sleep is altered. Sleep-related GER is very common in patients with daytime GER. Sleep-related GER can be diagnosed clinically as well as with esophageal pH testing integrated with polysomnography. Potential extraesophageal manifestations of sleep-related GER include sleep-related asthma, sleep-related laryngospasm, and a possible association with OSA. Furthermore, management of sleep-related GER includes conservative measures, medical therapies (H_2-receptor antagonists, PPIs, and prokinetic agents), and surgical fundoplication in selected patients. Nasal CPAP has shown efficacy in treating sleep-related GER, especially in patients with OSA.

ACKNOWLEDGMENTS

Financial support: Dr. Harding currently receives grant support and consultant fees from AstraZeneca LP.

REFERENCES

1. Nebel OT, Formes MF, Castell DO (1976) Symptomatic gastroesophageal reflux: incidence and precipitating factor. Dig Dis Sci 21:953–956.
2. A Gallup Survey on Heartburn Across America. The Gallup Organization, Princeton, NJ, 1988.

3. Shaker R, Castell DO, Schoenfeld PS, et al. (2003) Nighttime heartburn is an under-appreciated clinical problem that impacts sleep and daytime function: the results of a Gallup Survey conducted on behalf of the American Gastroenterological Association. Am J Gastroenterol 98:1487–1493.
4. Mittal RK, Balaban DH (1997) The esophagogastric junction. New Engl J Med 336:924–932.
5. Mittal RK, Holloway RH, Penagini R, et al. (1995) Transient lower esophageal sphincter relaxation. Gastroenterology 109:601–610.
6. Helm JF, Riedel DR, Teeter BC, et al. (1983) Determinants of esophageal acid clearance in normal subjects. Gastroenterology 85:607–612.
7. Moore JG (1991) Circadian dynamics of gastric acid secretion and pharmacodynamics of H_2 receptor blockade. Ann NY Acad Sci 618:150–158.
8. Elsenbruch S, Orr WC, Harnish MJ, et al. (1999) Disruption of normal gastric myoelectric functioning by sleep. Sleep 22:453–458.
9. Goo RH, Moore JG, Greenberg E, et al. (1987) Circadian variation in gastric emptying of meals in humans. Gastroenterology 93:515–518.
10. Kahrilas PJ, Dodds WJ, Dent J, et al. (1987) Effect of sleep, spontaneous gastroesophageal reflux, and a meal on upper esophageal sphincter pressure in normal human volunteers. Gastroenterology 92:466–471.
11. Orr WC, Johnson LF, Robinson MG (1984) The effect of sleep on swallowing, esophageal peristalsis, and acid clearance. Gastroenterology 86:814–819.
12. Schneyer LH, Pigmar W, Heyahar L (1956) Rate of flow on human parotid, sublingual, and submaxillary secretions during sleep. J Dental Res 35:109–114.
13. Orr WC, Johnson LF (1998) Responses to different levels of esophageal acidification during waking and sleep. Dig Dis Sci 43:241–245.
14. Orr WC, Elsenbruch S, Harnish MJ, et al. (2000) Proximal migration of esophageal acid perfusions during waking and sleep. Am J Gastroenterol 95:37–42.
15. Kahrilas PJ, Quigley EMM (1996) Clinical esophageal pH recording: a technical review for practice guideline development. Gastroenterology 110:1982–1996.
16. *Esophageal pH Monitoring*: *Practical Approach and Clinical Applications*. 2nd ed. (Richter JE, ed.) Williams & Wilkins, Baltimore, MD, 1997.
17. Harding SM, Richter JE, Guzzo MR, et al. (1996) Asthma and gastroesophageal reflux: acid suppressive therapy improves asthma outcome. Am J Med 100:395–405.
18. American Academy of Sleep Medicine (2005) *International Classification of Sleep Disorders Diagnostic and Coding Manual*. 2nd ed. American Academy of Sleep Medicine, Westchester, IL
19. Johnson LF, DeMeester TR (1974) Twenty-four hour pH monitoring of distal esophagus: a quantitative measure of gastroesophageal reflux. Am J Gastroenterol 62:325–332.
20. DeMeester TR, Johnson LF, Guy JO, et al. (1996) Patterns of gastroesophageal reflux in health and disease. Ann Surg 184:459–470.
21. Orr WC, Heading R, Johnson LF, et al. (2004) Review article: sleep and its relationship to gastro-oesophageal reflux. Aliment Pharmacol Ther 209(Suppl 9):39–46.
22. Orr WC (2005) Heartburn: another "danger" in the night? Chest 127:1486–1488.
23. Shaker R (2004) Nighttime GERD: clinical implications and therapeutic challenges. Best Pract Res Clin Gastroenterol 18:31–38.
24. Fass R, Quan SF, O'Connor GT, et al. (2005) Predictors of heartburn during sleep in a large prospective cohort study. Chest 127:1658–1666.
25. Chand N, Johnson DA, Tabangin M, et al. (2004) Sleep dysfunction in patients with gastro-oesophageal reflux disease: prevalence and response to GERD therapy, a pilot study. Aliment Pharmacol Ther 20:969–974.
26. Johnson DA, Orr WC, Crawley JA, et al. (2005) Effect of esomeprazole on nighttime heartburn and sleep quality in patients with GERD: a randomized placebo-controlled trial. Am J Gastroenterol 100:1914–1922.
27. Freidin N, Fisher MJ, Taylor W, et al. (1991) Sleep and nocturnal acid reflux in normal subjects and patients with reflux oesophagitis. Gut 32:1275–1279.
28. Khoury RM, Camacho-Lobato L, Katz PO, et al. (1999) Influence of spontaneous sleep positions on nighttime recumbent reflux in patients with gastroesophageal reflux disease. Am J Gastroenterol 94:2069–2073.
29. Fass R, Achem Sr, Harding S, et al. (2004) Review article: supra-oesophageal manifestationis of gastro-oesophageal reflux disease and the role of night-time gastro-oesophageal reflux. Aliment Pharmacol Ther 20(Suppl 9):26–38.

30. Harding SM (1999) Nocturnal asthma: role of nocturnal gastroesophageal reflux. Chronobiol Intl 16:641–662.
31. Harding SM (2005) Gastroesophageal reflux: a potential asthma trigger. Immunol Allergy Clin NA 25:131–148.
32. Gislason T, Janson C, Vermeire P, et al. (2002) Respiratory symptoms and nocturnal gastroesophageal reflux: a population-based study of young adults in three European countries. Chest 121:158–163.
33. Gunnbjornsdottir MI, Omenaas E, Gislason T, et al. (2004) Obesity and nocturnal gastro-esophageal reflux are related to onset of asthma and respiration and symptoms. Eur Respir J 24:116–121.
34. Sontag, SJ, O'Connell S, Miller TQ, et al. (2004) Asthmatics have more nocturnal gasping and reflux symptoms than non-asthmatics, and they are related to bedtime eating. Am J Gastrointesterol 99:789–796.
35. Jack CIA, Calverley PMA, Donnelly RJ, et al. (1995) Simultaneous tracheal and oesophageal pH measurement in asthmatic patients with gastro-oesophageal reflux. Thorax 50:201–204.
36. Cuttitta G, Cibella F, Visconti A (2000) Spontaneous gastroesophageal reflux and airway patency during the night in adult asthmatics. Am J Respir Crit Care Med 151:177–181.
37. Thurnheer R, Henz S, Knoblauch A (1997) A sleep-related laryngospasm. Eur Respir J 10:2084–2086.
38. Janson C, Gislason TR, De Backer W, et al. (1995) Daytime sleepiness, snoring and gastro-oesophageal reflux amongst young adults in three European countries. J Int Med 237:277–285.
39. Green BT, Broughton WA, O'Connor JB (2003) Marked improvement in nocturnal gastroesophageal reflux in a large cohort of patients with obstructive sleep apnea. Arch Intern Med 163:41–45.
40. Demeter P, Visy KV, Magyar P (2005) Correlation between severity of endoscopic findings and apnea-hypopnea index in patients with gastroesophageal reflux disease and obstructive sleep apnea. World J Gastroenterol 14:839–841.
41. Ozturk O, Ozturk L, Ozdogan A, et al. (2004) Variables affecting the occurrence of gastroesophageal reflux in obstructive sleep apnea patients. Eur Arch Otorhinolaryngol 261:229–232.
42. Penzel T, Becker HF, Brandenburg U, et al. (1999) Arousal in patients with gastro-oesophageal reflux and sleep apnoea. Eur Respir J 14:1266–1270.
43. Graf KI, Karaus M, Heinemann S, et al. (1995) Gastroesophageal reflux in patients with sleep apnea syndrome. Z Gastroenterol 33:689–693.
44. Ing AJ, Ngu MC, Breslin AB (2000) Obstructive sleep apnea and gastroesophageal reflux. Am J Med 108(Suppl 4A):120S–125S.
45. Senior BA, Khan M, Schwimmer C, et al. (2001) Gastroesophageal reflux and obstructive sleep apnea. Laryngoscope 111:2144–2146.
46. Berg S, Hoffstein V, Gislason T (2004) Acidification of distal esophagus and sleep-related breathing disturbances. Chest 125:2101–2106.
47. Morse CA, Quan SF, Mays MZ, et al. (2004) Is there a relationship between obstructive sleep apnea and gastroesophageal reflux disease. Clin Gastroenterol Hepatol 2:761–768.
48. Kim H-N, Vorona RD, Winn MP, et al. (2005) Symptoms of gastro-oesophageal reflux disease and the severity of obstructive sleep apnoea syndrome are not related in sleep disorders center patients. Aliment Pharmacol Ther 21:1127–1133.
49. Demeter P, Pap A The relationship between gastroesophageal reflux disease and obstructive sleep apnea. J Gastroenterol 39:815–820.
50. Lundell L (2002) Advances in treatment strategies for gastroesophageal reflux disease. In: *Basic Mechanisms of Digestive Diseases*: *The Rationale for Clinical Management and Prevention.* (Farthing MJG, Malfertheiner P, eds.) John Libbey Eurotex, Paris, France, pp. 13–22.
51. Hamilton JW, Boisen RJ, Yamamoto DT, et al. (1988) Sleeping on a wedge diminishes exposure of the esophagus to refluxed acid. Dig Dis Sci 33:518–522.
52. DeVault KR, Castell DO (1999) Updated guidelines for the diagnosis and treatment of gastroesophageal reflux disease: the Practice Parameters Committee of the American College of Gastroenterology. Am J Gastroenterol 94:1434–1442.
53. Sexton MW, Harding SM (2003) Sleep-related reflux: a unique clinical challenge. J Respir Dis 24:398–406.
54. Orr WC (2005) Night-time gastro-oesophageal reflux disease: prevalence, hazards, and management. Eur J Gastroenterol Hepatol 17:113–120.
55. Peghini PL, Katz PO, Bracy NA, et al. (1998) Nocturnal recovery of gastric acid secretion with twice-daily dosing of proton pump inhibitors. Am J Gastroenterol 93:763–767.
56. Fackler WK, Ours TM, Vaezi MF, et al. (2002) Long-term effect of H_2RA therapy on nocturnal acid break through. Gastroenterology 122:625–632.

57. Orr WC, Harnish MJ (2003) The efficacy of omeprazole twice daily with supplemental H_2 blockade at bedtime in the suppression of nocturnal oesophageal and gastric acidity. Aliment Pharmacol Ther 17:1553–1558.
58. Peters JH, Heimbucher J, Kauer WK, et al. (1995) Clinical and physiologic comparison of laparoscopic and open Nissen fundoplication. Am Coll Surg 180:385–393.
59. Spechler SJ, Lee E, Ahnen D, et al. (2001) Long-term outcome of medical and surgical therapies for gastroesophageal reflux disease: follow-up of a randomized controlled trial. JAMA 285:2331–2338.
60. Lundell L, Miettinen P, Myrvold HE, et al. (2001) Continued (55-year) follow up of a randomized clinical study comparing anti-reflux surgery and omeprazole in gastroesophageal reflux disease. J Am Coll Surg 192:172–181.
61. Vela MF, Tutuian R, Katz PO, et al. (2003) Baclofen decreases acid and non-acid post-prandial gastro-oesophageal reflux measured by combined multichannel intraluminal impedance and pH. Aliment Pharmacol Ther 17:243–251.
62. Wakelin DE, Sampliner RE (2005) Endoscopic anti-reflux procedures: A good wrap? Clin Gastroenterol Hepatol 3:831–839.

24 Circadian Rhythm Disorders

Lois E. Krahn, MD

CONTENTS

INTRODUCTION

Simply stated, everyday people should strive to fall asleep at the time when they are sleepiest. For most people this means having the major sleep period start in the evening and conclude at dawn. However, situations arise in which a person's sleep timing, or circadian rhythm of sleep, is not synchronized with other factors, potentially leading to sleep quality problems. The term *circadian* refers to a circuit or period that is about 24 hours long. Many physiological, biochemical, and behavioral activities have a circadian rhythm, with the sleep–wake cycle being the most easily recognized. The sleep–wake cycle is related to other circadian rhythms, such as core body temperature and concentrations of melatonin or cortisol, through a complex interaction of signals.

Patients with a circadian rhythm disorder have adequate quality and quantity of sleep, but are unable to sleep at the desired or expected time. As a consequence, they are awake or asleep at inappropriate times, possibly experiencing insomnia, excessive daytime sleepiness, or both. Circadian rhythm disorders can be conceptualized according to which component of the sleep–wake cycle is aberrant: the ability to develop periodicity (non-24-hour sleep–wake disorder), the motivation to perpetuate

From: *Current Clinical Practice: Primary Care Sleep Medicine: A Practical Guide*
Edited by: J. F. Pagel and S. R. Pandi-Perumal © Humana Press Inc., Totowa, NJ

periodicity (irregular sleep–wake disorder), or timing relative to the community in which the person lives (delayed and advanced sleep phase disorder, shift work, and jet lag sleep disorder).

CIRCADIAN INFLUENCES ON SLEEP–WAKE ACTIVITY

The sleep–wake rhythm is determined by several important factors. Two major processes, circadian rhythmicity (process C) and sleep homeostasis (process S), were initially recognized during temporal isolation studies that allowed the sleep–wake schedule to become dissociated from the body's temperature cycle. Sleep homeostasis represents the time elapsed since the last episode of sleep. As time passes, the pressure to sleep builds up and eventually reaches a point where sleep is irresistible because of the accumulated sleep debt. Once this debt has been satisfied, the pressure to sleep decreases; with time it again increases progressively. Circadian rhythmicity, which determines time points when sleep is more likely to occur based on the sleep–wake pacemaker, is the other important factor. The interplay of homeostatic and circadian factors determines sleep in rigorously controlled conditions like a temporal isolation chamber. In a community setting, many other factors including personal choice, work schedules, family responsibilities, physical activities, and exogenous substances such as hypnotics or caffeine play a contributory role to setting sleep onset and awakening.

Circadian rhythmicity is primarily determined by a group of cells in the suprachiasmatic nuclei (SCN) located in the hypothalamus, often called the biological clock. This pacemaker produces the circadian rhythm of sleep for the adult (one major sleep period per 24-hour period) that, with maturity, replaces the pattern of both daytime and night time sleep in infants. Isolation of these nuclei from the rest of the brain results in an abolition of circadian rhythms outside the small hypothalamic island, but neural circadian rhythm persists within the nuclei themselves. Although in more primitive animals like the fruit fly, a variety of body regions such as the limbs appear capable of setting the circadian rhythm, in mammals the circadian pacemaker is restricted to the SCN. Intriguing reports that a region on the human lower extremity can respond to light stimuli and determine circadian rhythms have not been replicated *(1)*.

The periodicity of the biological clock has been studied by means of temporal isolation experiments in which subjects were placed in an environment totally without time cues. Early experiments indicated that in such an environment, the sleep–wake cycle free-runs with subjects opting to go to sleep and waking approx 1 hour later every day. This suggested that the human biological pacemaker had an intrinsic periodicity of 24.9 hours, as compared with the environmental cycle of 24 hours. However, more recent work with rigorously controlled light conditions has shown that the actual periodicity of the human pacemaker is 24 hours 11 ± 8 minutes, with the earlier erroneous figure attributed to masking effects of low-level illumination used in the experiments *(2)*. Over time even this small mismatch between the periodicity of the environmental 24-hour clock and the intrinsic human sleep–wake cycle can still result in some people's internal sleep–wake phase becoming desynchronized from the community's predominant schedule. This potential desynchronization may explain the delayed sleep phase type of circadian rhythm sleep disorder (DSPD).

Intensive efforts have been made to understand the molecular mechanism of circadian rhythms and genetic influences on these influential cells. Several genes have been identified, although their exact role is still to be determined. In essence, protein gene products feed back to the nucleus, temporarily inhibiting their own genetic synthesis, thus establishing a biological rhythm with fixed periodicity. In the mouse, a gene (*Clock*) that controls the circadian sleep/wake rhythm has been identified *(3)*. When the *Clock* gene is mutated, the circadian rhythm of sleep, and in particular the ultradian rhythm of rapid eye movement (REM) sleep, is altered. In humans, a mutation has been reported in another circadian gene (*PER*), with the finding that the *hPER2* gene is dysfunctional in families with advanced sleep phase syndrome *(4)*.

The process of adapting the biological clock's intrinsic periodicity to the geosynchronous cycle of 24 hours is called entrainment. This is an adaptable and dynamic system, with several factors being able to alter the sleep–wake circadian rhythm. Such factors leading to entrainment are called *zeitgebers*, from the German term meaning "time givers." Bright light is indisputably the predominant zeitgeber, although social cues and food play a role. Whether a person's eyes are open or closed, light enters the eye and excites photoreceptor cells in the retina. Melanopsin, discovered in 2000, is a light-sensitive pigment found in those retinal ganglion cells that project to the SCN. Studies in mice with absent melanopsin show that this novel pigment is required for normal circadian phase setting *(5)*. The signal from the retinal ganglion cells is transmitted along the retinohypothalamic tract to the SCN in the anterior hypothalamus, thus directly causing entrainment. In addition, the signal is then transmitted down brainstem sympathetic pathways to the intermediolateral cell column of the upper thoracic spinal cord and from there to the superior cervical ganglion, which provides sympathetic input to the pineal gland. The degree to which exposure to light affects the sleep–wake rhythm depends on the timing, intensity, and duration of light exposure. In general, light exposure in the morning delays the sleep onset, whereas evening light does the reverse.

When persons are in the dark or dim light at night, the pineal gland secretes the hormone melatonin. Melatonin receptors are present in the SCN and thus the hormone might be involved in humoral feedback regulation of the pacemaker. When a person is exposed to bright natural or artificial light (10,000 l×, the intensity of unfiltered light from the sun) regardless of the time of day or night, melatonin secretion is promptly suppressed. The reverse situation, the absence of bright light, does not lead to melatonin release unless the darkness corresponds to the appropriate point on the circadian rhythm of melatonin, approx 16 hours after the cessation of the previous cycle's secretion. In healthy persons, melatonin is secreted from about 10 PM until 6 AM, depending on the timing of bedtime and light exposure. Because people with a normal sleep–wake circadian rhythm typically sleep during the night, by extension melatonin is often used as a marker of the circadian rhythm of sleep–wake activity. However, melatonin data must be interpreted carefully with awareness of the light conditions and medication use (β_1-adrenergic antagonists block the noradrenergic innervation of the pineal gland). Because of these factors, the initial rise of melatonin concentration at night in blood, saliva, or urine should be referred to as *dim-light melatonin onset*.

DIAGNOSTIC CONSIDERATIONS

Circadian rhythm disorders can be diagnosed based on a careful history of the patient's sleep–wake schedule. A detailed sleep diary covering several weeks can be helpful. Because many patients struggle to accurately complete a sleep diary, wrist actigraphy can be an extremely useful supplemental procedure. Poor recall, misperception of sleep/wake time, or deliberate distortion (e.g., an adolescent who does not want his parents to be aware of his late-night activities) may be factors that cause the sleep diary data to differ markedly from the information collected with the actigraph. In these cases, the actigraphic data may be more reliable than the patient self-report.

CIRCADIAN RHYTHM SLEEP DISORDER, DELAYED SLEEP PHASE TYPE (DELAYED SLEEP PHASE DISORDER)

Demographics

Patients with DSPD fall asleep later and awaken later than expected or desired. Of the circadian rhythm disorders, apart from jet lag and shift-related issues, sleep specialists and other clinicians are most likely to encounter this circadian-rhythm disorder. DSPD is common, although in-depth epidemiological studies are lacking. In one study of 10,000 Scandinavians followed with sleep logs, a prevalence of 0.72% was reported *(6)*. This number is suspected to be an underestimate because of the limitations of survey research that cannot eliminate the factors of poor recall, misperception, or distortion inherent in self-report questionnaire data. In this study, the mean age of onset was during adolescence at 15.4 years and the disorder was chronic (mean duration, 19.2 years). The condition rarely starts after the age of 30 years. The male-female mix is uncertain, but some studies note a male predominance. There are no reports of a familial predisposition.

Clinical Features

DSPD is characterized by initial sleep and awake times that are consistently later than desired. The total sleep time over the 24-hour period is normal. Many patients note that this sleep problem developed after a stretch of late-night studying or social activities. If the patient manages to arise at a socially acceptable hour, excessive daytime sleepiness is usually present during the morning hours. On vacation, when the patient is not trying to conform to any specified schedule, the wake-up time will be delayed. Patients with DSPD often recognize that they have the longstanding trait of being "night owls," feeling most alert and performing best late at night. Some individuals cope by selecting careers that involve evenings and avoid mornings, such as restaurant work. Students may compensate by taking night classes.

Because of the difficulty in falling asleep in the earlier part of the night, patients may seek for treatment for insomnia. Estimates are that 10% of patients seeking treatment for insomnia may have DSPD. Some of these patients are persuaded to seek help by bed partners or parents who are concerned about their inability to fall asleep. Others face consequences related to school or work because of their difficulty in getting up at the desired time and they seek assistance with falling asleep earlier. DSPD is often associated with psychiatric disorders, specifically depression. It is unclear if the adolescent first has psychiatric symptoms and then develops delayed sleep phase or if the circadian rhythm disorder leads to absenteeism, which in turn results in psychiatric, academic, and social problems. Patients and their families are often intensely frustrated by the condition.

Differential Diagnosis

The differential diagnosis includes major depression, with patients having an increased need to sleep, sometimes coexisting with an initial insomnia. If a patient pursues treatment for the mood disorder with improvement in mood and other symptoms but has persisting delayed sleep phase, then a coexisting circadian rhythm disorder should be suspected. Some patients with avoidant or schizoid personality disorder will seek out the solitude of night. A careful history should not only explore the person's sleep–wake schedule but also look for signs of deliberate avoidance of daytime interactions. Some people who are on vacation, disabled, or unemployed may voluntarily select a late-night schedule. Determining the motivation and effort expended to conform to the more conventional timetable is of value in differentiating them from true patients with DSPD.

Occasionally patients will appear to have a disorder of excessive daytime sleepiness such as narcolepsy or idiopathic hypersomnia. The assessment should include careful exploration of the presence of excessive sleepiness during the evening and night, with normal alertness during these times more likely indicating DSPD. Patients with DSPD may have sleep-onset REM periods during the first or second naps of the Multiple Sleep Latency Test, especially if the test's start time was not delayed in accordance with the patient's phase shift. This does not reflect REM sleep intruding into daytime alertness but rather the patient's final REM sleep of his or her major sleep period. Initial sleep latencies usually increase with successive naps in DSPD. In all the circadian-rhythm disorders, polysomnography may be indicated if there is suspicion that a coexisting sleep disorder such as obstructive sleep apnea may be present. When polysomnography is used, the start time of the sleep study may need to be adjusted.

Management

Patients must strive toward a consistent sleep–wake schedule, as staying up late deliberately on weekends and holidays can interfere with falling asleep as desired on weeknights. Patient motivation is an essential component in a successful treatment plan. If the patient does not actively embrace the practices necessary to correct the circadian rhythm disorder, treatment is unlikely to be effective. In some cases, patients espouse an intention to strive toward a phase shift but actually maintain a passive-aggressive attitude that can contribute significantly to family strain. In many cases, psychotherapy may be essential in giving the patient an opportunity to understand and modify the factors that may be contributing to late-night activity. Family as well as individual therapy may be useful in finding solutions to complex family and school problems.

The most commonly recommended treatment is to have the patient use bright-light therapy in the morning from 6 to 9 AM to adjust their sleep–wake cycle. When patients are adherent, this has been demonstrated to be effective *(7)*. Patients typically start at a later time, for example 9 AM, and as their ability to awake earlier improves, they advance the time of light exposure earlier in 30-minute increments. However, despite this, many patients have difficulty awakening in order to get light exposure from a light box or the sun. Adherence is often inconsistent, with patients complaining that they cannot find the necessary 30 minutes each morning for the treatment.

The recommended light intensity is 10,000 l×. Several different light units are available and the manufacturers' specifications should be followed concerning the distance the patient should sit from the light box. This varies depending on whether the unit has a single central light or two smaller units on either side of the patient. Patients should make light exposure their priority and engage in activities like reading, applying make-up, or eating breakfast only as long as their eyes are positioned adequately in front of the box. Many patients prefer to combine exposure to natural sunshine with exercise by jogging, biking, or running outside in clear weather. Patients should be reminded not to look directly at the sun to prevent eye damage. Potential side effects of light boxes include retinal burns, which are more likely to develop if the patient is taking anticholinergic medications that increase the pupillary diameter. Patients taking photosensitizing medications should not be advised to use phototherapy.

Patients should also be advised to avoid bright light, possibly by wearing sunglasses, from 4 PM until dusk. Other treatment options have included melatonin, which has been beneficial in several controlled trials *(8–10)*. Melatonin is given 1–3 hours (depending on the severity of the phase delay) before the desired bedtime and used on an ongoing basis. The dose of melatonin is typically low (3 mg). Melatonin has not been as rigorously tested for side effects as hypnotic agents. Because it is not considered a pharmaceutical agent by the US Food and Drug Administration, but is rather classified as a nutritional supplement available in health-food stores, patients may have difficulty verifying the purity of the product available for purchase. Safety data regarding chronic usage have not appeared in the medical literature, although no anecdotal reports of serious side effects have surfaced to date. In general, melatonin is only weakly sedating. Some preliminary studies have combined melatonin with phototherapy. This combined approach may be desirable when patients are suspected to have poor adherence with phototherapy and be more likely to take a tablet. Apart from the increased cost, there are no known risks in combining melatonin with light therapy. The melatonin receptor agonist, ramelteon, was approved in 2005 for the treatment of insomnia. Although in theory this selective agent for both the melatonin 1 and 2 receptor may be useful in DSPD, no clinical trial data have been published to date.

Most treatment plans for DSPD no longer emphasize the role of chronotherapy. This approach involved patients sequentially delaying their bedtime by 1–2 hours a night around the clock until they fell asleep at the desired time. Outcomes were poor because of the understandable difficulty in conforming to this complex regimen and the tendency for many patients to slip back into a delayed sleep phase pattern over time. Hypnotics and psychostimulants have not been found to be useful because the patient fundamentally gets adequate sleep but is not synchronized with the community. If the patient has coexisting major depression, antidepressant medications may be appropriate. Some clinicians opt to prescribe sedating antidepressants like mirtazapine, although these approaches are not based on evidence from clinical trials.

CIRCADIAN RHYTHM SLEEP DISORDER, ADVANCED SLEEP PHASE TYPE (ADVANCED SLEEP PHASE DISORDER)

Patients with this condition fall asleep and awaken at times earlier than desired. Patients may inappropriately fall asleep during evening activities and when awake during the second half of the night experience loneliness, or boredom when awake in the early morning. This condition is rare, especially when compared with DSPD. A survey of 10,000 Scandinavians did not find a single case of advanced sleep phase disorder *(6)*. This striking difference in prevalence between advanced and delayed sleep phase disorder is likely because the human sleep–wake circadian period of slightly more than 24 hours promotes phase delay. The condition likely becomes more common with age. In nursing homes and assisted-living facilities, the institutional routines frequently encourage bedtime in the early evening, sometimes because of reduced staffing at those times.

The differential diagnosis includes major depression, as both conditions can be characterized by insomnia in the early morning. The evaluation should include a sleep diary (completed by the patient or facility staff) and wrist actigraphy.

An autosomal-dominant familial form of advanced sleep phase disorder has been reported in three families. All affected patients fell asleep and wakened 4 hours earlier than expected and had melatonin and temperature rhythms that were also advanced by 3–4 hours. The circadian sleep–wake period was shortened to 23.3 hours. The genetic defect was traced to a mutation in the period (*PER*) gene named *hPER2*. Affected individuals have a mutation in the casein kinase 1 binding region of the *hPER2* gene with a serine-to-glycine mutation. This mutation interferes with the functioning of the clock component, causing a significant advance in the circadian period consistent with advanced sleep phase disorder *(4)*.

Treatment involves avoidance of morning bright light and a daytime schedule that encourages entrainment to a conventional sleep–wake schedule. Evening light therapy has also been successfully used in short-term studies *(11,12)*. Progressive earlier shifting of bed time by 3 hours every 2 days has been reported as having short-term utility in one case report *(13)*. One recent study examined therapy of advanced phase sleep disorder in a group of children with Smith-Magenis syndrome, a complex genetic disease caused by a deletion in chromosome 17p. Sleep, as well as melatonin phase, was delayed with the combined administration in the evening of controlled-release melatonin and in the morning a β_1-adrenergic antagonist, blocking the noradrenergic neurotransmission to the pineal gland that releases melatonin *(14)*.

CIRCADIAN RHYTHM SLEEP DISORDER, FREE-RUNNING TYPE (NONENTRAINED TYPE)

Non-24-hour sleep–wake syndrome, otherwise known as hypernychthemeral disorder, is a rare condition usually limited to visually impaired people, some of whom are also developmentally handicapped. These patients develop sleep patterns similar to those observed in subjects living without environmental time cues. They cannot benefit from the powerful entraining effect of light on the SCN, experiencing a free-running rhythm without a consistent phase. Clinically these patients may present with intermittent insomnia and excessive daytime sleepiness. For a brief time their sleep–wake activity may be synchronized with the community, but after several days it will again drift out of phase. In addition to idiosyncratic sleep–wake patterns, they may develop other unpredictable circadian rhythms, for example, melatonin secretion. Patients complain of undesired daytime sleep corresponding to diurnal melatonin that, in the absence of light perception, is not suppressed. The sleep–wake rhythm may also dissociate from the body's other circadian rhythms, such as temperature (internal desynchronization). Sleep initiation difficulties may worsen at times when the free-running circadian rhythm for sleep–wake activity corresponds to points of the temperature rhythm other than the nadir. Because many affected patients try to conform to a socially acceptable sleep–wake schedule, they awaken earlier than appropriate, resulting in insufficient sleep. However, even on vacation, when they are less likely to arise at a specified time, they do not develop a consistent sleep schedule.

In one recent study using polysomnography, actigraphy, and Braille sleep logs, sleep was studied in 26 totally blind patients and matched control subjects *(15)*. These patients were living in the community but still were observed to have multiple sleep complaints, presumably as a result of a free-running cycle. Patients who were employed had a longer major sleep period than those who were retired or unemployed. Patients who have a mental handicap or multiple disabilities may cope more poorly because of increased difficulty in conforming to social routines.

This condition should be suspected in any patient without light perception who has sleep complaints. Non-24-hour sleep–wake disorder should be differentiated from the other circadian-rhythm disorders, including DSPD. In DSPD, patients have initial insomnia and force themselves to arise at an inappropriately early time because of social obligations. In contrast to non-24-hour sleep–wake rhythm disorder, DSPD patients experience a stable sleep–wake cycle on vacation, albeit with a delayed pattern. Another diagnostic consideration is the irregular sleep–wake disorder in which patients with an inconsistent schedule are capable of entrainment but disregard the cues. A detailed sleep diary recording several weeks of functioning accompanied by wrist actigraphy can assist in distinguishing these syndromes. The medical and social consequences of a non-24-hour sleep–wake rhythm have not been well studied but would be expected to include professional and family difficulties.

Few therapeutic options have been studied. Melatonin has been explored as a means to entrain circadian rhythms. Low-dose melatonin is typically administered at 8 PM (expected to be near the time of the dim-light melatonin onset) to achieve an 11 PM effect *(16)*. A sleep diary should be used before starting melatonin, allowing the treatment to begin only after the major sleep period shifts to night. Assessing whether bright light suppresses melatonin may be worthwhile in some blind persons, as occasionally the retinohypothalamic pathway remains intact despite the absence of sight. In such cases, bright light may be used for entrainment purposes. Other schedule cues, such as social activities and exercise, have therapeutic value in this lifelong disorder.

CIRCADIAN RHYTHM SLEEP DISORDER, IRREGULAR SLEEP–WAKE TYPE (IRREGULAR SLEEP–WAKE RHYTHM)

Irregular sleep–wake rhythm or chaotic sleep–wake rhythm is a state in which patients permit their sleep–wake rhythms to become desynchronized. Patients have the capacity to be entrained but voluntarily disregard the day–night transitions in their community, overriding their internal sleep–wake rhythm. Irregular sleep–wake rhythms are most common in adolescents and young adults. In most cases the state develops in the second decade and the duration is highly variable. The incidence and prevalence of the disorder is unknown.

Clinical Features

In this condition, patients have an average amount of sleep tallied over a 24-hour period but there is marked day-to-day variability in length and timing of the major sleep period. Patients can have insomnia and excessive daytime sleepiness because of their extremely variable sleep schedule. Unlike patients with non-24-hour sleep–wake disorder, these patients are capable of entraining to a regular sleep–wake rhythm. Reasons for the unconventional sleep–wake schedule can include social activities, hobbies (including Internet usage), schoolwork, and absence of sleep–wake discipline.

Irregular sleep–wake cycles are associated with psychiatric disorders, which may either predispose to the circadian dysfunction or occur as a result of it. The condition may also occur in patients with neurological disorders such as dementia, delirium, head injury, and coma emergence, where cognitive, behavioral, or environmental issues, such as a facility's erratic bathing schedule for residents, promote irregular sleep–wake rhythms. Patients with chemical dependency states including intoxication, dependence, and withdrawal may similarly be unwilling, or as long as they are influenced by the exogenous substance, unable to sustain sleep–wake rhythmicity.

The consequences of this condition depend on its severity. A pattern of staying up late on weekend nights may cause no impairment beyond some mild sleep deprivation. For people with a flexible occupation, like writing or internet-based pursuits, fewer adverse consequences may arise from their choice to have irregular hours. However, for individuals who have family or occupational responsibilities, an irregular sleep–wake rhythm may seriously interfere with their functioning. Excessive daytime sleepiness and insomnia develop because of timing issues. Inattention or irritability as a result of sleep deprivation can impair work and school performance and can result in motor vehicle accidents.

Assessment and Management

Obtaining an accurate history of the patient's actual sleep–wake cycle can be difficult because of poor recall, distortion, or denial. Recognizing the irregular schedule is necessary to avoid an inappropriate and misleading diagnosis of a chronic fatigue state.

Assessment involves careful tracking of the sleep–wake schedule using a sleep diary completed each day. Wrist actigraphy can be very useful to get more objective observations from patients who may be unable or unwilling to accurately describe their schedule.

The patient's motivation to change is a major determinant of treatment outcome. Psychotherapy may be important to help a patient appreciate the adverse consequences of this lifestyle and to examine reasons why the patient might resist change. The first step is to have a consistent schedule even if it has a pronounced abnormal phase. Over time, a sleep–wake schedule with an abnormal phase can be shifted using the modalities described earlier in this chapter, including phototherapy and social cues. Melatonin has not been extensively studied but has potential to be beneficial in this circadian-rhythm disorder.

CIRCADIAN RHYTHM SLEEP DISORDER, JET LAG TYPE (JET LAG DISORDER)

Clinical Features

With the development of long-distance transmeridian travel, a new sleep disorder has emerged. Jet lag (otherwise known as time-zone change syndrome) represents an acute problem in which travelers' sleep–wake circadian rhythms become out of phase with the light–dark cycle at their destination. The magnitude of the problem increases as travelers cross more time zones. In general, without measures to accelerate adjustment, 1 day is required to adjust to every hour of time zone change. Longitudinal (north-south) travel may result in sleep debt related to obtaining quality sleep on board a plane, but does not challenge a traveler with adapting to a new time zone.

In contrast to shift workers, the entrainment process is facilitated for travelers with jet lag, as they are attempting to adapt to the sleep–wake cycle of the destination community. Most people can more readily phase-delay than phase-advance the timing of their major sleep period, probably because of the more than 24-hour periodicity of the human circadian pacemaker. Thus, east-to-west travel is typically easier to adjust to than the equivalent travel from west to east. Travelers who make frequent long-distance trips can develop a more chronic condition because they have not adequately adapted before a further change in sleep–wake schedule occurs. When people such as airline personnel face frequent circadian adjustments because of work schedules, jet lag overlaps with shift-work sleep disorder.

The consequences of jet lag are similar to other sleep–wake rhythm disorders, with excessive daytime sleepiness, insomnia, disturbed nocturnal sleep, and occupational problems relating to inadequate alertness. The effect of jet lag on other circadian rhythms is less well known. Some travelers tolerate transmeridian travel without significant jet lag, but the reasons for individual variations are not well understood. No sex-related differences exist for jet lag, but the ability to adapt sleep–wake rhythms decreases with age.

Treatment

Treatment options are controversial and no one strategy is clearly preferred. Numerous research studies have been conducted but most have significant limitations, primarily study design issues, including controlling light exposure and assuring subject adherence with the protocol. Few experimental models exist for jet lag that account for all of the variables encountered in the real world of travel. For example, a protocol might call for three successive days of bright light exposure at a consistent time after arrival at one's destination, steps that would be inconvenient for most tourists or business travelers.

The most commonly used strategies are optimizing sleep hygiene, manipulating one's sleep–wake schedule, taking melatonin, using phototherapy, and cautious use of hypnotics. The traveler should be urged to obtain sleep of sufficient quality and quantity. A daytime flight eliminates the need to get adequate sleep in an uncomfortable setting. Helpful measures include using a bedroom at the destination that is dark, quiet, and a comfortable temperature. Relaxation techniques may hasten sleep onset at an unfamiliar hour. Alcohol use is not recommended. Dietary measures have been proposed, such as a presleep tryptophan-rich carbohydrate diet (promoting sedation mediated by serotonin and therefore melatonin production) and protein intake on awakening (increasing alertness by means of tyrosine), but these programs are not supported by convincing evidence. Herbal remedies, other than melatonin, have limited usefulness.

One helpful approach is to try to adapt the time of the major sleep period as quickly as possible to the new schedule. For example, if a traveler arrives at 6 AM in Europe after a west-to-east transatlantic flight, the person is phase-delayed as much as 6–7 hours behind the time at the destination. For example, the traveler's sleep–wake rhythm may be at 1–2 AM although he has arrived in time for morning activities in Europe. The traveler needs to phase-advance and should avoid sleeping until as close to the desired bedtime as possible. For westward flights, the circadian challenge is the opposite. The person needs to adapt to the advanced sleep phase by phase-delaying his sleep–wake schedule in order to conform to the destination's time.

Meals and exercise at the destination should be timed carefully to serve as social cues that encourage and reinforce an appropriate sleep–wake cycle. Some experts advocate naps before, during, and after transmeridian travel to prevent developing a significant sleep debt. These naps should be timed carefully to allow sufficient sleep pressure to build up so that the traveler can still initiate sleep at the desired bedtime at the destination. Caffeine use should be carefully tracked so as to minimize caffeine-related insomnia.

Hypnotics, traditionally the short-acting benzodiazepines such as triazolam, have been shown to be of some benefit in jet lag. These compounds decrease sleep latency, reduce awakenings, and increase total sleep time. A more recently available but less studied option are the nonbenzodiazepine agents like zolpidem, zaleplon, and eszopiclone. The half-life of any hypnotic should be relatively short to avoid a hangover effect. Potential side effects of both these classes of hypnotics include amnesia, whereas cognitive impairment may occur with the benzodiazepines.

Because bright light is known to exert the strongest influence on the SCN, this modality has clear potential for resetting the sleep–wake circadian rhythm to match the schedule of the destination. Numerous studies have led to jet lag algorithms. The intent is to get light exposure before the concurrent melatonin peak and temperature nadir if a phase advance is desired. The light exposure should come after these circadian markers if a phase delay is sought. Use of carefully timed light exposure may accelerate phase adjustments from 1 to 3 hours change per day. This strategy, although scientifically based on the physiology of the SCN, is difficult to implement in real-life travel. There are no simple tools for determining the melatonin peak or measuring core body temperature. The duration of an episode of phototherapy, the number of successive daily sessions, the light spectrum, and the effects of age and individual differences are unknown. Nonetheless, awareness of the effects of light on circadian rhythms is important because at a minimum, travelers should avoid bright light exposure at critical times. If phase advance is desired, morning bright light exposure should be minimized (potentially by using wraparound sunglasses) and bright light should be avoided in the evening if a phase delay is desired.

Melatonin has been the subject of intense interest as a tool for the prevention or treatment of jet lag. Some, but not all, studies show the value of this compound as a chronotherapeutic agent for improving jet lag subjectively *(17,18)*. Melatonin should be administered at a 12-hour phase difference from light therapy. If provided before the nadir of the core body temperature, melatonin will advance the sleep–wake circadian rhythm. If administered after this pivotal point, rhythms will delay. Experts advise travelers to start using melatonin during the early evening before departure for eastward trips and thereafter at the desired bedtime at the destination. For westward travel, after arrival at the destination, melatonin should be administered at 11 PM or even later to promote a phase delay.

CIRCADIAN RHYTHM SLEEP DISORDER, SHIFT-WORK TYPE (SHIFT-WORK SLEEP DISORDER)

Clinical Features

An increasing number of people, 20% of the work force in some countries, are employed in jobs that involve working shifts. The type of shift varies but can encompass early morning start times, evening shifts, night work, split 24-hour schedules, and on-call responsibilities. Workers with rotating schedules—as opposed to straight second (evening) or third (night) shift—are at higher risk for complications because their sleep–wake circadian rhythm is constantly adapting to a new timetable. In general, older persons find it harder to adapt to shift changes than younger ones.

Shift workers have high rates of either insomnia or excessive daytime sleepiness. Insomnia and/or excessive daytime sleepiness become clinically significant by interfering with functioning for a subset of shift workers or an estimated 2–5% of the total population. Because of environmental factors, such as neighborhood noise or sunlight, initiating or maintaining sleep during the day can be difficult. Many shift workers get 2–4 hours of insufficient sleep nightly, because they sacrifice daytime sleep to spend time with family, do leisure activities, or run errands. Having a coexisting sleep disorder, such as obstructive sleep apnea, increases the probability of excessive daytime sleepiness. Shift work puts individuals at high risk for several problems. Working when not fully alert poses the risk of performance difficulties relating to inadequate vigilance. Research into fatigue reveals that patients can experience cognitive or motor impairment *(19)*.

Many industrial or transportation incidents, including the Exxon Valdez and the Three Mile Island nuclear power accident, have occurred at night, suggesting that worker fatigue may have been a contributing factor. Missing opportunities to interact with family or friends because of the shift work or recovery sleep can lead to social problems and family strain. Young children in particular may have difficulty understanding that a parent must be allowed to get adequate sleep after returning home from work. Recent work has found an increase in common respiratory infections in shift workers, third shift more than second, with the hypothesis that fatigue renders employees vulnerable to infection *(20)*.

Treatment

Several strategies have been identified to assist workers who must incorporate shift work into their lifestyles. Some people have an affinity for functioning well at certain times, for example, people with a tendency toward a delayed sleep phase may actually cope satisfactorily with an evening work schedule provided that they can sleep late the following morning. Meals should be timed to promote sleep. Hunger or foods that cause dyspepsia may fragment sleep. The workplace environment should be carefully planned to take into account worker's safety and sleep needs. Bright lights and a slightly cool air temperature may improve alertness. Ideally attention should be given to the type of tasks undertaken by employees, especially on the night shift, with monotonous duties interspersed with more stimulating activities.

The sleeping environment at home may need to be modified. A person may wish to wear wraparound dark glasses as he drives home at dawn from work. A quiet and dark bedroom is more important to a shift worker than others. Special window coverings may be required. The telephone should be switched off and messages collected with an answering machine. Family members should be urged not to awaken someone in the midst of their major sleep period. Sleep hygiene should be optimized.

Studies have shown that workers cope better when switching from one shift to another if they delay, rather than advance, their work and sleep time. For instance, if they move from evening to night shift, most individuals adjust more easily to the change. Preparing for an approaching shift change by gradually shifting bedtime and wake time back by 2 hours starting several days before the switch has been found to be beneficial. However, family responsibilities often complicate careful sleep schedule adjustments of this type. Other effective coping strategies include taking a break during work hours. Recent work has focussed on the transportation industry, specifically airline personnel, where a 30-minute nap partway through the shift increases productivity, reduces fatigue, and improves employee satisfaction.

Long-haul aircraft have now been designed to include bunks or reclining seats for scheduled naps *(21)*.

Some employers and employees prefer work schedules that use permanent shift assignments. Night-shift workers should endeavor to keep to a consistent sleep–wake schedule even on days when they do not work. Reverting to night time sleep over a weekend or even a single day off presents adjustment problems similar to those faced by workers assigned to rotating shifts. Again, family and social responsibilities make it difficult for people to follow an exclusive night activity schedule. Workers with on-call schedules present a slightly different problem, as they cannot predict when they will be required to perform a task. Typically the time block for on-call workers is longer than for most other shift workers (e.g., 24 hours) and they cannot plan their sleep–wake schedule in advance. Naps may be especially important under these circumstances. Although in general people are urged to have a major sleep period each 24-hour day as opposed to several shorter stretches of sleep, naps are reasonable if that is the only means by which adequate sleep can be obtained.

Other medications have been examined to help shift workers initiate sleep at the desired time. Regular use of long-acting benzodiazepines creates the risk of physical dependence as well as a hangover effect, especially with longer-acting agents. Short-term use of a newer nonbenzodiazepine hypnotic like zaleplon or zolpidem is preferable to a benzodiazepine. Caution must be taken even with these agents, as they have not been studied or approved for long-term use. Shift workers should first fully explore means to get adequate sleep by means of careful schedule changes, making sufficient sleep a priority, and taking naps if indicated. The hypnotics provide symptomatic relief without addressing the underlying circadian rhythm disturbance inherent in shift work.

In 2003 the Food and Drug Association approved modafinil for the treatment of excessive daytime sleepiness associated with shift work. A recent multisite clinical trial enrolled 209 employees with chronic sleep disturbance who worked at least five night shifts with 6 hours or more between 10 PM and 8 AM *(22)*. Over a 3-month period they received either modafinil (200 mg) or placebo taken 30–60 minutes before the start of their shift. Subjects given modafinil resulted in a modest improvement in the clinical symptoms and the duration of their initial sleep onset. Their attention during a night time testing session improved based on vigilance testing. Because participants had residual excessive daytime sleepiness and decreased performance, the results of this study were not dramatic; however, these data indicate the potential of modafinil in combination with other approaches for shift work sleep disorder.

Caffeine may be useful to boost alertness but should be avoided close to bedtime in order not to interfere with sleep onset. As in jet lag, bright light therapy delivered at precise times may be a useful option. Melatonin has been explored as a possible chronotherapeutic agent, although it is not currently widely used. Very recently, the melatonin agonist ramelteon has shown promise in pilot studies *(23)*.

Alcohol should be avoided as a means of inducing sleep because of its detrimental effects on the patency of the upper airway and tendency to reduce the quality of non-REM sleep. In general, because of the risk of dependence and chronic sleep deprivation, there is agreement that prescribed psychostimulant medications are not an appropriate means to treat shift work sleep disorder. As with the hypnotics, patient should be discouraged from what might become long-term use of a habituating medication and instead be encouraged to rely on scheduling issues and naps. As much as possible, getting adequate sleep needs to be the priority.

REFERENCES

1. Campbell S, Murphy P (1998) Extraocular circadian phototransduction in humans. Science 279:396–399.
2. Czeisler C, Duffy J, Shanahan T, et al. (1999) Stability, precision, and near-24-hour period of the human circadian pacemaker. Science 284:2177–2181.
3. Naylor E, Bergmann B, Krauski K, et al. (2000) The circadian clock mutation alters sleep homeostasis in the mouse. J Neurosci 20:8138–8143.
4. Toh K, Jones C, He Y, et al. (2001) An hPer2 phosphorylation site mutation in familial advanced sleep phase syndrome. Science 291:1040–1043.
5. Hattar S, Lucas RJ, Mrosovsky N, et al. (2003) Melanopsin and rod-cone photoreceptive systems account for all major accessory visual functions in mice. Nature 424:75–81.
6. Schrader H, Bovim G, Sand T (1993) The prevalence of delayed and advanced sleep phase syndromes. J Sleep Res 2:51–55.
7. Cole R, Smith J, Alcala Y, et al. (2002) Bright-light mask treatment of delayed sleep phase syndrome. J Biol Rhythms 17:89–101.
8. Arendt J, Deacon S, English J, et al. (1995) Melatonin and adjustment to phase shift. J Sleep Res 4:74–79.
9. Kayumov L, Brown G, Jindal R, et al. (2001) A randomized, double-blind, placebo-controlled crossover study of the effect of exogenous melatonin on delayed sleep phase syndrome. Psychosom Med 63:40–48.
10. Nagtegaal JE, Kerkhof GA, Smits MG, et al. (1998) Delayed sleep phase syndrome: a placebo-controlled cross-over study on the effects of melatonin administered five hours before the individual dim light melatonin onset. J Sleep Res 7:135–143.
11. Campbell S, Dawson D, Anderson MW (1993) Alleviation of sleep maintenance insomnia with timed exposure to bright light. J Am Geriatr Soc 41:829–836.
12. Murphy P, Campbell S (1996) Enhanced performance in elderly subjects following bright light treatment of sleep maintenance insomnia. J Sleep Res 5:165–172.
13. Moldofsky H, Musisi S, Phillipson E (1986) Treatment of a case of advanced sleep phase syndrome by phase advance chronotherapy. Sleep 9:61–65.
14. De Leersnyder H, Bresson J, de Blois M, et al. (2003) Beta 1-adrenergic antagonists and melatonin reset the clock and restore sleep in a circadian disorder, Smith-Magenis syndrome. J Med Genet 40:74–78.
15. Leger D, Guilleminault C, Santos C, et al. (2002) Sleep/wake cycles in the dark: sleep recorded by polysomnography in 26 totally blind subjects compared to controls. Clin Neurophysiol 113:1607–1614.
16. Lewy A, Bauer V, Hasler B, et al. (2001) Capturing the circadian rhythms of free-running blind people with 0.5 mg melatonin. Brain Res 918:96–100.
17. Petrie K, Dawson AG, Thompson L, et al. (1993) A double-blind trial of melatonin as a treatment for jet lag in international cabin crew. Biol Psychiatr 33:526–530.
18. Spitzer RL, Terman M, Williams JB, et al. (1999) Jet lag: clinical features, validation of a new syndrome-specific scale, and lack of response to melatonin in a randomized, double-blind trial. Am J Psychiatr 156:1392–1396.
19. Wright S, Lawrence L, Wrenn K, et al. (1998) Randomized clinical trial of melatonin after night-shift work: efficacy and neuropsychologic effects. Ann Emerg Med 32:334–340.
20. Mohren DC, Jansen NW, Kant IJ, et al. (2002) Prevalence of common infections in employees on different work shifts. J Occup Environ Med 44:1003–1011.
21. Rosekind M, Smith R, Miller D, et al. (1995) Alertness management: strategic naps in operational settings. J Sleep Res 4:62–66.
22. Czeisler CA, Walsh JK, Roth T, et al. (2005) Modafinal for excessive sleepiness associated with shift-work sleep disorder. N Engl J Med 353:476–486.
23. Nickelsen T, Samel A, Vejvoda M, et al. (2002) Chronobiotic effects of the melatonin agonist LY 156735 following a simulated 9h time shift: results of a placebo-controlled trial. Chronobiol Int 19:915–936.

25 Bruxism

Donald A. Falace, DMD

CONTENTS

INTRODUCTION

Bruxism is generally defined as the grinding, clenching, or gnashing of the teeth and can occur when awake as well as during sleep. Bruxing when awake, along with other oral habits such as jaw or mouth posturing, cheek biting, and nail biting, often occur without cognitive awareness, especially during periods of concentration, or stressful situations. Once the activity is brought to the attention of the individual it often can be stopped or modified. Bruxism during sleep is distinct from bruxism when awake and occurs in relationship to arousals. Furthermore, it is beyond volitional control. It is also likely that the etiology differs between diurnal and sleep bruxism *(1)*. Whether bruxism occurs during the day when awake or at night during sleep, the occasional outcomes of tooth wear and jaw pain are familiar to most dentists.

The terminology used to describe bruxism differs somewhat in dentistry and medicine. In dentistry, bruxism, whether it occurs during sleep or when awake, has traditionally been viewed as a form of parafunctional activity, as distinguished from normal functional activity of the teeth and jaws such as chewing, speaking, or swallowing *(2)*. However, from a medical perspective, bruxism occurring during sleep is separated from diurnal bruxism and is classified as a sleep disorder. In the first edition of the *International Classification of Sleep Disorders*, sleep bruxism was classified as a parasomnia, which is an undesirable movement occurring during sleep *(3)*. Subsequently, in the second edition, *International Classification of Sleep Disorders*-2, bruxism was redesignated as a sleep-related movement disorder: a specific subset of parasomnias, primarily characterized by relatively simple, usually stereotyped movements that disturb sleep, and are less complex than other parasomnias. Bruxism for which no cause

From: *Current Clinical Practice: Primary Care Sleep Medicine: A Practical Guide*
Edited by: J. F. Pagel and S. R. Pandi-Perumal © Humana Press Inc., Totowa, NJ

can be attributed is termed *primary*, whereas bruxism occurring as a result of medication or a medical problem is termed *secondary (4)*.

EPIDEMIOLOGY

The true prevalence of bruxism is difficult to determine as estimates are most often based on self-report of awareness, witnessed reports of occurrence by a parent or spouse, or a clinical finding of tooth wear. With sleep bruxism, this is especially problematic, as subjects are typically unaware of the activity, thus necessitating the use of polysomnography or other recording technology to provide definitive evidence. In addition, the occurrence of bruxism can be variable over time, making the determination of active bruxism difficult at any given point in time *(1,5)*. Thus, a finding of tooth wear is not necessarily indicative of current tooth grinding. Bruxism occurs in all ages and in both sexes. The mean reported prevalence of sleep bruxism is 8%; it is greatest in children under 11 years of age (19%), and falls to a low of 3% after the age of 60 years *(6,7)*. With daytime bruxism, the prevalence of reported awareness in adults is 20% *(8)*.

PATHOPHYSIOLOGY

Over the years, there has been much speculation and controversy over the cause of sleep bruxism. Dentists have long believed that undesirable occlusal factors cause bruxism, with occlusal adjustment or dental reconstruction recommended as treatment *(9–11)*. Subsequently, however, studies have failed to show a significant role of occlusion in the genesis or treatment of sleep bruxism *(12–16)*. This continues to be a subject of some controversy in dentistry, however, with some dentists still recommending occlusal adjustment as a treatment for bruxism in spite of the lack of evidence of effectiveness *(17)*.

Psychological stress has often been postulated as a cause of nocturnal bruxism. The exact role of stress remains unclear. Early reports found an association between daytime stress and nocturnal tooth grinding *(18,19)*. Subsequent reports have continued to include increased psychological stress as a probable contributing factor *(1,8,20)*. However, other studies fail to show a consistent effect of stress or personality types *(16,21)*. It has been noted that rigorous evidence is lacking to support the notion that sleep bruxism is an anxiety-related disorder *(22)*. Thus, the exact relationship between psychological stress and sleep bruxism remains to be defined. In addition to stress and anxiety, other reported risk factors include sleep apnea, loud snoring, daytime sleepiness, alcohol, caffeine, and smoking *(20)*. Although data are not definitive, it appears that bruxism is exacerbated by the use of certain medications, such as the selective serotonin reuptake inhibitors, dopamine agonists, and calcium-channel blockers *(23,24)*.

More recently, investigation of the causation and regulation of bruxism has focused on the central nervous system. Studies have demonstrated the occurrence of spontaneous bursts of activity in the masticatory musculature (rhythmic masticatory muscle activity) during sleep that may or may not be followed by tooth contact, and that occur with a frequency of four to eight episodes per hour during sleep *(25)*. These events are markers of microarousals and are found in normal control subjects as well as individuals with tooth grinding *(13)*. However, bruxers have more frequent events with higher amplitudes as compared with controls, although their sleep macrostructure is normal *(26,27)*. Intriguingly, it has been shown that rhythmic masticatory muscle activity, and subsequent tooth contact, are *preceded* by increased cortical electroencephalogram activity and an increase in heart rate, suggesting that sleep bruxism is an oromotor manifestation associated with microarousals *(28)*. This suggests that sleep bruxism is initiated by central factors rather than peripheral factors.

SLEEP AND BRUXISM

Interestingly, subjects with sleep bruxism do not differ from control individuals in sleep architecture or the usual parameters used to measure sleep *(29,30)*. Bruxing has been reported to occur in all stages of sleep, but is most often found in stages 1 and 2 of nonrapid eye movement (REM) sleep *(26,29,30)*. One small study reported that severe bruxing occurred predominately in REM sleep *(31)*. Saber et al. *(32)* found that only 5–10% of sleep bruxism occurred during REM sleep in a group of young bruxers. It has also been observed that most bruxing events occur when in the supine position, which is also the position in which most events of obstructive sleep apnea occur *(22,33)*. The exact correlation between sleep apnea and bruxism is not clear, but a recent large epidemiological study found that sleep apnea was the most common risk factor for sleep bruxism *(20)*. Oksenberg and Arons *(34)* investigated the effect of continuous positive airway pressure on a group of sleep apnea patients who also had sleep bruxism. They reported that successful treatment with continuous positive airway pressure eliminated both the sleep apnea and sleep bruxing activity. Oksenberg and Arons *(34)* and Sjoholm et al. *(35)* reported that bruxing events rarely occur during apneic episodes, but rather are related to disturbed sleep. In a study of schoolchildren with diagnosed sleep apnea scheduled to undergo tonsillectomy and adenoidectomy, 45.6% were reported to have sleep bruxism. After surgery, none was found to have sleep apnea and sleep bruxism was reported in only 11.8% *(36)*. Thus, there appears to be a strong correlation between sleep apnea and sleep bruxism in both adults and children.

DIAGNOSIS OF SLEEP BRUXISM

A clinical diagnosis of sleep bruxism is generally made based on the

1. The self-report of awareness by the patient or by the bed partner.
2. The presence of wear on teeth.
3. Jaw pain or discomfort upon awakening.

Tooth wear may be isolated to one or two teeth (Fig. 1A), usually canines and incisors, or it can be generalized to the entire dentition (Fig. 1B). The degree of wear can vary as well, ranging from minor wear facets to the loss of all or most of the clinical crowns. However, the presence of tooth wear is not well correlated with current bruxing activity *(37)*. In addition, patients with sleep bruxism may complain of generalized cold sensitivity of their teeth *(38,39)*. Occasionally, significant masseter hypertrophy may also be seen (Fig. 2) as well as radiographic evidence of bone deposition at the angles of the mandible. Patients with bruxism will often have scalloping of the lateral borders of the tongue, presumably as a result of habitual tongue pressure exerted against the inner surfaces of the teeth associated with parafunctional activity. Other intraoral signs of parafunction include a pronounced linea alba and cheek or lip biting. In spite of the presence of pronounced tooth wear and hypertrophy of the masseter muscles, patients with sleep bruxism may be completely asymptomatic or have only minor symptoms. Only about 20% of patients with sleep bruxism report pain upon awakening *(22,40)*. About 20–50% of patients with daytime clenching or grinding, report an

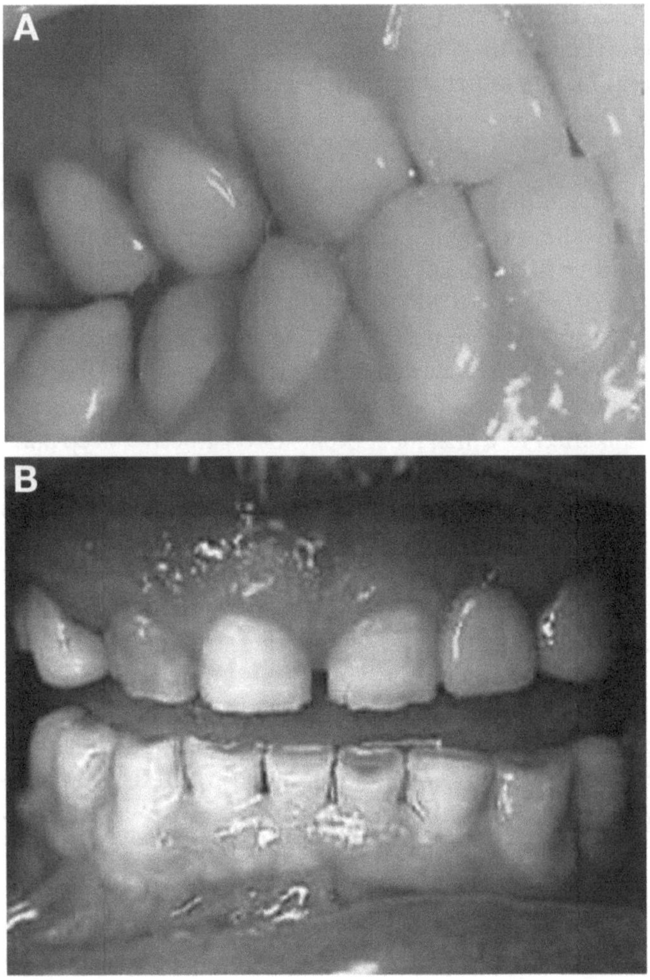

Fig. 1. (A) Mild, localized tooth wear. **(B)** Severe, generalized tooth wear. Photographs courtesy of Jeff Okeson, DMD, Lexington, KY.

awareness of their habit *(41–44)*. Patients with symptomatic daytime clenching or grinding typically report discomfort that occurs during or at the end of the day as opposed to having pain upon awakening. A definitive diagnosis of sleep bruxism requires the use of polysomnography. This is usually not necessary except in isolated cases or for research purposes. Lavigne and colleagues *(22)* have published detailed criteria for the definitive laboratory diagnosis of sleep bruxism.

MANAGEMENT OF BRUXISM

Although there is no definitive cure for bruxism, a number of approaches have been used to manage the problem with varying degrees of success. Three primary methods of management are used: behavioral modification, occlusal appliances, and medications. Behavioral modification includes a broad variety of methods including sleep hygiene education, cognitive awareness, habit reversal, biofeedback training, physical therapy, massed practice, and hypnosis *(22,45)*. These approaches all generally attempt to reduce stress and improve relaxation skills.

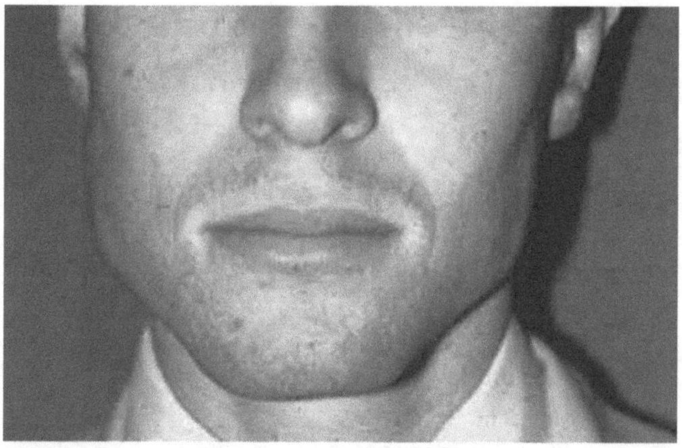

Fig. 2. Masseter hypertrophy in a patient with severe bruxism. Photograph courtesy of Jeff Okeson, DMD, Lexington, KY.

The most common method of treatment for sleep bruxism by dentists is the use of an occlusal appliance (also known as splints, biteguards, mouthguards, or stabilization appliances). Many types of appliances have been advocated, including hard or soft, upper or lower, full coverage or partial coverage, flat plane or with guidance. Most available data are for the full-coverage, maxillary hard appliance (Fig. 3). Clinical experience has shown that oral appliances do result in improvement in many patients with symptomatic sleep bruxism and that they protect the dentition from further damage. Why patients improve while using an appliance has been a subject of controversy. Conventional wisdom held that the reason for the symptom improvement was that appliances stopped and/or prevented bruxing activity by stabilizing the occlusion. However, it has been demonstrated that whereas signs or symptoms of bruxism are reduced by use of appliances, bruxing activity continues *(46,47)*. There has also been controversy over which type of splint is more efficacious. One small study suggests that a hard, full-coverage splint is superior to a soft splint, and that a soft splint may actually increase bruxing activity *(48)*. Partial-coverage appliances—for example, nociceptive trigeminal inhibition, tension suppression system (NTI-TSS Inc; Mishawaka, IN)—that cover only a few maxillary anterior teeth have been advocated for a variety of temporomandibular problems, including bruxism. Recently, these appliances have been shown to be inferior to full-coverage appliances in symptom relief and to have the potential to allow the unintended extrusion of posterior teeth with extended use *(49)*.

One of the most intriguing findings is that sham or placebo appliances covering only the palate with no occlusal coverage have been shown to be equally effective in relieving symptoms of bruxism, as appliances that cover the occlusal surfaces *(50,51)*. These findings question the role of occlusal influences of an appliance, and suggest that other mechanisms are involved. Of concern is a recent pilot study demonstrating that full-coverage occlusal appliances were associated with aggravation of respiratory disturbance in some patients with sleep apnea *(52)*. Conversely, it has recently been observed that the use of a double-arch occlusal device to advance the mandible for the treatment of sleep apnea was found to decrease sleep bruxism in addition to improving the sleep apnea *(53)*. These findings will need further investigation to determine their significance.

A variety of medications have been used to treat sleep bruxism, most commonly benzodiazepines (e.g., diazepam, clonazepam), muscle relaxants (e.g., cyclobenzaprine,

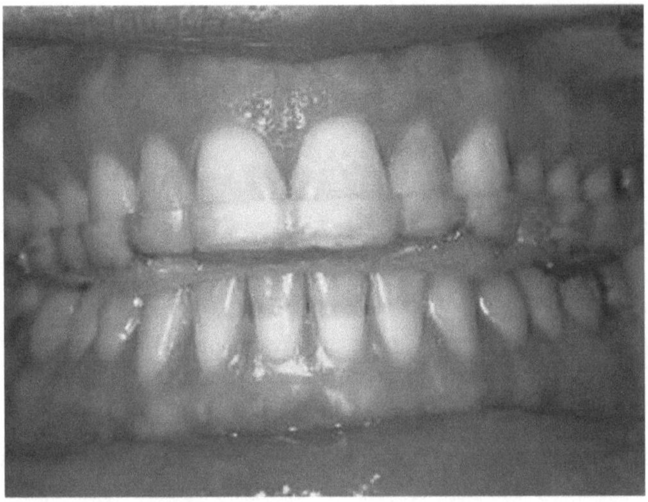

Fig. 3. Acrylic occlusal splint. Photograph courtesy of Jeff Okeson, DMD, Lexington, KY.

methocarbamol), and tricyclic antidepressants (e.g., amitriptyline). Clinically, many patients report benefit from the use of these medications, but supportive data for their use and efficacy are generally lacking *(54–57)*. The use of these medications should be limited to short-term administration. Other medications, such as L-DOPA and clonidine, have been suggested as being effective or possibly effective *(58,59)*.

CONCLUSIONS

Bruxism is a common benign disorder that is variably considered to be a form of either parafunction, parasomnia, or movement disorder. It is found in all age groups but is most prevalent in young children. The cause of sleep bruxism is unclear but is associated with arousals with distinct EEG and physiological findings. There appears to be a strong association with sleep apnea. The diagnosis of sleep bruxism is most commonly based on self-report, morning jaw discomfort, or the presence of tooth wear. Definitive diagnosis requires the use of polysomnography. The management of sleep bruxism is often multifaceted and includes behavioral modification, occlusal appliances, and various medications.

REFERENCES

1. Rugh JD, Harlan J (1988) Nocturnal bruxism and temporomandibular disorders. Adv Neurol 49:329–341.
2. Okeson J (2003) *Management of Temporomandibular Disorders and Occlusion*. 5th ed. St. Louis, MO, Mosby.
3. American Sleep Disorders Association (1990) *International classification of sleep disorders: diagnostic and coding manual*. American Academy of Sleep Medicine Rochester, MN.
4. American Academy of Sleep Medicine (2005) *International Classification of Sleep Disorders*. 2nd ed. Westchester, IL.
5. Lavigne GJ, Guitard F, Rompre PH, et al. (2001) Variability in sleep bruxism activity over time. J Sleep Res 10:237–244.
6. Laberge L, Tremblay RE, Vitaro F, et al. (2000) Development of parasomnias from childhood to early adolescence. Pediatrics 106:67–74.
7. Lavigne GJ, Montplaisir JY (1994) Restless legs syndrome and sleep bruxism: prevalence and association among Canadians. Sleep 17:739–743.

8. Goulet J, Lund JP, Montplaisir J, et al. (1993) Daily clenching, nocturnal bruxism, and stress and their association with TMD symptoms. J Orofac Pain 7:120.
9. Dawson PE (1998) *Evaluation, Diagnosis and Treatment of Occlusal Problems.* 2nd ed. St. Louis, MO, Mosby.
10. Shore N (1959) *Occlusal Equilibration and Temporomandibular Joint Dysfunction.* JB Lippincott, Philadelphia, PA.
11. Ramfjord S, Ash M (1971) *Occlusion.* 3rd ed. WB Saunders, Philadelphia, PA.
12. Rugh JD, Barghi N, Drago CJ (1984) Experimental occlusal discrepancies and nocturnal bruxism. J Prosthet Dent 51:548–553.
13. Kato T, Thie NM, Huynh N, et al. (2003) Topical review: sleep bruxism and the role of peripheral sensory influences. J Orofac Pain 17:191–213.
14. Lobbezoo F, Naeije M (2001) Bruxism is mainly regulated centrally, not peripherally. J Oral Rehabil 28:1085–1091.
15. Manfredini D, Landi N, Tognini F, et al. (2004) Occlusal features are not a reliable predictor of bruxism. Minerva Stomatol 53:231–239.
16. Watanabe T, Ichikawa K, Clark GT (2003) Bruxism levels and daily behaviors: 3 weeks of measurement and correlation. J Orofac Pain 17:65–73.
17. Christensen GJ (2005) The major part of dentistry you may be neglecting. J Am Dent Assoc 136:497–499.
18. Rugh JD, Solberg W (1975) Electromyographic studies of bruxism behavior before and after treatment. J Calif Dent Assoc 3(9):56–59.
19. Rugh JD (1981) Psychological stress in orofacial neuromuscular problems. Int Dent J 31:202–205.
20. Ohayon MM, Li KK, Guilleminault C (2001) Risk factors for sleep bruxism in the general population. Chest 119:53–61.
21. Pierce CJ, Chrisman K, Bennett ME, et al. (1995) Stress, anticipatory stress, and psychologic measures related to sleep bruxism. J Orofac Pain 9:51–56.
22. Lavigne G, Manzini C, Takafumi K (2005) Sleep bruxism. In: *Principles and Practice of Sleep Medicine.* 4th ed. (Kryger MH, Roth T, Dement WC, eds.) WB Saunders, Philadelphia, PA, pp. 946–959.
23. Lavigne GJ, Soucy JP, Lobbezoo F, et al. (2001) Double-blind, crossover, placebo-controlled trial of bromocriptine in patients with sleep bruxism. Clin Neuropharmacol 24:145–149.
24. Winocur E, Gavish A, Voikovitch M, et al. (2003) Drugs and bruxism: a critical review. J Orofac Pain 17:99–111.
25. Lavigne GJ, Kato T, Kolta A, et al. (2003) Neurobiological mechanisms involved in sleep bruxism. Crit Rev Oral Biol Med 14:30–46.
26. Bader GG, Kampe T, Tagdae T, et al. (1997) Descriptive physiological data on a sleep bruxism population. Sleep 20:982–990.
27. Lavigne G, Manzini C (2000) Bruxism In: *Principles and Practice of Sleep Medicine.* 3rd ed. (Kryger MH, Roth T, Dement WC, eds.) WB Saunders, Philadelphia, PA, pp. 773–785.
28. Kato T, Rompre P, Montplaisir JY, et al. (2001) Sleep bruxism: an oromotor activity secondary to micro-arousal. J Dent Res 80:1940–1944.
29. Macaluso GM, Guerra P, Di Giovanni G, et al. (1998) Sleep bruxism is a disorder related to periodic arousals during sleep. J Dent Res 77:565–573.
30. Lavigne GJ, Rompre PH, Montplaisir JY (1996) Sleep bruxism: validity of clinical research diagnostic criteria in a controlled polysomnographic study. J Dent Res 75:546–552.
31. Ware JC, Rugh JD (1988) Destructive bruxism: sleep stage relationship. Sleep 11:172–181.
32. Saber M, Guitard F, Rompre P, et al. (2003) Correlation between slow wave activity, rhythmic masticatory muscle activty/bruxism and microarousals across sleep. J Dent Res 26:A320–A321.
33. Miyawaki S, Lavigne GJ, Pierre M, et al. (2003) Association between sleep bruxism, swallowing-related laryngeal movement, and sleep positions. Sleep 26:461–465.
34. Oksenberg A, Arons E (2002) Sleep bruxism related to obstructive sleep apnea: the effect of continuous positive airway pressure. Sleep Med 3:513–515.
35. Sjoholm TT, Lowe AA, Miyamoto K, et al. (2000) Sleep bruxism in patients with sleep-disordered breathing. Arch Oral Biol 45:889–896.
36. DiFrancesco RC, Junqueira PA, Trezza PM, et al. (2004) Improvement of bruxism after T & A surgery. Int J Pediatr Otorhinolaryngol 68:441–445.
37. Baba K, Haketa T, Clark GT, et al. (2004) Does tooth wear status predict ongoing sleep bruxism in 30-year-old Japanese subjects? Int J Prosthodont 17:39–44.
38. Yip KH, Chow TW, Chu FC (2003) Rehabilitating a patient with bruxism-associated tooth tissue loss: a literature review and case report. Gen Dent 51:70–74.

39. Wilson TG (2002) Bruxism and cold sensitivity. Quintessence Int 33:559.
40. Lavigne GJ, Rompre PH, Montplaisir JY, et al. (1997) Motor activity in sleep bruxism with concomitant jaw muscle pain: a retrospective pilot study. Eur J Oral Sci 105:92–95.
41. Melis M, Abou-Atme YS (2003) Prevalence of bruxism awareness in a Sardinian population. Cranio 21:144–151.
42. Watts MW, Tan EK, Jankovic J (1999) Bruxism and cranial-cervical dystonia: is there a relationship? Cranio 17:196–201.
43. Glass EG, McGlynn FD, Glaros AG, et al. (1993) Prevalence of temporomandibular disorder symptoms in a major metropolitan area. Cranio 11:217–220.
44. Duckro PN, Tait RC, Margolis RB, et al. (1990) Prevalence of temporomandibular symptoms in a large United States metropolitan area. Cranio 8:131–138.
45. Pierce CJ, Gale EN (1988) A comparison of different treatments for nocturnal bruxism. J Dent Res 67:597–601.
46. Yap AU (1998) Effects of stabilization appliances on nocturnal parafunctional activities in patients with and without signs of temporomandibular disorders. J Oral Rehabil 25:64–68.
47. Sheikholeslam A, Holmgren K, Riise C (1993) Therapeutic effects of the plane occlusal splint on signs and symptoms of craniomandibular disorders in patients with nocturnal bruxism. J Oral Rehabil 20:473–482.
48. Okeson JP (1987) The effects of hard and soft occlusal splints on nocturnal bruxism. J Am Dent Assoc 114:788–791.
49. Magnusson T, Adiels AM, Nilsson HL, et al. (2004) Treatment effect on signs and symptoms of temporomandibular disorders: comparison between stabilisation splint and a new type of splint (NTI); a pilot study. Swed Dent J 28:11–20.
50. Dube C, Rompre PH, Manzini C, et al. (2004) Quantitative polygraphic controlled study on efficacy and safety of oral splint devices in tooth-grinding subjects. J Dent Res 83:398–403.
51. Dao TT, Lavigne GJ, Charbonneau A, et al. (1994) The efficacy of oral splints in the treatment of myofascial pain of the jaw muscles: a controlled clinical trial. Pain 56:85–94.
52. Gagnon Y, Mayer P, Morisson F, et al. (2004) Aggravation of respiratory disturbances by the use of an occlusal splint in apneic patients: a pilot study. Int J Prosthodont 17:447–453.
53. Guitard F, Landry M, Rompre PH, et al. (2005) Effect of double arch device and occlusal splint in sleep bruxism patients. Sleep 28:A258.
54. Kato T, Thie NM, Montplaisir JY, et al. (2001) Bruxism and orofacial movements during sleep. Dent Clin North Am 45:657–684.
55. Raigrodski AJ, Mohamed SE, Gardiner DM (2001) The effect of amitriptyline on pain intensity and perception of stress in bruxers. J Prosthodont 10:73–77.
56. Raigrodski AJ, Christensen LV, Mohamed SE, et al. (2001) The effect of four-week administration of amitriptyline on sleep bruxism: a double-blind crossover clinical study. Cranio 19:21–25.
57. Mohamed SE, Christensen LV, Penchas J (1997) A randomized double-blind clinical trial of the effect of amitriptyline on nocturnal masseteric motor activity (sleep bruxism). Cranio 15:326–332.
58. Lobbezoo F, Lavigne GJ, Tanguay R, et al. (1997) The effect of catecholamine precursor L-dopa on sleep bruxism: a controlled clinical trial. Mov Disord 12:73–78.
59. Huynh N, Rompre P, Montplaisir J, et al. (2005) Comparison of various treatments for sleep bruxism using the “number needed to treat” method. Sleep 28:A258.

26 Restless Legs Syndrome and Periodic Limb Movements

Michael J. Thorpy, MD

CONTENTS

INTRODUCTION

Restless legs syndrome (RLS), a common sensory-motor disorder is characterized by uncomfortable sensations in the limbs, especially at rest and at bedtime *(1)*. This paresthesia usually involves an irresistible urge to move the limbs, which provides temporary relief. The symptoms occur most often in the legs but can involve the arms or, in severe cases, the whole body. Although RLS occurs while the individual is awake, difficulty falling asleep, and sleep disruption as a result of periodic limb movements occurs *(2)*. The pathophysiology of RLS is not well-understood; however, iron and central dopaminergic systems have been implicated *(3)*.

RLS was described and named in 1945 by a Swedish neurologist, Karl-Axel Ekbom who estimated the prevalence to be 5% *(4)*. Recent studies suggest a prevalence of between 3 and 15% of the general population and as high as 24% in primary care patients *(5,6)*. Not all patients require treatment; it is estimated that approx 3% require pharmacological treatment. As diagnostic criteria have only recently been established, many cases go undiagnosed and untreated *(7)*. Standardized criteria for the diagnosis were updated in 2003 by the International Restless Legs Syndrome Study Group *(1)*.

Treatment options for primary RLS are limited, and only one medication that has been approved by the US Food and Drug Administration (FDA) is available (ropinirole). Dopamine agonists are considered the treatment of choice for primary RLS, providing 90–100% relief of RLS symptoms *(3–5)*. Alternative pharmacotherapeutic medications include anticonvulsants, opioids, and benzodiazepines *(4)*. Secondary RLS can occur; when it results from iron-deficiency anemia, it may be managed with iron replacement therapy.

From: *Current Clinical Practice: Primary Care Sleep Medicine: A Practical Guide*
Edited by: J. F. Pagel and S. R. Pandi-Perumal © Humana Press Inc., Totowa, NJ

GENETICS AND PATHOPHYSIOLOGY

There are two forms of RLS: primary (idiopathic) and secondary. Primary RLS may represent a genetic cause, as 50–92% of individuals with primary RLS report a positive family history *(8–10)*. There is a high concordance of RLS in monozygotic (MZ) twins *(11)*. A study evaluated RLS symptoms in 1937 MZ and dizygotic (DZ) twins pairs; 933 MZ pairs, and 1004 DZ pairs *(12)*. Concordance rates for RLS symptoms were higher for MZ than DZ twins. Additive genetic effects combined with unique environmental factors provide the best model for RLS symptoms. Heritability was estimated to be 54% for restless legs and 60% for leg jerking. These results suggested a substantial genetic contribution to the symptomatology of RLS.

An autosomal dominant mode of inheritance has been proposed *(3)*. Three loci have been reported for RLS, on chromosomes 12q, 14q, and 9p (RLS-1, RLS-2, and RLS-3), with a recessive (RLS-1) and autosomal dominant (RLS-2, RLS-3) mode of inheritance, respectively. The overall contribution of these loci to this disorder is not known *(13)*. Using markers on chromosome 12q, a study of five kindreds was consistent with linkage to chromosome 12q. The results support the presence of a major RLS-susceptibility locus on chromosome 12q. At least one additional locus may be involved in the origin of this prevalent condition *(14)*.

Secondary RLS is associated with several medical, neurological, and metabolic conditions such as disorders that result in iron deficiency, pregnancy, and end-stage renal disease *(15)*. Possible mechanisms of primary RLS pathophysiology include abnormal iron metabolism and functional alterations in central dopaminergic neurotransmitter systems, which may lead to altered spinal cord function. Pharmacological evidence that primary RLS is highly responsive to dopaminergic agents suggests an underlying defect in dopaminergic function *(4,9,16,17)*. Neuroimaging studies such as positron emission tomography and single-photon emission computed tomography suggest that reduced dopamine D_2 receptor-binding and nigrostriatal presynaptic dopaminergic hypofunction may contribute to the syndrome *(18,19)*. Single-photon emission computed tomography imaging of striatal pre- and postsynaptic dopamine transmission has shown that striatal dopamine transporter binding does not differ between the two groups; however, dopamine D_2 receptor-binding is significantly lower in RLS patients. Central dopamine function appears to be involved in RLS pathophysiology, and the mechanism probably involves a decrease in the number or affinity of dopamine D_2 receptors *(20)*.

Inadequate iron stores or abnormal metabolism of iron may decrease brain dopamine production and contribute to primary RLS *(21,22)*. Reflecting low brain iron levels in patients with RLS, cerebrospinal fluid (CSF) from patients with primary RLS had significantly lower ferritin and higher transferritin levels compared with control subjects' CSF *(21)*. Deficiencies in iron concentrations were correlated with the severity of primary RLS symptoms. Regions of the brain with iron deficiencies included the substantia nigra and the putamen. Histopathology studies from the brains of patients with primary RLS showed that iron and H-ferritin staining were markedly decreased in the RLS substantia nigra *(23)*. L-Ferritin staining was strong in that study; however, the cells staining for L-ferritin in RLS brains were morphologically distinct from those in the control brains. H- and L-subunits of ferritin are expressed from different chromosomes and have different functions. More recent studies have found and shown that both H- and L-ferritin are significantly decreased in early- but not late-onset RLS *(24)*. There is a strong correlation between the age of symptom onset and CSF ferritin values; the earlier the age, the lower the ferritin level *(25)*.

Abnormal iron metabolism may be directly related to the mechanism of altered central neurotransmitter systems, as dopamine production requires ferritin as a cofactor for tyrosine hydroxylase, the rate-limiting enzyme in dopamine production *(15)*. Animal data indicate that in iron-deficient states, excessive amounts of tyrosine hydroxylase are produced. Normally, dopamine would follow production of this enzyme, and feedback processes would signal cells to slow production. However, with decreased iron available, there may be a disassociation within the feedback process. Autopsies from individuals with RLS have shown increased tyrosine hydroxylase levels in substantia nigra tissue. Localized abnormalities within spinal pathways may arise in primary RLS from alterations in central dopamine production causing disinhibition (activation) of the normal CNS pacemaker. Case studies in patients with a temporal relationship to spinal cord injury and onset of RLS suggest that disinhibition of spinal pathways may be involved in symptom development *(26)*.

Secondary RLS occurs in association with conditions or disorders that result in iron deficiency, including pregnancy and end-stage renal disease *(15)*. Approximately 5% of patients with symptoms of RLS have iron-deficiency anemia; in many, the symptoms will reverse with adequate iron replacement therapy. Several comorbid conditions, including primary sleep disorders, Parkinson disease, neuropathies, rheumatoid arthritis, and metabolic disturbances have been associated with RLS, but a pathophysiological relationship between any of the conditions and RLS has not been determined. Several medications can worsen or cause symptoms of RLS, including antidepressants, antihistamines, and dopamine receptor blockers. Tricyclic antidepressants and selective serotonin-reuptake inhibitors may contribute to symptoms of RLS. Switching to a different medication in the same or a different class may alleviate the problem. Buproprion, which has some dopaminergic activity, may be less likely to exacerbate periodic leg movements than other antidepressants *(27)*. Buproprion has been reported to ameliorate symptoms in patients with RLS *(28)*.

A literature review on the association between RLS and attention-deficit/hyperactivity disorder (ADHD) has shown that up to 44% of subjects with ADHD have been found to have RLS or RLS symptoms, and up to 26% of subjects with RLS have been found to have ADHD or ADHD symptoms. Several mechanisms have been proposed to explain this association: sleep disruption associated with RLS might lead to inattentiveness, moodiness, and paradoxical overactivity; diurnal manifestations of RLS such as restlessness and inattention might mimic ADHD symptoms; alternatively, RLS might be comorbid with idiopathic ADHD; or people with RLS and a subset of individuals with ADHD might share a common dopamine dysfunction. Limited evidence suggests that some dopaminergic agents such as levodopa/carbidopa, pergolide, and ropinirole may be effective in children with RLS associated with ADHD symptoms *(29)*.

PREVALENCE AND EPIDEMIOLOGY

The prevalence of RLS in the general population is thought to be between 3 and 15%, is higher in women, and increases with age *(5–7)*. Berger and colleagues *(7)* surveyed individuals aged 20–79 years; among 4107 patients, they found an overall prevalence of RLS of 10.6%. The prevalence increased with age, and women had a twofold higher rate of RLS than men. The percentage of primary care patients with RLS may be substantially higher than in the general public, as 25% of adults evaluated in a rural primary care clinic meet all four of the standard criteria for RLS *(6)*. The patients who met the criteria were older and more likely to be female. The diagnosis of RLS is typically made in midlife. In a series of 54 patients with RLS, the mean age of onset was 34 ± 20 years *(10)*; however, onset of symptoms can occur in childhood and early adulthood. Forty five percent of patients with RLS report that symptoms first occurred before the age of 20 years *(30)*. Correct diagnosis may be significantly delayed in patients with early onset, as the average age at the time of correct diagnosis was 50 years.

Primary RLS is usually familial *(9,10)*. In patients with primary RLS, 94% had a positive family history of RLS, and 23.6% of first-degree relatives reported symptoms of RLS. Patients with a definite family history of RLS are younger at the age of onset of symptoms compared with patients who have a negative family history *(9)*.

CLINICAL FEATURES AND DIAGNOSIS

The diagnosis rate for RLS is low *(7)*. In an international study, less than 25% of patients meeting the criteria for RLS had been given the diagnosis *(23)*. The International Restless Legs Syndrome Study Group updated the criteria for the clinical diagnosis of RLS in 2003 *(1)*. These criteria are important for standardizing the diagnosis for research and are helpful to the clinician; however, patients may have difficulty describing the symptoms of RLS. The clinical criteria of RLS are as follows:

1. A desire to move the limbs (with or without paresthesia), and the arms may be involved.
2. The urge to move or the unpleasant sensation improves with activity, and symptoms are worse with rest or inactivity.
3. The urge to move or the unpleasant sensations are partially or totally relieved with movement.
4. The symptoms have a circadian variation, occurring most often in the evening or at night when the patient lies down.

The patient typically complains of discomfort in the legs, usually both legs simultaneously, and may describe the sensation as "creepy-crawly." However, other presentations occur such as deeper sensations in the muscles, a deep sensation in the bones, a sharp, lancing pain, or burning. Symptoms often occur daily, and sleep problems or disruption may be presenting complaints.

RLS often occurs in association with periodic limb movement disorder (PLMD), which is distinct from RLS and occurs during sleep *(3)*. Patients are usually unaware of periodic limb movements during sleep, but bed partners may report the symptoms. Approximately 80% of patients with RLS will have evidence of PLMD during polysomnographic studies. PLMD includes stereotypical, slow, periodic movements of the leg with flexion, usually of the ankle, knee, and hip *(15)*. The movements can occur in one leg or in both legs simultaneously, or alternate from one leg to the other. As with RLS symptoms, the movements can also occur in the arms. More than 15 episodes per hour is considered clinically significant, but some patients may have many hundreds of episodes in a night (American Academy of Sleep Medicine). Periodic leg movement during sleep recorded by polysomnography may be idiopathic or associated with sleep apnea, neurodegenerative diseases, spinal cord lesions, stroke, narcolepsy, or antidepressant or neuroleptic drugs.

The diagnosis of RLS should be differentiated from that of paresthesias and dysesthesias related to peripheral neuropathy, peripheral vascular disease (including varicose veins), arthritic and muscular pain, neuroleptic-induced akathisia, and the discomfort of painful legs/moving toes *(3,5)*. Akathisia, which is caused by earlier neuroleptic use, usually produces widespread body movements without a circadian variation.

TREATMENT

Nonpharmacological Management

Management of RLS symptoms with nonpharmacological therapy should be considered first; however, patients with moderate to severe symptoms often require drug therapy. Nonpharmacological treatment of RLS includes improving sleep hygiene with a regular sleep–wake cycle, avoiding caffeine, alcohol, and nicotine use, and moderate exercise daily. RLS disrupts sleep and inadequate sleep may contribute to increased severity of symptoms; therefore, patients need to be advised to go to bed and wake up at a regular time and only be in bed for an appropriate amount of time, usually less than 8 hours *(3,15)*. Excessive exercise may exacerbate symptoms and should be avoided, but relaxing exercise before bedtime may be helpful *(3)*. Relaxation techniques, including hot or thermal baths, leg vibration, massage, and biofeedback may be helpful, but these have not been well studied. Anecdotal information suggests that acupuncture may provide symptom relief. Treatment of secondary RLS requires managing the underlying disorder and discontinuing medications that may worsen symptoms.

Iron Therapy

Correcting iron deficiency can usually be accomplished with 325 mg of ferrous sulfate and 100 mg of vitamin C *(3)*. If the serum ferritin level is less than 50 μg/L or iron saturation is less than 16%, treatment of iron deficiency is warranted. Without evidence of iron deficiency, oral iron supplements are ineffective. Reversal of iron deficiency and improvement in RLS symptoms require time, and treatment should continue until the serum ferritin increases to more than 50 μg/L or iron saturation is more than 20%. Many patients who have iron deficiency may have a primary or idiopathic cause of their symptoms, with the iron deficiency occurring coincidentally. Adverse effects with oral iron therapy, which are frequent but not usually severe, include constipation and gastric discomfort. Rarely, hemochromatosis can occur.

Repeated IV doses of iron provide effective supplemental treatment of RLS in patients with severe or difficult-to-treat iron loss. Subjects were given a single 1000-mg infusion of iron, and supplemental 450-mg iron gluconate infusions were given if symptoms returned and the ferritin level was less than 300 μg/L *(31)*. RLS symptoms return on average 6 months after the initial 1000-mg infusion. Some subjects require multiple courses of supplemental iron. After the initial 1000-mg iron infusion, the ferritin decline is often substantially higher than the predicted value of less than 1 μg/L/week. This rate of ferritin decline decreases toward normal with repeated IV iron treatments. The slower the rate of ferritin decline, the more prolonged the symptom improvements. High ferritin levels are not in themselves a guarantee of sustained clinical improvements.

Pharmacological Treatment

Although 15% of the general population may be affected by RLS, which can have a significant impact on quality of life, until recently there have been no FDA-approved

Table 1
Drugs Used To Manage RLS

Drug	*Starting dose (mg)*	*Maximum daily dose (mg)*	*Common adverse effects*	*Serious adverse effects*
Dopaminergic agonists			Class effects: nausea, vomiting, orthostatic hypotension, hallucination, augmentation of symptoms, insomnia	
Levodopa	50	200 at bedtime		
Pramipexole	0.125	2; can be divided into 2–3 doses		
Ropinirole	0.25	6; can be divided into 2–3 doses		
Anticonvulsant				
Gabapentin	300	2400 divided into 3 doses 1500 single dose	Sedation, dizziness, fatigue, somnolence, ataxia	
Opioids			Sedation, constipation, nausea, and vomiting occur with all agents in this class	Dependence
Oxycodone	5	20–30, divided into 2–3 doses		
Propoxyphene	100–200	600, divided into 2–3 doses		
Methadone	5–10	25		
Benzodiazepine			Tolerance, sedation	
Clonazepam	0.25	2 at bedtime		

Adapted from ref. *5*.

medications for the syndrome *(2,32)*. As the pathophysiology suggests, dopaminergic medications such as ropinirole or pramipexole have the highest efficacy in RLS and are first-line treatment. The anticonvulsant gabapentin is second-line therapy, and opioids may be used as third-line therapy. Benzodiazepines, particularly clonazepam, may provide some relief. Drug selection should be individualized and include consideration of a patient's comorbid conditions as well as adverse effects (Table 1). Combinations of medications from different classes may be required.

Dopaminergic Medications

The efficacy of levodopa in RLS was first described in 1982 in patients who were given levodopa (200 mg nightly) and had complete resolution of symptoms *(33)*. Several small studies supported these findings, including beneficial effects of levodopa in patients with severe symptoms. Levodopa is effective in doses much lower than that needed for treating Parkinson disease, usually 100 mg daily. The disadvantages of levodopa therapy are augmentation and rebound, and patients can develop tolerance.

Augmentation is the occurrence of more severe and more widespread distribution of symptoms that develop earlier in the evening *(33,34)*. More than 80% of patients receiving levodopa for RLS develop augmentation. Rebound or the recurrence of symptoms in the early morning hours, occurs in approx 25% of patients treated with levodopa. Sustained-release formulations delay rebound until about 7 hours after dosing, compared with 3–4 hours after immediate release of levodopa *(33,34)*.

Dopamine Agonists

Dopamine agonists control the symptoms of RLS with low doses and less risk of augmentation; however, tolerance may develop more quickly. Pergolide is a semisynthetic ergot alkaloid with agonist activity at D_1 and D_2 dopamine receptors. It has been investigated for use in RLS, but safer options are now available *(35)*. The most serious concerns with pergolide are pulmonary fibrosis and cardiac dysfunction *(36–39)*. Pramipexole, a D_3 dopamine receptor agonist was developed for treatment of Parkinson disease *(16)*. The efficacy of pramipexole was evaluated in 10 patients with RLS treated in a 10-week, double-blind, placebo-controlled, crossover trial. Pramipexole therapy was initiated at 0.375 mg/day, increased to 0.75 mg/day after 1 week, and then 1.5 mg/day after the second week *(16)*. Compared with placebo, pramipexole therapy significantly decreased subjective leg restlessness during daytime, in the evening, at bedtime, and during the night *(16)*. The number of periodic leg movements while awake (PLMWs) was significantly decreased with pramipexole treatment *(16)*. The results of a pramipexole dose-finding and efficacy study of 109 patients with RLS indicated that dosing should be individualized with 0.5 mg and 0.75 mg pramipexole daily *(40)*.

Ropinirole is the most extensively studied dopamine agonist, with several studies supporting the efficacy of this synthetic nonergoline derivative in RLS. Doses needed to control symptoms are much lower (1.5–6 mg daily) than the 24-mg total daily dose often needed for Parkinson disease. Several open-label and small randomized trials using ropinirole to treat the symptoms of RLS have been performed *(17,41)*. The initial doses were 0.25 mg of ropinirole; at study end, the average daily dose was 2.8 mg, with doses of up to 6 mg. A preliminary report from a randomized, double-blind study ($n = 65$) indicated that ropinirole was effective in decreasing the periodic leg movements per hour of sleep index associated with RLS in many patients *(42)*.

Three large, multicenter, 12-week, double-blind, placebo-controlled studies have evaluated the efficacy of ropinirole in RLS. One was completed in 10 European countries *(43)*, one was a European study including the United States *(44)*, and one was solely in the United States *(45)*. The primary end point for all of the studies was the International Restless Legs Scale (IRLS) score. The mean IRLS total scores were significantly lower with ropinirole compared with placebo *(42)*. The mean daily dose at 12 weeks in each study was 1.9, 1.8, and 2.1 mg, respectively, with a median dose of 1.5, 1.5, and 2 mg. There was also a study looking at the effect of ropinirole on periodic limb movements *(46)*. Subjects had at least 5 periodic limb movements per hour of sleep; after 12 weeks of treatment, there was a 62% reduction in the mean periodic limb movements with arousal per hour with ropinirole, vs 32% with placebo.

A dopamine agonist, rotigotine has been studied in a transdermal patch formulation in Europe. At 34 centers, 371 patients with moderate-severe RLS were studied; an improvement in the IRLS of more than 6 points was found in 70–88% of rotigotine-treated patients, compared with 62% of those treated with placebo *(47)*. Doses were

2.25–9 mg/day. Another study found 4.5 mg to be the preferred dose *(48)*. The most frequent adverse events were nausea, skin reactions, and headaches.

Apomorphine, a combined opioidergic and dopaminergic agonist was studied in nine patients with RLS who were pretreated with oral domperidone for 3 days *(49)*. A modified suggested immobilization test was carried out between 8 PM and 1 AM under the following conditions of IV drug administration: baseline–apomorphine–apomorphine plus naloxone–apomorphine plus metoclopramide. Compared with baseline, apomorphine resulted in a rapid and significant improvement in subjective RLS symptoms and an almost immediate cessation of PLMW, measured by the PLMW index. Apomorphine may be an effective treatment for idiopathic RLS. Its effectiveness may reflect both to its dopaminergic and its opioidergic activity, as it is not diminished significantly by blocking only one of these pathways.

Anticonvulsants

Gabapentin is the preferred treatment for patients who cannot take a dopamine agonist. The mechanism of gabapentin in relieving the symptoms of RLS is unknown, but efficacy is supported by clinical studies. In an open-label evaluation of eight patients, four patients reported response *(50)*. Doses in patients responding ranged from 300 to 2400 mg daily. Doses of up to 2400 mg/day may be necessary. In a randomized trial, gabapentin was compared with placebo in 24 patients with RLS *(51)*. IRLS scores were significantly better with gabapentin treatment than with placebo treatment. The mean daily dose of gabapentin was 1855 (± 105.6) mg. Gabapentin was also effective in 11 of 12 hemodialysis patients with RLS in a randomized, double-blind, placebo-controlled, crossover study *(52)*. The dose of gabapentin was 200–300 mg with each dialysis session. Carbamazepine may be effective in RLS, but is a less desirable alternative to gabapentin because of the risk of severe adverse effects and drug interactions.

Opioids

Oxycodone and propoxyphene have been studied in open-label or short-duration (2 weeks) studies of RLS symptom management *(3)*. Methadone has been shown to be useful in treating patients who are refractory to treatment with dopamine agonists *(53)*. Methadone (5–40 mg/day; final dose, 15.6 ± 7.7) was given to 29 patients with RLS who failed to respond to dopaminergics. Of the 27 patients who met inclusion criteria, 17 remained on methadone for 23 ± 12 months (range, 4–44 months) at a dose of 15.5 ± 7.7 mg/day. All patients who continued taking methadone reported at least a 75% reduction in symptoms. None developed augmentation. Methadone should be considered in RLS patients with an unsatisfactory dopaminergic response.

The benzodiazepine clonazepam has been evaluated in RLS and may be beneficial in patients with sleep disturbances who do not respond to other medications *(3)*.

Individualized Treatment

Drug selection should be individualized and consideration given to comorbid conditions and concomitant medications. Dopamine agonists are first-line therapy in the management of RLS symptoms (Fig. 1), generally providing relief in 70–100% of patients and reducing the frequency of periodic leg movements of sleep. Levodopa can be used as needed for episodic RLS, it causes augmentation and rebound when used chronically, although these effects can occur (but to a lesser extent) with any of the dopamine agonists. Individual patient considerations include age, the severity and

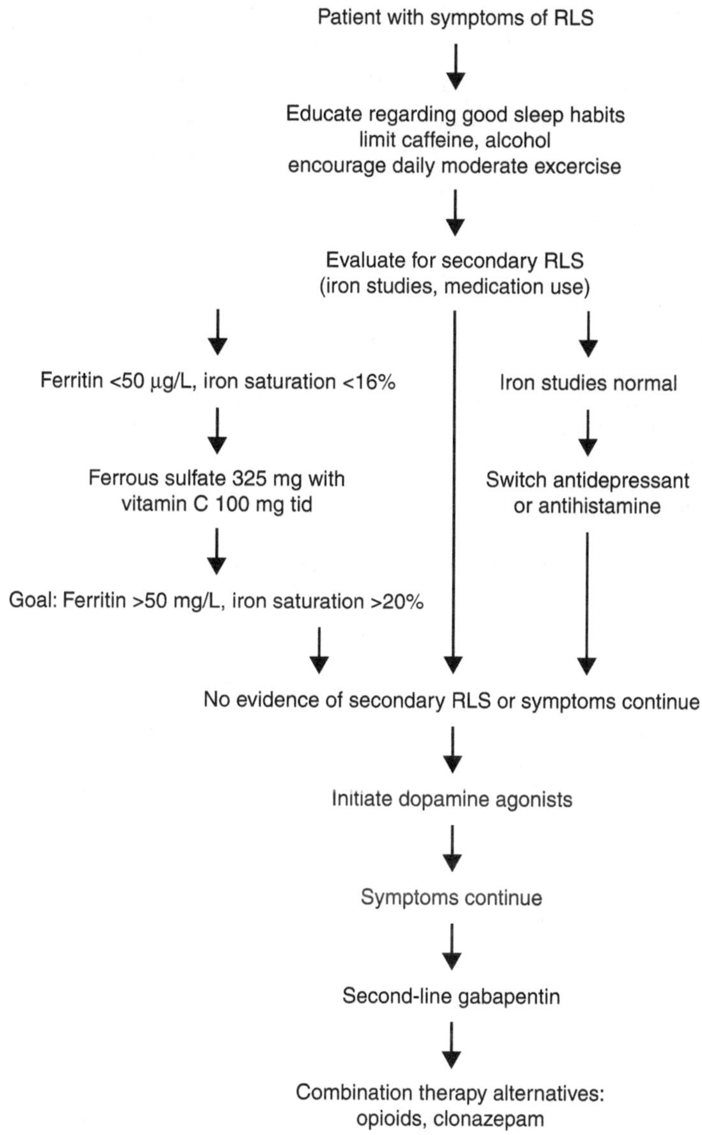

Fig. 1. Algorithm for the management of symptoms in RLS.

frequency of symptoms, medication dose, augmentation, and rebound. Gabapentin is the preferred agent for patients who cannot tolerate dopamine agonists. Although clinical studies are not available, combination therapy is often needed. Adjunct therapy may include opioids or benzodiazepines.

CONCLUSIONS

RLS is a common disorder that can have a significant effect on quality of life and should be suspected in any patient who complains of leg discomfort during the evening or at bedtime, or who has sleep-onset insomnia and nocturnal restlessness. Although the prevalence increases with age, individuals can have onset of symptoms in childhood, and the diagnosis is often missed, delayed, or ascribed to other conditions such as growing pains or ADHD. Secondary causes of RLS should be investigated, including evaluation of anemia, and iron stores, and medications that can cause or worsen symptoms. The pathophysiology of RLS is thought to involve abnormal brain iron metabolism and central dopaminergic systems. Dopamine agonists are first-line therapy, including low-dose levodopa, pramipexole, and ropinirole, which has been the most widely studied in controlled clinical trials. Alternative or adjunct therapy includes gabapentin, opioids, and clonazepam.

REFERENCES

1. Allen RP, Picchietti D, Hening WA, et al. (2003) Restless legs syndrome: diagnostic criteria, special considerations, and epidemiology; a report from the restless legs syndrome diagnosis and epidemiology workshop at the National Institutes of Health. Sleep Med 4:101–119.
2. Hening W, Allen R, Walters AS, et al. (2003) Prevalence of restless legs syndrome (RLS) and impact of symptoms on the quality of life of sufferers [abstract SC 338]. Eur J Neurol 10(Suppl 1):43.
3. Hening W, Allen R, Earley C, et al. (1999) The treatment of restless legs syndrome and periodic limb movement disorder: an American Academy of Sleep Medicine Review. Sleep 22:970–998.
4. Chesson AL, Wise M, Davila D, et al. (1999) Practice parameters for the treatment of restless legs syndrome and periodic limb movement disorder. Sleep 22:961–968.
5. Earley CJ (2003) Restless legs syndrome. New Engl J Med 348:2103–2109.
6. Nichols DA, Allen RP, Grauke JH, et al. (2003) Restless legs syndrome symptoms in primary care: a prevalence study. Arch Intern Med 163:2323–2329.
7. Berger K, Luedemann J, Trenkwalder C, et al. (2004) Sex and the risk of restless legs syndrome in the general population. Arch Intern Med 164:196–202.
8. Trenkwalder C, Paulus W (2004) Why do restless legs occur at rest? Pathophysiology of neuronal structures in RLS: neurophysiology of RLS (part 2). Clin Neurophysiol 115:1975–1988.
9. Winkelmann J, Wetter TC, Collado-Seidel V, et al. (2000) Clinical characteristics and frequency of the hereditary restless legs syndrome in a population of 300 patients. Sleep 23:597–602.
10. Ondo W, Jankovic J (1996) Restless legs syndrome: clinicoetiologic correlates. Neurology 47:1435–1441.
11. Ondo WG, Vuong KD, Wang Q (2000) Restless legs syndrome in monozygotic twins: clinical correlates. Neurology 55:1404–1406.
12. Desai AV, Cherkas LF, Spector TD, et al. (2004) Genetic influences in self-reported symptoms of obstructive sleep apnoea and restless legs: a twin study. Twin Res 7:589–595.
13. Winkelmann J, Lichtner P, Putz B, et al. (2006) Evidence for further genetic locus heterogeneity and confirmation of RLS-1 in restless legs syndrome. Mov Disord 21:28–33.
14. Desautels A, Turecki G, Montplaisir J, et al. (2005) Restless legs syndrome: confirmation of linkage to chromosome 12q, genetic heterogeneity, and evidence of complexity. Arch Neurol 62:591–596.
15. Parker KP, Rye DB (2002) Restless legs syndrome and periodic limb movement disorder. Nurs Clin North Am 37:655–673.
16. Montplaisir J, Nichols A, Denesle R, et al. (1999) Restless legs syndrome improved by pramipexole: a double-blind randomized trial. Neurology 52:938–943.
17. Ondo W (1999) Ropinirole for restless legs syndrome. Mov Disord 14:138–140.
18. Ruottinen HM, Partinen M, Hublin C, et al. (2000) An FDOPA PET study with periodic limb movement disorder and restless legs syndrome. Neurology 54:502–504.
19. Turjanski N, Lees AJ, Brooks DJ (1999) Striatal dopaminergic function in restless legs syndrome: 18F-dopa and 11C-raclopride PET studies. Neurology 52:932–937.
20. Michaud M, Soucy JP, Chabli A, et al. (2002) SPECT imaging of striatal pre- and postsynaptic dopaminergic status in restless legs syndrome with periodic leg movements in sleep. J Neurol 249:164–170.
21. Earley CJ, Connor JR, Beard JL, et al. (2000) Abnormalities in CSF concentrations of ferritin and transferring in restless legs syndrome. Neurology 54:1698–1700.
22. Allen RP, Barker PB, Wehrl F, et al. (2001) MRI measurement of brain iron in patients with restless legs syndrome. Neurology 56:263–265.
23. Connor JR, Boyer PJ, Menzies SL, et al. (2003) Neuropathological examination suggests impaired brain iron acquisition in restless legs syndrome. Neurology 61:304–309.

24. Clardy SL, Earley CJ, Allen RP, et al. (2006) Ferritin subunits in CSF are decreased in restless legs syndrome. J Lab Clin Med 147:67–73.
25. Earley CJ, Connor JR, Beard JL, et al. (2005) Ferritin levels in the cerebrospinal fluid and restless legs syndrome: effects of different clinical phenotypes. Sleep 28:1069–1075.
26. Hartmann M, Pfister R, Pfadenhauer K (1999) Restless legs syndrome associated with spinal cord lesions [letter]. J Neurol Neurosurg Psychiatry 66:688–697.
27. Yang C, White DP, Winkelman JW (2005) Antidepressants and periodic leg movements of sleep. Biol Psychiatry 58:510–514.
28. Kim SW, Shin IS, Kim JM, et al. (2005) Bupropion may improve restless legs syndrome: a report of three cases. Clin Neuropharmacol 28:298–301.
29. Cortese S, Konofal E, Lecendreux M, et al. (2005) Restless legs syndrome and attention-deficit/hyperactivity disorder: a review of the literature. Sleep 28:1007–1013.
30. Walters AS, Hickey K, Maltzman J, et al. (1996) A questionnaire study of 138 patients with restless legs syndrome: the "Night-Walkers" survey. Neurology 46:92–95.
31. Allen R, Hening W, Montplaisir J, et al. (2003) Diagnosis, treatment and referral of patients with symptoms for restless legs syndrome (RLS): the RLS epidemiology, symptoms and treatment (REST) primary care study [abstract SC 339]. Eur J Neurol 10(Suppl 1):43.
32. Earley CJ, Heckler D, Allen RP (2005) Repeated IV doses of iron provides effective supplemental treatment of restless legs syndrome. Sleep Med 6:301–305.
33. Comella CL (2002) Restless legs syndrome: treatment with dopaminergic agents. Neurology 58(Suppl 1):S87–S92.
34. Stiasny K, Wetter TC, Trenkwalder C, et al. (2001) Restless legs syndrome and its treatment by dopamine agonists. Parkinsonism Relat Disord 7:21–25.
35. Winkelmann J, Wetter TC, Stiasny K, et al. (1998) Treatment of restless legs syndrome with pergolide: an open clinical trial. Mov Disord 3:566–569.
36. Bleumink GS, van der Molen-Eijgenraam M, Strijbos JH, et al. (2002) Pergolide-induced pleuropulmonary fibrosis. Clin Neuropharmacol 25:290–293.
37. Danoff SK, Grasso ME, Terry PB, et al. (2001) Pleuropulmonary disease due to pergolide use for restless legs syndrome. Chest 120:313–316.
38. Horvath J, Fross RD, Kleiner-Gisman G, et al. (2004) Severe multivalvular heart disease: a new complication of the ergot derivative dopamine agonists. Mov Disord 19:656–662.
39. Baseman DG, O'Suilleabhain PE, Reimold SC, et al. (2004) Pergolide use in Parkinson disease is associated with cardiac valve regurgitation. Neurology 63:301–304.
40. Partinen M, Hirvonen K, Alakuijala A, et al. (2004) Pramipexole is safe and efficacious in the treatment of idiopathic restless legs syndrome: results of a large randomized double-blind, placebo-controlled, dose-finding study [abstract 657]. Sleep 27(Abstract Suppl):A293–A294.
41. Adler CH, Hauser R, Sethi K, et al. (2003) Ropinirole is beneficial for restless legs syndrome: a placebo-controlled crossover trial [abstract]. Neurology 60(Suppl 1):A439.
42. Allen RP, Becker P, Bogan R, et al. (2003) Restless legs syndrome: the efficacy of ropinirole in the treatment of RLS patients suffering from periodic leg movements of sleep [abstract]. Sleep 26(Abstract Suppl):A341.
43. Trenkwalder C, Garcia-Borreguero D, Montagna P, et al. (2004) Ropinirole in the treatment of restless legs syndrome: results from TREAT RLS 1 study, a 12-week, randomised, placebo-controlled study in 10 European countries. J Neurol Neurosurg Psychiatry 75:92–97.
44. Walters AS, Ondo WG, Dreykluft T, et al. (2004) Ropinirole is effective in the treatment of restless legs syndrome: TREAT RLS 2; a 12-week, double-blind, randomized, parallel-group, placebo-controlled study. Mov Disord 19:1414–1423.
45. Walters AS, Ondo W, Sethi K, et al. (2003) Ropinirole versus placebo in the treatment of restless legs syndrome (RLS): a 12-week multicenter double-blind placebo-controlled study in 6 countries [abstract 0866.N]. Sleep 26(Abstract Suppl):A344.
46. Allen R, Becker PM, Bogan R, et al. (2004) Related ropinirole decreases periodic leg movements and improves sleep parameters in patients with restless legs syndrome. Sleep 27:907–914.
47. Oertel WH, Benes H, Geisler P, et al. (2005) Rotigotine patch efficacy and safety in the treatment of moderate to severe idiopathic restless legs syndrome: results from a multi-national double-blind placebo-controlled multi-center dose-finding study. 1st Congress World Association of Sleep Medicine (WASM): Advancing Sleep Health Worldwide. Berlin, Oct. 15–18, 2005. Sleep Med 6(suppl 2):159.
48. Stiasny-Kolster K, Kohnen R, Schollmayer E, et al. (2004) Patch application of the dopamine agonist rotigotine to patients with moderate to advanced stages of restless legs syndrome: a double-blind, placebo-controlled pilot study. Mov Disord 19:1432–1438.

49. Tribl GG, Sycha T, Kotzailias N, et al. (2005) Apomorphine in idiopathic restless legs syndrome: an exploratory study. J Neurol Neurosurg Psychiatry 76:181–185.
50. Adler CH (1997) Treatment of restless legs syndrome with gabapentin. Clin Neuropharmacol 20:148–151.
51. Garcia-Borreguero D, Larrosa O, de la Llave Y, et al. (2002) Treatment of restless legs syndrome with gabapentin: a double-blind, cross-over study. Neurology 59:1573–1579.
52. Thorp ML, Morris CD, Bagby SP (2001) A crossover study of gabapentin in treatment of restless legs syndrome among hemodialysis patients. Am J Kidney Dis 38:104–108.
53. Ondo WG (2005) Methadone for refractory restless legs syndrome. Mov Disord 20:345–348.

27 Introduction to Polysomnography

Bashir A. Chaudhary, MD, FCCP, FACP, FAASM

CONTENTS

INTRODUCTION

A typical polysomnogram (Current Procedural Terminology code 95810) includes recording of an electroencephalography (EEG), an electro-oculogram (EOG), an electromyogram (EMG) of chin muscles, oronasal airflow, chest and abdominal movements, leg movements, snoring, and oximetry. Following is a discussion of some of the aspects of polysomnography.

ELECTROENCEPHALOGRAPHY

Brain electrical activity is recorded through surface electrodes placed on the skull in accordance with an internationally accepted method. These electrical signals pass from the electrodes and through amplifiers, where they are modified before being recorded on paper (analog) or digital recorders.

INTERNATIONAL 10–20 SYSTEM

The 10–20 system was developed in 1958 to standardize the placement of electrodes for EEG recording. The system is termed *10–20* because electrodes are placed either

From: *Current Clinical Practice: Primary Care Sleep Medicine: A Practical Guide*
Edited by: J. F. Pagel and S. R. Pandi-Perumal © Humana Press Inc., Totowa, NJ

at 10 or 20% of the total distance between two skull landmarks. The use of percents instead of absolute distances allows for variation in head sizes. Based on specific anatomic correlates, this system of electrode placement allows for comparison of electrical activity from different areas of the brain and serial comparison of follow-up EEGs in a single patient; also, it is consistent from one patient to another. The four landmarks used are nasion (the indentation between the forehead and the nose), inion (the ridge at the back of the skull), and two preauricular points (indentations just above the tragus cartilage). The nomenclature gives each electrode a site pertaining to a certain area of the brain (F = frontal; P = parietal; T = temporal; C = central; O = occipital; A = auricular) with the exception of the "z" electrode, which refers to the midline or zero line. The subscript numbers refer to the right (even numbers) and the left (odd numbers) side of the brain. The numbered subscripts also define the electrode location in relation to the midline. The smaller the subscript, the closer the electrode position is to the midline.

The standard scoring channel for sleep stages is the central channel (C_3/A_2 or C_4/A_1). Usually both of these channels are used to minimize the possibility of electrode displacement during the recording. Sleep spindles, K-complexes, vertex waves, and δ-waves are clearly recorded from these channels. α-rhythms are better seen in occipital channels and these occipital channels are helpful in defining sleep onset.

AMPLIFIERS

The amplitudes (voltage) of the EEG signals recorded at the scalp are too small and must be increased to make them suitable for interpretation. Modern amplifiers, in addition to amplifying the signal, have calibration devices and contain filters to reduce unwanted EEG frequencies. Sometimes, amplifiers are arbitrarily referred to as preamplifiers if they receive small inputs (micro- and millivolts) and amplifiers if they receive larger inputs (volts). An amplifier multiplies an input signal with a constant, which is usually in the range of 2–1000. This amplification factor is referred to as *gain*. The gain can also be expressed as V (out)/V (in).

Differential alternating-current amplifiers used for EEG monitoring receive voltage input from two sources (grid 1 [G1] and grid 2 [G2]); the difference between the two voltages is passed through. For example, if the input at G1 is –70 μV and the input from G2 is –10 μV, the difference, i.e., 60 μV, will be amplified and passed further. Signals common to both inputs, for example, the noise from a 60-Hz line current are called *in phase* or *common mode* and are not passed further. The ability of an amplifier to amplify the difference in voltage and to reject the voltage common to both inputs is expressed as the *common-mode rejection ratio*. Good EEG amplifiers have common-mode rejection of 10,000 or more.

The ability of a recording system to respond (i.e., pen deflection) to a given input signal is a function of its *sensitivity*. Sensitivity describes the amount of voltage needed to produce a fixed amount of pen deflection and is usually expressed in microvolts/centimeter. The usual sensitivity setting for sleep stages in adults is 50 μV/cm. That is, in order to have a pen deflection of 1 cm, an input of 50 μV is needed. If the amount of pen deflection needs to be increased, then the number of microvolts needed to produce 1 cm of pen deflection has to be decreased. This will give a lower numerical value for sensitivity (e.g., 25 μV/cm). Similarly, if the amplitude of the EEG waves is too high, as is often the case in children, this amplitude may have to be decreased by increasing the number of microvolts needed to produce 1 cm of pen deflection. This change (e.g., 75 μV/cm) will give a higher numeric number for sensitivity even though the amplitude for pen deflection is being decreased. Because the ECG signal is very strong compared with the EEG signal, the sensitivity of the ECG signal has to be very high. The typical sensitivity setting for the ECG signal is 1–10 mV/cm (mV/cm is 1000 times more than a μV/cm).

The relationship of sensitivity, voltage, and pen deflection is similar to the relationship of voltage, current, and resistance in Ohm's law (voltage = current × resistance). In the EEG, sensitivity represents resistance and pen deflection represents current. If the resistance (sensitivity) goes up, then the current (pen deflection) will decrease provided there is no change in voltage. Amplifiers not only increase the size of the input signal but also are able to filter out undesirable signals. Three main types of filters used include low-frequency filters (LFFs), notch filters, and high-frequency filters (HFFs).

HFFs are used to attenuate frequencies higher than the desired frequency (e.g., muscle activity–related artifacts). These filters are also called *low-pass filters*. Most frequencies of interest in EEG range from 0.16 to 100 Hz. The usual high frequency during the sleep stages is less than 20 Hz. An HFF setting of 35 Hz is generally considered adequate for sleep stages. The main concern is in patients who might have seizures. The upper frequency of spike discharge (with a 20-ms base) is 50 Hz. Spikes by definition have a base of 20–70 ms, with frequency of 14–50 Hz. In such cases the HFF may be set at a higher frequency (e.g., at 70 Hz). A filter does not have a static or single level of attenuation. The HFF usually attenuates the designated frequency by 80% and this percent increases progressively for frequencies higher than the designated frequency of the HFF.

LFFs are used to attenuate undesirable frequencies in the lower frequency range. These filters are also called *high-pass filters*. These filters attenuate the signal at the designated frequency by 20%. For example, a LFF set at 0.3 Hz will attenuate a 0.3 Hz signal of 100–80 μV. EEG frequencies lower than the designated frequency of the LFF are progressively attenuated more. The *time constant* is another form of expressing filtration of low frequencies. The time constant is defined as the time it takes for a square wave signal to drop to 37% of the original baseline. Frequently, time constant and LLF are used interchangeably, although the numeric values are not the same. A time constant of 1 second represents an LFF of 0.1 and a time constant of 0.3 second represents an LFF of 0.5.

Notch filters are designed to sharply attenuate a narrow-frequency bandwidth within the range of 50 or 60 Hz. Notch filters are also known as 60-Hz filters. These filters are used to eliminate the noise from electric power lines. Routine use of notch filters is not appropriate because they can mask frequencies that may be of interest in seizure monitoring. This filter can also hide high electrode impedance and poor signal transmission. In EMG channels, the notch filter may excessively attenuate the muscle tone, leading to misinterpretation of the sleep stage. Electrical interference can be minimized if the power cords are kept away from the circuit. Low impedance of the electrodes also helps in minimizing the electric line noise. By convention, the display of EEG signals using differential amplifiers is that negative waveforms cause an upward deflection and positive waveforms cause a downward deflection.

ELECTRO-OCULOGRAPHY

In EOG, the eye movements are recorded from electrodes placed near the outer canthus of each eye. The right outer canthus electrode (ROC) is attached about 1 cm above and out from the outer canthus of the right eye. The left outer canthus electrode (LOC) is attached about 1 cm below and out from the outer canthus of the left eye. Additional electrodes may be attached during multiple sleep latency testing to better appreciate the eye movements. These electrodes are usually referred to the same auricular electrode (e.g., ROC/A_1 and LOC/A_1). It is desirable to refer each electrode to the opposite side (ROC/A_1, LOC/A_2), which equalizes the amplitude of both eyes' movements and maximizes the amplitudes of both eyes' movements.

Placement of electrodes just above one eye and just below the opposite eye produces out-of-phase deflections for conjugate eye movements. This is helpful in distinguishing artifacts coming to ROC and LOC from other channels. δ-waves are frequently seen in these channels but can be distinguished by being in the same direction (i.e., in phase). The small electropotential difference that normally exists between the front and the back of the eye is responsible for the eye movements recorded during polysomnography. The eyeball is like a dipole in which the cornea is positive and the retina is negative. When the eyes move to one side, the electrode placed on the same side as the eye movement will record a positive deflection (downward), whereas the other electrode will record a negative deflection (upward) because the other eye is going away from that electrode.

Eye movements can be divided into slow eye movements (SEMs) and rapid eye movements (REMs). There are no well-defined criteria to distinguish SEMs from REMs. The frequency of SEMs is usually less than 0.5 Hz and the duration of the entire waveform of REMs is less than 1 second. Another feature that helps in distinguishing these two types of eye movements is that the duration of initial deflection of REMs is less than 200 ms. The main reason for recording the eye movements is to establish the presence of REM sleep. REM sleep cannot be diagnosed without the presence of REMs. The frequency of REMs per hour of REM sleep is designated as *REM density* and is a reflection of REM sleep intensity. The presence of SEMs usually means that sleep stage 1 either has begun or is about to begin; hence it is helpful in defining the sleep onset.

ELECTROMYOGRAPHY

In routine polysomnography, EMG is recorded from chin muscles and anterior tibialis muscles. The chin EMG is recorded from an electrode placed over the chin and an electrode placed under the chin and is described as mental-submental derivation. Usually two but at times three electrodes about 1–2 cm apart are attached under the chin. The EMG is recorded bipolarly and a combination of any two electrodes can be used. The third electrode serves as the backup electrode and is particularly helpful for studies extending to the daytime, when there is a higher likelihood of electrodes coming off during eating and talking. The limb electrodes are attached about 2–4 cm apart over the anterior tibialis muscle on both legs. Additional electrodes are attached in certain situations. EMG from the masseter muscle is helpful in the evaluation of bruxism. In patients suspected of having periodic limb movements (PLMs), electrodes may also be attached to the upper limbs, as PLMs of sleep occur in all four limbs.

Chin-muscle EMG is recorded mainly to distinguish REM sleep from non-REM (NREM) sleep. Reduction of muscle tone is one of the requirements for diagnosing REM sleep. PLMs of sleep are diagnosed from limb EMG channels. Sometimes intercostal EMG is used to determine respiratory effort. The normal EMG frequency is between 20 and 200 Hz and generally is more than 40 Hz. The use of a 60-Hz filter can substantially reduce the amplitude of the EMG signal. Conversely, reduction in muscle tone may be difficult to detect in the presence of significant 60-Hz artifact.

RESPIRATORY MEASUREMENT

Respiratory effort can be measured in many ways, including esophageal pressure monitoring, flow monitoring by pneumotachometer, flow monitoring by thermistor and thermocouple, nasal pressure monitoring, intercostal EMG monitoring, and inductive plethysmography. As yet there is no consensus as to which method of monitoring is the best method for polysomnography.

Thermistors and thermocouples detect airflow indirectly and semiquantitatively by sensing the temperature change during breathing. The sensors sense the temperature difference between the cooler inspiration and warmer expiration. The change in temperature of the sensor is associated with a change in resistance. A thermistor measures this as a change in resistance and a thermocouple as a change in electromotive force. These sensors are well tolerated by the patients. The correlation between the temperature change and the flow is relatively poor. Although apneas are detected reliably, hypopneas are usually underestimated.

Pneumotachometers, placed in tightly fitted masks, measure total oronasal airflow by detecting changes in pressure between inspiration and expiration. In central sleep apnea, respiratory effort and hence pressure change is absent. Monitoring of airflow by this method requires a tightly fitting mask, which can cause discomfort and disruption of sleep. Because of these problems, mask pneumotachometry has not become popular for clinical studies.

Nasal pressure can be measured through nasal cannulas placed inside the nares and connected to pressure transducers. Airflow is estimated by measuring nasal airway pressure, which decreases during inspiration and increases during expiration. The flattened contour of inspiratory flow is suggestive of upper airway resistance. Nasal pressure monitoring is more sensitive but less specific than thermistors. This technique underestimates the degree of airflow reduction in patients with nasal obstruction and hence is not recommended in patients who are mouth breathers. Newer cannulas have been introduced that can detect both nasal and oral airflow.

Series and Marc compared the detection of sleep-related breathing using thermistory, inductive plethysmography, and nasal pressure cannulas and found that in 9% of the patients, measurements of nasal pressure were inadequate because of impaired ventilation. Nasal pressure cannulas were similar in detecting respiratory events. One advantage of nasal cannulas was the detection of inspiratory flow limitation, which was missed by thermistory.

Respiratory inductive plethysmography measures the volume changes in the chest and abdomen during a breathing cycle. The sum of these measurements provides an estimate of tidal volume. During disordered breathing, there is asynchronous breathing (paradoxical chest wall and abdominal movements) that can be detected. This method does not allow for accurate distinction between apneas and hypopneas in the absence of an airflow measurement. This technique has been suggested for identification of upper airway resistance syndrome by looking at the ratio of the peak inspiratory flow to mean flow. The loops generated by his technique may also be useful for titration of continuous positive airway pressure. The American Academy of Sleep Medicine in 1999 made recommendations regarding various methods of airflow measurement. Only measurement

Table 1
EEG Rhythms

Rhythms	*Frequency (cps)*
β	≥14
α	8–13
θ	4–7
δ	<4
μ	7–11

by the pneumotachometer was given an A grade, whereas nasal pressure and respiratory inductive plethysmography were given B grades. Thermal sensors and expired CO_2 measurements were graded D.

SCORING CRITERIA

The main categories of scoring during polysomnography include sleep stages, respiratory events, leg movements, and arousals. Many other parameters, such as oximetry, ECG, snoring, continuous positive airway pressure titration, and effect of posture are also evaluated.

SLEEP STAGES

Depending on the frequency (i.e., cycles per second), the EEG waves are divided into rhythms such as β-, α-, θ-, δ-, and μ-rhythms (Table 1). From the awake state, we go into the sleep state, divided into NREM sleep, which is further subdivided into four stages, stage 1 being the most superficial and stage 4 the deepest and REM sleep. Sleep stages are scored in 30-second segments (epochs) based on EEG, EOG, and EMG.

The awake stage (stage 0) is characterized by low-amplitude, mixed-frequency EEG. When the eyes are closed, the α-rhythm becomes prominent and then diminishes at sleep onset. Eye movements are present and muscle tone is high. Stage 1 sleep is characterized by a change from α-activity into θ-activity. Vertex waves are frequently present during stage 1 sleep. Sleep onset is defined by the presence of sleep for at least three consecutive epochs of stage 1 sleep. SEMs are usually present at sleep onset. Muscle tone usually diminishes at sleep onset compared with the awake stage.

Stage 2 sleep is characterized by the continuation of the same low-amplitude, mixed-frequency EEG of stage 1 sleep and the appearance of two markers. Sleep spindles and K-complexes define the presence of Stage 2 sleep. Sleep spindles have a frequency of 12–14 cps and duration of 0.5–1.5 seconds. Incipient (mini, baby) spindles are less than 0.5 second in duration and are seen in stage 1 sleep that precedes stage 2 sleep. Sleep spindles occur with a frequency of 3–8 spindles/minute in normal adults. K-complexes have sharp upward (negative) deflection followed by a downward (positive) component and are at least 0.5 second in duration. Amplitude is not a criterion for defining a K-complex. The usual frequency of K-complexes during stage 2 sleep is about 1–3/minute. The muscle tone is lower than in the awake stage and eye movements are uncommon.

Stage 3 and 4 sleep is called δ-sleep and is characterized by the presence of high voltage (75 μV or higher) waves with slow frequency (2 cps or slower). A δ-wave should be at least 0.5 second in duration. Stage 3 sleep is defined by the presence of δ-waves that occupy at least 20% of an epoch. Stage 4 sleep is defined by the presence of δ-waves that occupy at least 50% of an epoch. Occasional sleep spindles may be present in δ-sleep. K-complexes may be present but are difficult to distinguish from δ-waves. Muscle tone is usually still high, but might be so low that it resembles the muscle tone of REM sleep. Eye movements are usually absent, but δ-waves are frequently seen in eye channels because of the high voltage of δ-waves.

REM sleep has three cardinal features:

1. Low-amplitude, mixed-frequency EEG.
2. Bursts of REMS.
3. Loss of muscle tone.

The background EEG is similar to that seen in stage 1 or stage 2 sleep. Although an EEG pattern called "sawtooth" waves (because of the notched morphology) is frequently seen during this stage, the presence of this pattern alone does not define REM sleep. The frequency of sawtooth waves is in the θ-range. α-rhythm is commonly present in REM sleep and its frequency is 1–2 cps lower than in the awake stage. The EOG shows bursts of REMs. The EMG shows loss of muscle tone. There are occasional muscle twitches. REM sleep is divided into phasic and tonic components based on the presence or absence of eye movements and muscle twitches. The occasional presence of a sleep spindle does not change stage REM sleep; however, if two spindles bracket more than one half of the epoch, that epoch is scored as stage 2 sleep.

RULES OF STAGE 2 AND REM SLEEP

Two rules commonly used in sleep stages are the 3-minute stage 2 rule and the stage REM rule. Sleep spindles and K-complexes are transient phenomena and long periods of sleep may occur without these markers of stage 2 sleep. After an epoch has been scored as stage 2 sleep, the next 3 minute are also scored as stage 2 sleep even in the absence of sleep spindles and K-complexes, as long as there are no markers of another stage of sleep and muscle tone remains low. If there is an increase in the muscle tone or the 3-minute limit is exceeded, the sleep stage is changed to stage 1.

There is a similar rule for extension of stage REM sleep. Once stage REM has been established, the stage REM is extended both forward and backwards, even in the absence of REMs, until there is evidence of another stage of sleep, as long as there is no change in EMG and EEG. How long can this stage of REM be extended? In contrast to the "stage 2 rule," which extends stage 2 sleep for the next 3 minute in the absence of sleep spindles and K-complexes, there is no time limit for stage REM sleep. The author often describes this "REM rule" as "REM rules." When one rules, one rules without time limits.

MOVEMENT TIME

Movements occur frequently during sleep and obscure EEG and EOG recordings. It becomes difficult to ascertain whether the patient is awake or asleep. If this occurs for 15 second or more, the epoch is scored as movement time.

SLEEP-DISORDERED BREATHING

Sleep-disordered breathing includes apneas, hypopneas, and respiratory effort-related arousals. There has been great deal of controversy about the definition of these events. In 1999, a task force of the American Academy of Sleep Medicine made recommendations for the definition of these terms for clinical research. A follow-up report by the Clinical Practice Review Committee of the American Academy of Sleep Medicine published guidelines for scoring hypopneas in adults. The Center of Medicare and Medicaid Services recently adopted these guidelines for clinical purposes.

Apnea is defined as cessation of airflow for more than 10 seconds. The reduction in airflow should be 80–100% compared with baseline. Baseline is defined as the mean amplitude of stable breathing and oxygenation in the preceding 2 minutes or the mean amplitude of the three largest breaths in the preceding 2 minutes.

Hypopnea is defined as a 30% or more decrease (compared with baseline) in airflow or thoracoabdominal movements associated with 4% or more oxygen desaturation.

A *respiratory effort-related arousal* event is defined as a sequence of breaths characterized by increasing respiratory effort leading to an arousal from sleep. This is usually diagnosed with an esophageal balloon measuring progressively more negative pressure.

AROUSALS

Cortical arousals (i.e., those seen on EEG) indicate sleep disruption and are important in defining upper airway resistance syndrome and in determining the clinical impact of nocturnal myoclonic episodes. Arousals were a part of the criteria used to define hypopneas; however, the recent recommendations of the Center of Medicare and Medicaid Services did not include arousals as part of the definition of hypopneas.

Arousal is defined as an abrupt shift in EEG frequency that may include θ, α, and/or frequencies higher than 16 but not spindles. Because this change in EEG activity lasts less than 15 seconds, it does not change the sleep stage. If the change in EEG activity lasts 15 seconds or more, the epoch is scored as awake stage. The American Sleep Disorders Association (now called the American Academy of Sleep Medicine) suggested the following rules for scoring of arousals:

1. There should be at least 10 second of continuous sleep before an arousal.
2. There should be 10 second of continuous sleep before a second arousal.
3. An arousal should be at least 3 seconds long.
4. Arousal in NREM sleep can be scored without EMG elevation.
5. Arousals in REM sleep must have concurrent elevation of chin EMG.
6. Arousals should not be scored based on submental EMG alone.
7. Artifacts, K-complexes, and δ-waves are not arousals unless there is a change in EEG.
8. Pen-deflection artifacts are not arousals unless there is a change in EEG.
9. Nonconcurrent, but contiguous EEG and EMG changes that last less than 3 seconds individually but more than 3 seconds together are not arousals.
10. α-Sleep is not arousal.
11. Transition from one sleep stage to another sleep stage is not arousal.

Some authors use a different duration criterion (e.g., 1.5 seconds) for defining an arousal. Arousals are also seen during normal sleep and there is no consensus at the present time about the normal frequency of arousals. An arousal index (number of arousals per hour of sleep) of less than 10 is generally considered within the normal range. Arousal indices of more than 20 (or 25) may be abnormal.

PERIODIC LIMB MOVEMENTS

Limb movements are recorded from one or both anterior tibialis muscles. Sometimes, the recordings are also made from upper extremities. A limb movement is a burst of muscle activity that lasts for 0.5–5 seconds (mean duration, 105–2.5 seconds). The amplitude of a movement should be at least 25% of the movement recoded during calibration. Limb movements are called periodic when they occur in a stereotypic manner at intervals of 20–40 seconds. Random aperiodic limb movements are not counted. A PLM sequence is four or more movements that are separated by at least 5 seconds but not more than 90 seconds. The total number of limb movements divided by the number of hours of sleep is called PLM index. Limb movements with arousals are counted separately and the PLM with arousal index is calculated.

Leg movements associated with termination of apneas or hypopneas are generally not considered a part of periodic limb movements of sleep. On the other hand, leg movements associated with arousals may be a marker of upper airway resistance syndrome. Leg movements without arousals are very common in patients taking antidepressants. Muscle twitches with a shorter duration are called *fragmentary myoclonus*. Bursts of brief muscle twitches are also commonly seen in phasic REM sleep.

REFERENCES

1. *A Manual of Standardized Terminology: Techniques and Scoring System for Sleep Stages of Human Subjects*. (Rechtschaffen A, Kales A, eds.) UCLA Brain Information Service/ Brain Research Institute, Los Angeles, CA, 1968.
2. Carskadon MA, Rechtschaffen A (2000) Monitoring and staging of human sleep. In: *Principles and Practice of Sleep Medicine*. 3rd ed. (Kryger M, Roth T, Dement W, eds.) WB Saunders, Philadelphia, PA, pp. 1197–1215.
3. Keenan SA (1999) Polysomnographic technique: an overview. In: *Sleep Disorders Medicine: Basic Science, Technical Consideration, and Clinical Aspects*. (Chokroverty S, ed.) 2nd ed. Butterworth-Heinemann, Boston, MA, pp. 149–174.
4. Tyner FS, Knott JR, Mayer WB *Fundamentals of EEG Technology: volume* 1. *Basic Concepts and Methods*. Raven Press, New York, NY, 1983.
5. Jasper H (1958) The ten twenty electrode system of the International Federation. EEG Clin Neurophysiol 10:371–375.
6. Radtke RA (1990) Sleep disorders. In: *Current Practice of Clinical EEG*. 2nd ed. (Daly DD, Pedly TA, eds.) Raven Press, New York, NY, pp. 561–592.
7. Series F, Marc I (1999) Nasal pressure recording in the diagnosis of sleep apnoea hypopnea syndrome. Thorax 54:506–510.
8. Whyte KF, Gugger M, Gould GA, et al. (1991) Accuracy of respiratory inductive plethysmography in measuring tidal volume during sleep. J Appl Physiol 71:1866–1871.
9. Santamaria J, Chiappa KH (1987) *The EEG of Drowsiness*. Demos, New York, NY.
10. Loube DI, Andrada TF (1999) Comparison of nocturnal respiratory parameters in upper airway resistance and obstructive sleep apnea syndrome patients. Chest 115:1217–1222.
11. Series F, Marc I (1995) Accuracy of breath-by-breath analysis of flow-volume loop in identifying sleep-induced flow limited breathing cycles in sleep apnoea-hypopnoea syndrome. Clin Sci 88:707–712.
12. Berg S, Haight JSJ, Yap V, et al. (1997) Comparison of direct and indirect measurements of respiratory airflow: implications for hypopneas. Sleep 20:60–64.
13. Gaillard J-M, Blois R (1981) Spindle density in sleep of normal subjects. Sleep 4:385–391.
14. Sleep-related breathing disorders in adults: recommendations for syndrome definition and measurement techniques in clinical research; The Report of an American Academy of Sleep Medicine Task Force. (1999) Sleep 22:667–689.

15. Meoli AL, Casey KR, Clark RW, et al. (2001) Hypopnea in sleep-disordered breathing in adults. Sleep 24:469–470.
16. EEG arousals: scoring rules and examples; a preliminary report from the Sleep Disorders Atlas Task Force of the American Sleep Disorders Association. (1992) Sleep 15:173–184.
17. Recording and scoring leg movements: the Atlas Task Force. (1993) Sleep 16:748–759.
18. Butkov N (1996) *Atlas of Clinical Polysomnography* vol 2. Synapse Media, OR, Ashland, pp. 286–301.

28 Portable Monitoring

Charles W. Atwood, Jr., MD, FCCP

CONTENTS

INTRODUCTION

The field of sleep medicine has grown up around the main test used to measure disorders of sleep: the polysomnogram (PSG). The PSG is a comprehensive, technology-heavy test that requires special facilities, specially trained technologists, and careful scoring of the record to yield a meaningful result. Almost since PSG came into widespread clinical use, the field of sleep medicine has sought alternatives to PSG that would give an accurate measure of sleep apnea. As obstructive sleep apnea (OSA) is the most common reason that a PSG is performed, it is reasonable to focus on OSA in developing non-PSG techniques for accurately diagnosing this particular disorder.

Why are alternatives to PSG desirable? First, there is the concern about access to sleep medicine clinical services. Not all communities have sleep laboratories. Some segments of the population do not have access to full PSG capabilities, whether it is because of geography, particular financial limitations of the patient, or the particular insurance plan covering that patient. In some communities, there are long waiting times for sleep laboratory testing. A second reason is cost. PSGs are expensive and are not covered by all insurance plans. Paying out of pocket for a PSG would be prohibitively expensive for many patients. A final reason is that some patients prefer to have testing at home, if it is available. From a clinician's standpoint, in some cases, this may be preferred over sleeping in the sleep laboratory, especially because most patients do not sleep as well in the sleep laboratory as they do at home. Sleeping at the home is the natural

From: *Current Clinical Practice: Primary Care Sleep Medicine: A Practical Guide*
Edited by: J. F. Pagel and S. R. Pandi-Perumal © Humana Press Inc., Totowa, NJ

environment; sleep clinicians would want to know what the patient's sleep is like in the normal, as opposed to the sleep laboratory, condition.

TERMINOLOGY OF PORTABLE SLEEP APNEA MONITORING

Out-of-sleep laboratory monitoring for OSA goes by several different names. Some have referred to it as ambulatory monitoring. This is somewhat of a misnomer, because the testing is not ambulatory (unless the patient is sleepwalking). What is meant here is that the test takes place at a nonmedical site. Strictly speaking, this is not necessarily true, because portable sleep apnea testing can be performed in medical settings. In fact, this is a common approach in some settings, such as certain facilities in England and some US Veteran's Administration (VA) Hospitals. Some refer to this testing as "portable sleep testing." This is also a misnomer, because, in most cases, no sleep is recorded. Typically, several respiratory parameters and electrocardiogram or a related measure of heart rate are recorded, such as the tachogram. Some refer to these monitors as cardiopulmonary monitors. This is an accurate name, based on the signals recorded, but somewhat misses the point of the testing, which is to test for sleep apnea, not cardiopulmonary function. The author believes that the term *portable sleep apnea monitors* (*PSAM*) or *portable sleep apnea testing* is the most accurate label given to this type of device or the activity for which it is used.

TYPES OF MONITORS

The types of sleep apnea monitoring devices available have been classified by the number and complexity of the signals they record *(1)*.

1. Type 1: standard in-laboratory PSG.
2. Type 2: miniaturized, comprehensive PSG that can be performed outside of the sleep laboratory.
3. Type 3: devices that record cardiopulmonary signals; these are used for portable sleep apnea testing.
4. Type 4: continuous single or dual parameter testing, such as oximetry, or two signal devices, such that measure oximetry and airflow.

EVIDENCE-BASED REVIEW OF THE LITERATURE OF PSAM

A comprehensive literature review was published in *CHEST (1)* in 2003. It is an authoritative reference for this discussion. Students of portable monitoring should read it and be familiar with it. Another important paper to be aware of is a companion document published in *Sleep (2)* the same year. This is a practice guideline, based on the evidence published in the *CHEST* paper. In this evidence-based review, the authors comprehensively described the literature on PSAM. Because type 2 monitors are rarely used in clinical (as opposed to research) practice, the following summary is limited to types 3 and 4 monitors. The author provides a brief summary of the findings of the evidence review and the practice guideline.

TYPE 3 MONITORS

Sleep-Laboratory Based

There were nine studies of sleep-laboratory-based comparisons of type 3 monitors and PSG. Eight of the studies were considered to have good quality evidence. The studies were analyzed using sensitivity, specificity, and likelihood ratios. The results of the likelihood ratios showed that seven of the eight studies reviewed had low likelihood ratios and, thus, very high sensitivities. All of the studies had some subjects with negative PSAM results. These were subject to being false-negatives. However, the false-negative rate was quite low, ranging from 4 to 8%. The conclusion of this analysis was that type 3 monitors were reasonably accurate in a sleep laboratory environment for ruling in and ruling out OSA.

Home-Based Testing

Four studies examined the ability of PSAM to rule in and rule out OSA when the study is performed at the patient's home and unattended by sleep laboratory technologists. In this situation, the evidence was found to be less robust than the evidence found for the technologist-attended, laboratory-based studies. There was higher variability in the sensitivity, specificity, and likelihood ratios.

Conclusions

The authors of the evidence-based review concluded that type 3 monitors used in a technologist-attended setting were able to both increase and decrease the likelihood of an abnormal apnea-hypopnea index. In the unattended, home-based, testing scenario, the evidence was not conclusive, mainly because of the limited number of studies and the higher variability of results.

TYPE 4 MONITORS

Sleep-Laboratory Based

A limited number of studies that use oximetry alone, or combined oximetry with another signal were analyzed. Some had reasonably high and low likelihood ratios, whereas others did not. Again, moderate variability was found.

Home-Based Testing

A smaller number of studies with mixed results were found. Some used oximetry alone, whereas others used oximetry with another signal. The results from these few studies were heterogeneous and inconclusive.

Conclusions

The panel conclusion was that the utility of using oximetry, either alone or added to another signal, such as airflow, to rule in or rule out OSA, was not demonstrated.

WHAT DATA ARE NEEDED TO DETERMINE IF PSAM HAS A ROLE IN OSA DIAGNOSTIC TESTING?

The studies that have been performed to date have been limited to relatively small sample studies of sleep clinic populations. These tend to be white, middle-aged men. Studies of patients older than 65 years are notably lacking. Other important aspects of diagnostic device validation studies are also limited in the present studies, including few patients with important comorbid conditions, such as chronic obstructive pulmonary disease or congestive heart failure, and few ethnic minorities or women have been included in studies. Finally, the test-retest response has not been established in PSAMs to an adequate degree.

The design of studies so far has been appropriate to developing an early understanding of how these monitors may fit into a diagnostic framework. There is reasonable evidence that the PSAMs record sleep apnea adequately, when compared head-to-head with PSG. This is a necessary step but not a sufficient one for PSAM to become accepted as a viable technology. The field is now ready for outcome studies to test the use of portable monitors against sleep-laboratory-based PSG, with patient outcomes as the measure of interest. Such studies are now starting to be developed.

HOW CAN PSAM FIT INTO A RATIONAL APPROACH TO OSA DIAGNOSIS, GIVEN THE UNCERTAINTY ABOUT ITS UTILITY?

Portable sleep apnea testing is controversial. Because of the relatively limited amount of clinical trial evidence supporting its use, some professional societies and many health insurance companies do not recognize it as a legitimate method of diagnosing OSA. Unarguably, the scientific evidence supporting its widespread clinical use has not been developed. Nonetheless, despite the lack of conclusive evidence of its utility in diagnosing OSA, especially in the home setting, PSAM is widely used. The volume of home portable studies is not known.

The decision to develop this type of clinical practice use without conclusive evidence of utility is usually driven by reimbursement. In areas where managed care organizations control reimbursement decisions, PSAM may be viewed as a less expensive alternative to full PSG and, therefore, may gain acceptance despite there being no cost-effectiveness studies at all for PSAM. PSAM may be less expensive, but whether it is cost effective is simply unknown. For example, future studies may find that the negative test rate is high, and that negative studies will generate confirmatory PSGs. Depending on the OSA prevalence in the population, the prestudy probability may be such that low-likelihood patients should have full PSG instead of indeterminate portable test followed by a definitive PSG.

One possible approach to using PSAM in clinical practice is to reserve it for high-likelihood individuals. In a high-pretest probability environment, the available evidence suggests that false-positive PSAM results are low, indicating that a positive PSAM is diagnostic for OSA. In this scenario, the patient then goes for a trial of positive pressure therapy. PSAM-negative patients in this setting may go for a confirmatory PSG or may return to the clinician for clinical re-evaluation. If the patient has not seen a sleep clinician before the PSAM, then a referral to a specialist may be indicated.

Another approach to using PSAM may be as a triage tool for areas where PSG resources are unavailable or scarce. If a patient has a highly positive PSAM, then that person goes for treatment more urgently than if the PSAM is low or borderline. A variant on this approach, used in conjunction with a validated questionnaire about sleep apnea, was shown to reduce the need for PSG by a modest amount *(3)*. This is an approach suited to a managed care or VA model.

In the VA system, PSAM is widely used in several ways. One common way is to do home-based PSAM. In some cases, PSG is available, on a limited basis, if the PSAM is negative or nondiagnostic but a high clinical suspicion for OSA is still present. Another approach is to use PSAM monitors in a sleep lab environment, instead of full PSG. This method is consistent with the previous validation studies for type 3 monitors. The author's VA practice operates in this way for approx 60% of the diagnostic sleep studies. This approach allows sleep laboratory technologists to do more diagnostic sleep studies with very little extra effort. Yet, the patients are in a monitored environment, and the technologists can respond to requests for assistance. Furthermore, the technologists can contribute their own observations to the night's recordings, which are frequently insightful and helpful. This approach works best in clinical practices or locations where maximizing reimbursement is not a primary goal.

THE FUTURE OF PORTABLE MONITORING

The American Academy of Sleep Medicine, the American Thoracic Society, and the American College of Chest Physicians jointly sponsored and performed the original evidence-based review and the practice parameter paper *(1,2)*. Future efforts by these three professional societies may examine how PSAM fits into clinical practice, with less than strong evidence for its utility. This real-world approach to PSAM should produce valuable insights into how best to use this technology in a rapidly changing health care landscape. Although the future of PSAM is not clear at this point, it is likely to be discussed, studied, and utilized for years to come.

REFERENCES

1. Flemons WW, Littner MR, Rowley JA, et al. (2003) Home diagnosis of sleep apnea: a systematic review of the literature: an evidence review cosponsored by the American Academy of Sleep Medicine, the American College of Chest Physicians, and the American Thoracic Society. Chest 124:1543–1579.
2. Chesson AJ, Berry R, Pack A (2003) Practice parameters for the use of portable monitoring devices in the investigation of suspected obstructive sleep apnea. Sleep 26:907–913.
3. Gurubhagavatula I, Maislin G, Pack A (2001) An algorithm to stratify sleep apnea risk in a sleep disorders clinic population. Am J Respir Crit Care Med 164:1904–1909.

29 Correct CPT Coding, Billing, and Documentation in Sleep Medicine

Barbara A. Phillips, MD, MSPH, FCCP

CONTENTS

DIAGNOSTIC DEFINITIONS AND TECHNIQUES FOR SLEEP STUDIES

The gold standard for the diagnosis of obstructive sleep apnea syndrome (OSAS) remains to be overnight polysomnography (PSG). A nocturnal PSG includes recordings of airflow, ventilatory effort, oxygen saturation, electrocardiogram, body position, electromyography, and electroencephalography. In standard, laboratory-based PSG, a technician is present for the entire study to completely monitor the patient. A single overnight study is generally sufficient to diagnose OSAS. In many instances, the level of Sleep-disordered breathing (SDB) is severe enough that the diagnosis of OSAS can be established early in the study. In this event, a "split-night" study may be performed, where the second half of the study is used to titrate treatment (positive airway pressure) for OSAS. The Centers for Medicare and Medicaid Services (CMS, formerly called the Health Care Financing Administration) has recently endorsed the performance of split-night PSG but requires that the diagnostic portion of the test last at least 2 hours of sleep, to avoid artificially inflating the severity of the SDB. (*See* Appendix for sample split-night study protocol.)

The apnea/hypopnea index (AHI) is the most commonly used criterion to establish the diagnosis of OSAS and to quantify its severity. The AHI is defined as the sum of episodes of apnea and hypopneas divided by the hours of sleep. Recently, some unanimity in the criteria for defining apneas and hypopneas has been achieved, largely as a result of the

From: *Current Clinical Practice: Primary Care Sleep Medicine: A Practical Guide*
Edited by: J. F. Pagel and S. R. Pandi-Perumal © Humana Press Inc., Totowa, NJ

Sleep Heart Health Study (SHHS). In adults, apneas and hypopneas require at least a 10-second reduction of airflow (to 30% of baseline for apneas and to 70% of baseline for hypopneas). In the SHHS, the definitions of both apneas and hypopneas required an oxygen desaturation of 4% or more, of note, the definition of apnea, promulgated by the American Academy of Sleep Medicine (AASM) and by the CMS, do not require oxygen desaturation (although the definition of hypopnea does). In obstructive apneas and hypopneas, reduction of airflow occurs despite continued ventilatory efforts. In central apneas, respiratory effort is not detectable during the reduction in airflow.

According to the AASM, the OSA/hypopnea syndrome (OSAHS) exists when a patient has five or more obstructed breathing events per hour of sleep, with the appropriate clinical presentation.

PAYMENT FOR DIAGNOSTIC STUDIES

Currently, there are six current procedural terminology (CPT) sleep codes: 95805, 95806, 95807, 95808, 95810, and 95811. The most frequently used are 95810 (diagnostic PSG, with four or more channels) and 95811 (split-night study). These can be billed as a "global fee" for the study *in toto* or can be broken down into the professional component (26 modifier) and the technical component modifier. Currently, the physician fee for overnight PSG (95810) under Medicare is $178.78, and the technical component is $604.39. The AASM has been the primary entity working to achieve the appropriate reimbursement of these codes by working with membership and providing reports to the CMS, Relative Value Committee, and Practice Expense Advisory Committee. The CMS issued a final rule that will increase payments to more than 875,000 physicians and other health care professionals for services under the Medicare Physician Fee Schedule, by an average of more than 1.5% for the 2004 calendar year.

These increases were part of the Medicare Prescription Drug, Improvement, and Modernization Act and replaced payment rates published in November that would have reduced payment by an average of about 4.5%. On January 1, 2004, the new, higher rates became effective. Physicians in some rural and other areas will see an additional increase in payments, as a result of the Medicare Prescription Drug, Improvement, and Modernization Act provision requiring the CMS to change how it adjusts payments to recognize area cost differences. This provision will increase Medicare payment to physicians in some areas of the country by as much as 4.8%. A separate provision, affecting physicians in Alaska, will result in more than a 52% increase in average physician fee schedule payments for 2004.

The AASM accredits full-service sleep disorder centers and sleep-related breathing laboratories. Full-service sleep disorder centers require an American Board of Sleep Medicine board-certified medical director or center director and are capable of treating all sleep disorders. Sleep-related breathing laboratories require that a board-certified pulmonologist serve as the medical director or laboratory director and that they only treat patients with sleep-related breathing disorders. All other requirements of accreditation are centered on these differences. Either facility can be hospital-based or freestanding. At present, the AASM has accredited more than 500 facilities. Some insurers, some states, and some regional Medicare plans require that sleep centers be AASM-accredited, in order to reimburse for PSG studies performed there. A list of these is virtually impossible to create, because it varies constantly, as well as varying by insurer and region.

PAYMENT FOR TREATMENT

The CMS reimburses for continuous positive airway pressure (CPAP) treatment for patients with an AHI greater than 15, or with an AHI greater than 5 plus hypertension, stroke, sleepiness, ischemic heart disease, or "mood disorders." As noted earlier, the CMS endorsed the performance of split-night PSG (and pays slightly more for it than for simple PSG) but requires that the diagnostic portion of the test last for at least 2 hours of sleep to avoid artificially inflating the severity of the SDB. It also requires some measure of patient compliance for continued payment for CPAP after 4 months of use, though it is not very specific what this should be. (*See Additional Reading* for one actual policy and the appendix for a sample appeal letter if CPAP is denied on the basis of compliance.) Medicare and most managed care insurance companies buy two masks a year: one at the time of the initial setup and another 6 months into therapy. The Federal Drug Administration has labeled these masks as single patient use only; therefore, they cannot be returned or reused. Medicare prohibits dispensing free equipment to patients in which home medical equipment companies cannot exchange masks or give a second mask for free. Legally, they must bill for the supplies they distribute.

CONTROVERSIES AND FUTURE PREDICTIONS

Although there is now some consistency about the definitions of SDB, considerable variation in recording technique for measures of airflow and respiratory effort remains. The use of a pressure transducer as a means of assessing nasal airflow is more accurate than is thermistry and will probably supplant it. In the meantime, the innate inaccuracy and variability of current measurement techniques have almost certainly resulted in varying sensitivity for detection of SDB events.

Prediction Formulae

Several investigators have developed prediction formulae based from findings in the history or physical examination. Among the most useful of such findings are a history of witnessed apneas, male gender, body mass index, and neck circumference. In general, these formulae are sensitive but not specific compared with PSG. Whereas there is growing evidence that "classic" sleep apneics (sicker, heavier, men) can be diagnosed clinically without formal in-laboratory PSG, there are many patients who do not fit the stereotypical prototype of the obstructive sleep apneic. These include Asians, women, and older individuals. However, prediction formulae probably do have a place in the expedited diagnosis and/or triage of patients with suspected SDB.

Ambulatory Monitoring and Screening

Controversy exists about where sleep studies are best done and about the role of screening. Proponents of home testing suggest enhanced patient convenience, reduced cost, and increased accessibility as benefits of home testing. Opponents point out that with home studies, split-night studies cannot be done, equipment problems cannot be corrected, "live" assessments are not possible, and non-OSAHS disorders cannot be detected. Ironically, the best data available about the consequences and definitions of SDB actually come from portable monitoring, which is what was used in the SHHS. Numerous reports from the SHHS and from clinical series indicate that portable monitoring is reproducible with acceptable data loss and reasonable correlation with in-laboratory PSG. Better yet, portable-monitoring findings can predict the adverse outcomes of SDB.

Ambulatory monitors that measure as many channels as do in-laboratory PSG have been available for some time. The SHHS, using rigid protocols and a central reading system, has demonstrated that home monitoring can produce reliable data with acceptable rates of data loss. Similarly, because of the resources already invested in "full-service" sleep laboratories, organized sleep medicine has been slow to address new information about home monitoring that has emerged from the SHHS and other research. Indeed, the American Thoracic Society has joined the AASM and American College of Chest Physicians in producing a literature review and a practice parameters document that discount the utility of portable monitoring.

Several other tools have been developed to aid in the diagnosis or screening of SDB. Although currently not accepted by "mainstream" sleep specialists, these techniques do have a physiological basis and some diagnostic utility. Among them are measures of movement, such as actigraphy and static beds assessment. Also being developed, particularly by cardiologists, are measures of heart rate variability and pulse pressure, including Holter monitoring.

It is likely that the emphasis on in-laboratory PSG, in general, and on the AHI, in particular, will diminish in the future. Data are accumulating that the AHI is a poor "gold standard," because it does not take into account how long the apneas or hypopneas last, how much sleep is disturbed, how much oxygen desaturation there is, and whether there are associated problems, like cardiac arrhythmias. Further, measures and definitions of SDB are not standard between countries and communities. For example, reports of SDB use definitions of hypopnea that require varying (or no) degrees of oxygen desaturation. There is evidence that upper airways resistance syndrome and even simple snoring can cause many of the sequelae of OSA; in-laboratory PSG does not usually take this into account, and the sleep community has been unable to convince most insurers to pay for treatment of these ill-defined forms of SDB. Further, there remains an enormous debate about the cutoff between a "normal" and an "abnormal" AHI.

On top of these problems, waiting times for in-laboratory PSG in most countries average more than a month. As data accumulates that sleep apnea causes car wrecks, heart disease, and death, physicians are becoming increasingly uncomfortable with requiring patients to wait weeks or months for testing—and then weeks or months before titration and definitive treatment. In-laboratory PSG typically costs two or three times what a CPAP machine does. CPAP treatment is safe, cheap, and effective. The risks of delays or failure to treat sleep apnea include car wrecks and death. Although many patients will still require in-laboratory PSG, it is likely that screening tools and clinical prediction formulae will increasingly become used to triage patients with obvious severe SDB to early treatment with autotitrating CPAP.

REFERENCES

General

1. American Academy of Sleep Medicine (2000) *International Classification of Sleep Disorders (ICSD)* [revised]. Diagnostic and coding manual. American Academy of Sleep Medicine, Westchester, IL.
2. Buysse DJ (2003) Clinicians use of the international classification of sleep disorders: results of a national survey. Sleep 26:48–51.

Diagnosis/Definitions

3. American Academy of Sleep Medicine Task Force (1999) Sleep-related breathing disorders in adults: recommendations for syndrome definition and measurement techniques in clinical research. Sleep 22:667–689.
4. Hosselet JJ, Norman RG, Ayappa I, et al. (1998) Detection of flow limitation with a nasal cannula/pressure transducer system. Am J Respir Crit Care Med 157:1461–1467.
5. Meoli AL, Casey KR, Clark RW, et al. (2001) Hypopnea in sleep-disordered breathing in adults. Sleep 24:469–470.
6. Stradling JR, Davies RJ (2004) Obstructive sleep apnoea/hypopnoea syndrome: definitions, epidemiology, and natural history. Thorax 59:73–78.

Portable Monitoring

7. Chesson AL Jr, Berry RB, Pack A, et al. (2003) Practice parameters for the use of portable monitoring devices in the investigation of suspected obstructive sleep apnea in adults. Sleep 26:907–913.
8. Davila DG, Richards KC, Marshall BL, et al. (2003) Oximeter's acquisition parameter influences the profile of respiratory disturbances. Sleep 26:91–95.
9. Golpe R, Jimenez A, Carpizo R (2002) Home sleep studies in the assessment of sleep apnea/hypopnea syndrome. Chest 122:1156–1161.
10. Quan SF, Griswold ME, Iber C, et al. (2002) Short-term variability of respiration and sleep during unattended nonlaboratory polysomnography: the Sleep Heart Health Study. Sleep 25:843–849.

Prediction Models

11. Kushida CA, Efron B, Guilleminault C (1997) A predictive morphometric model for the obstructive sleep apnea syndrome. Ann Intern Med 127:581–587.
12. Netzer NC, Stoohs RA, Netzer CM, Clark K, Strohl KP (1999) Using the Berlin Questionnaire to identify patients at risk for the sleep apnea syndrome. Ann Intern Med 131:485–491.
13. Rowley JA, Aboussouan LS, Badr S (2000) The use of clinical prediction formulae in the evaluation of obstructive sleep apnea. Sleep 23:929–938.

Autotitrating CPAP

14. Ayas NT, Patel SR, Malhotra A, et al. (2004) Auto-titrating versus standard continuous positive airway pressure for the treatment of obstructive sleep apnea: results of a meta-analysis. Sleep 27:249–253.
15. Hudgel DW, Fung C (2000) A long-term randomized, cross-over comparison of auto-titrating and standard nasal continuous airway pressure. Sleep 23:645–648.
16. Littner M, Hirskowitz M, Davila D, et al. (2002) Practice parameters for the use of auto-titrating continuous positive airway pressure devices for titrating pressures and treating adult patients with obstructive sleep apnea syndrome. Sleep 25:143–147.
17. Massie CA, McArdle N, Hart RW, et al. (2003) Comparison between automatic and fixed positive airway pressure in the home. Am J Respir Crit Care Med 167:20–23.
18. Randerath W, Schraeder O, Galetke, et al. (2001) Autoadjusting CPAP therapy based on impedance efficacy, compliance and acceptance. Am J Crit Care Med 163: 652–657.

Web Sites

19. CDC Web site. Available at: http://www.cdc.gov/nchs/about/otheract/icd9/abticd10.htm. *Describes ICD 10 and links to other relevant sites.*
20. American Academy of Sleep Medicine. Available at: http://www.aasmnet.org. *The primary advocate for sleep physicians and their patients.*
21. Centers for Medicare and Medicaid Services. Available at: http://cms.hhs.gov/. *Formerly called the HCFA.* Cpap.Com Web site. Available at: http://www.cpap.com/.

Additional Reading
From the CMS Website

Article ID Number	A12530
Article Type	Basic Article
Article Title	CPAP and Respiratory Assist Devices–Apnea/Hypopnea Index
Primary Geographic Jurisdiction	Alaska American Samoa Arizona California–Entire State Guam Hawaii Iowa Idaho Kansas Missouri–Entire State Montana North Dakota Nebraska Nevada Oregon South Dakota Utah Washington Wyoming Northern Mariana Islands
DMERC Region	Region D
Article Covers	
Article Publication Date	03/17/2003
Article Beginning Effective Date	04/01/2003
Article Text	Changes in the CPAP and Respiratory Assist Devices local medical review policies, effective July 1, 2002, represented significant liberalizations in the criteria for qualification for these devices when used in the treatment of obstructive sleep apnea. However, based upon inquiries from suppliers, there are several basic points that merit emphasis. The AHI refers to the average number of apneas and hypopneas per hour and must be based on a minimum of 2 hours of sleep off a positive pressure device, recorded by PSG using actual recorded hours of sleep. The definition for apnea and hypopnea are included in the policies. Leg movement, snoring, respiratory event related arousals (RERAs), and other sleep disturbances that may be included by some polysomnographic facilities are not considered to meet the AHI definition in the Respiratory Assist Devices local medical review policies. Some facilities use the term Respiratory Disturbance Index (RDI) to describe a calculation that includes these other sleep disturbances. For that reason, the term RDI is being removed from the two policies. Claims for items based upon an index that does not score apneas and hypopneas separately from other sleep disturbance events, will be denied as not medically necessary. Only an AHI as defined in the policy and that meets coverage criteria qualifies for use of a KX modifier.

	PSG studies often take the form of split night studies in which a diagnostic portion of the study with the patient not on any device is followed by a therapeutic portion of the study in which a CPAP device is used to determine the response to treatment and to help select optimal pressure settings. Qualification for a CPAP device must be calculated based on a minimum of 2 hours of sleep without a device being worn. In other words, there must be a minimum of 2 hours of recorded sleep off CPAP in order to calculate the AHI and make the diagnosis of obstructive sleep apnea. The AHI may not be extrapolated or projected. If the date of service is for the fourth month or after in the capped rental cycle, compliance information must be obtained. For CPAP devices, this requirement was effective with the effective date of the policy, July 1, 2002, and applies to all beneficiaries on a CPAP device as of that date. Should suppliers choose to obtain this information through telephone, suppliers must document, at a minimum, the date of the call and to whom they spoke. For respiratory assist devices (RADs), the compliance requirements differ significantly from those for CPAP devices. Refer to the RAD policy for information on coverage criteria and documentation requirements for those devices. Suppliers are reminded that polysomnographic studies must be performed in a facility based sleep study laboratory. These facilities must be qualified suppliers of Medicare services, or a hospital certified to do such tests and must comply with all applicable state regulatory requirements. Durable Medical Equipment supliers may NOT perform the sleep studies.
Coverage Topic	Durable Medical Equipment
Other Comments	This article was published in the Spring 2003 DMERC Dialog.
Related Documents	This Article has no related documents.

APPENDIX

Sample Letter 1: Appeal for Denial of CPAP

Date:
To: Medical Director for Appeals
Insurance Company
CC: Home medical equipment companies
Patient
Primary MD

Re:
SS no.:
Birth date:
Date:
Dear Medical Director/Appeals:

I have received notice that you have denied payment for CPAP for the above-named patient. This is my official letter of appeal. It is also a notice to you that I am not liable for any adverse consequences that [he/she] suffers because of an arbitrary insurance company-based decision, based on an outdated algorithm by someone of whom has never seen or evaluated this patient.

This denial does not take into account recent developments in our understanding of the risks of sleep apnea. It places your members at medical risk and directly exposes you to liability.

Even "mild" (defined as an AHI or respiratory disturbance index of ≥5) sleep apnea is an independent risk factor for hypertension, death, congestive heart failure, stroke, cardiovascular disease, automobile accidents, cognitive impairment, reduced quality of life, increased health care costs, and cardiac arrhythmias. CPAP has been shown to reverse all of these consequences. In fact, CPAP is extraordinarily effective treatment. In *intention-to-treat* (not hours of use) models, it reduces cardiovascular risk, reduces mortality, reduces the risk of automobile accidents, and improves cognitive function. Please see the reference list below. Further, CPAP is cheap and harmless. Pepperell *(19)* estimates that the effect of CPAP on blood pressure is equivalent to monotherapy with antihypertensives. Certainly, CPAP is cheaper than treating the complications of untreated sleep apnea.

Frankly, I think you are doing a disservice to your member patients. You owe it to them to make decisions that are based on evidence, not arbitrary algorithms. Denial of CPAP treatment that has been prescribed by a physician who has seen and examined a patient is inappropriate and dangerous.

With this letter, I am urgently appealing your adverse decision concerning CPAP coverage. I am requesting an urgent appeal, because I believe that delay places this patient's health in serious jeopardy and exposes you to liability. Our mutual patients (and those in the cars and on the roads with them) are at risk.

I urge you to review the recent data on this topic (referenced below) and to visit the CMS website at your earliest opportunity. The AASM also has an excellent website at www.aasmnet.org.

I am sure that you understand and appreciate my need to send you a "form letter." After all, you sent me one. Writing an individual letter for each of these denials increases the cost of health care and takes my time away from patient care.

Sincerely,

Board Certified in Internal Medicine, Pulmonary Medicine, Critical Care Medicine, and Sleep Medicine

Sample Letter 2: Appeal for CPAP Denial Based on Compliance

Dear Dr ________:

I received your letter in which you deny payment for CPAP coverage for the above-named patient, because he has not used CPAP for the arbitrary amount of time that you have decreed. I believe this is bad medicine, legally questionable, and ultimately more expensive in the long run. The reasons for this are as follows:

1. CPAP is extraordinarily effective treatment. In *intention-to-treat* (not hours of use) models, it reduces cardiovascular risk, reduces mortality, reduces the risk of automobile accidents, and improves cognitive function *(1–19)*. Most studies showing a beneficial effect of CPAP have seen this benefit based on whether patients were prescribed CPAP, not on hours of use.
2. As long as the patient has a CPAP machine, there is a chance that he/she will use it and derive some benefit. When payment for CPAP treatment is denied, that chance goes to zero.
3. To my knowledge, most other medical treatments are "covered," regardless of use. This would include most prescription medication, home oxygen, and so on. CPAP appears to be unique in this regard. I think that this group of patients (sleep apnea patients) might have grounds for legal remedy, because they are being singled out as a class.
4. CPAP is cheap and harmless. Pepperell *(19)* estimates that the effect of CPAP on blood pressure is equivalent to monotherapy with antihypertensives. Certainly, CPAP is cheaper than treating the complications of untreated sleep apnea.

Frankly, I think you are doing a disservice to your member patients. You owe it to them to make decisions that are based on evidence, not arbitrary algorithms.

Sincerely,

REFERENCES (SAMPLE LETTERS 1 AND 2)

1. He J, Kryger MH, Zorick FJ, et al. (1988) Mortality and apnea index in obstructive sleep apnea: experience in 385 male patients. Chest 94:9–14.
2. Wright J, Johns R, Watt I, et al. (1997) The health effects of obstructive sleep apnoea and the effectiveness of treatment with continuous positive airway pressure: a systematic review of the research evidence. BMJ 314:851–860.
3. Jenkinson C, Davies RJ, Mullins R, et al. (1999) Comparison of therapeutic and subtherapeutic nasal continuous positive airway pressure for obstructive sleep apnea: a randomized prospective parallel trial. Lancet 353:2100–2105.
4. Peker Y, Hedner J, Norum J, et al. (2002) Increased incidence of cardiovascular disease in middle-aged men with obstructive sleep apnea: a 7-year follow-up. Am J Respir Crit Care Med 166:159–165.
5. Suzuki M, Otsuka K, Guilleminault C (1993) Long-term nasal continuous positive airway pressure can normalize hypertension in obstructive sleep apnea patients. Sleep 16:545–549.
6. Hack M, Davies RJ, Mullins R, et al. (2000) Randomized prospective parallel trial of therapeutic versus subtherapeutic nasal continuous positive airway pressure on simulated steering performance inpatients with obstructive sleep apnoea. Thorax 55:224–231.
7. Findley L, Smith C, Hooper J, et al. (2000) Treatment with nasal CPAP decreases automobile accidents in patients with sleep apnea. Am J Respir Crit Care Med 161:857–859.
8. Loredo J, Ancoli-Israel S, Dimsdale JE (1999) Effect of continuous positive airway pressure vs placebo on sleep quality in obstructive sleep apnea. Chest 116:1545–1549.
9. Engelman HM, Kingshott RN, Wraith PK, et al. (1999) Randomized placebo-controlled crossover trial of continuous positive airway pressure for mild sleep apnea/hypopnea syndrome. Am J Respir Crit Care Med 159:461–467.

10. Bardwell WA, Ancoli-Israel S, Berry CC, et al. (2001) Neuropsychological effects of one-week continuous positive airway pressure treatment in patients with obstructive sleep apnea: a placebo-controlled study. Psychosom Med 63:579–584.
11. Redline S, Adams N, Strauss ME, et al. (1998) Improvement of mild sleep-disordered breathing with CPAP compared with conservative therapy. Am J Respir Crit Care Med 157:858–865.
12. Dimsdale JE, Loredo JS, Profant J (2000) Effect of continuous positive airway pressure on blood pressure: a placebo trial. Hypertension 35:144–147.
13. Akashiba T, Minemura H, Yamamoto H, et al. (1999) Nasal continuous positive airway pressure changes blood pressure "non-dippers" to "dippers" in patients with obstructive sleep apnea. Sleep 22:849–853.
14. Faccenda JF, Mackay TW, Boon N, et al. (2001) Randomized placebo-controlled trial of continuous positive airway pressure on blood pressure in the sleep-apnea-hypopnea syndrome. Am J Respir Crit Care Med 163:344–348.
15. Bahammam A, Delaive K, Ronald J, et al. (1999) Health care utilization in males with obstructive sleep apnea syndrome two years after diagnosis and treatment. Sleep 22:740–747.
16. Engelman HM, Martin SE, Dreary IJ, et al. (1997) Effect of CPAP therapy on daytime function in patients with mild sleep apnoea/hypopnoea syndrome. Thorax 52:114–119.
17. Harbison J, O'Reilly P, McNicholas WT (2000) Cardiac rhythm disturbances in the obstructive sleep apnea syndrome: effects of nasal continuous positive pressure. Chest 118:591–595.
18. Sanner BM, Klewer J, Trumm A, et al. (2000) Long-term treatment with continuous positive airway pressure improves quality of life in obstructive sleep apnoea syndrome. Eur Respir J 16:118–122.
19. Pepperell JCT, Ramdassingh-Dow S, Crosthwaite N, et al. (2002) Ambulatory blood pressure after therapeutic and subtherapeutic nasal continuous positive airway pressure for obstructive sleep apnoea: a randomised parallel trial. Lancet 359:204–214.

Sample Letter 3: for Denial of Humidification

I am writing on behalf of my patient, _________, whom I have seen and examined as a treating physician. I have also reviewed polysomnographic data on this patient that demonstrates clinically significant OSAHS. As you know, CPAP is the treatment of choice for this condition and has been shown to reduce the rate of automobile accidents, improve cognitive function, normalize mortality, and lower blood pressure in patients with OSAHS. As you probably also know, patient compliance with CPAP is poor, averaging about 50% *(1)*. In the past year, two peer-reviewed articles have demonstrated something that those of us caring for these patients already knew: heated humidification improves patient compliance with CPAP *(2,3)*. I am attaching the abstracts of these papers to this letter.

In particular, my patient is having extreme difficulty tolerating his CPAP, even with a cool humidifier, because of severe nasal congestion during the day.

WITH THIS LETTER, I AM DECLARING AS A LICENSED PHYSICIAN WHO HAS SEEN AND EXAMINED THE PATIENT THAT HEATED HUMIDIFICATION ATTACHED TO CPAP IS MEDICALLY NECESSARY AND APPROPRIATE AND LIKELY TO IMPROVE OUTCOME. I AM REQUESTING INSURANCE REIMBURSEMENT FOR THIS TREATMENT.

Thank you for your consideration of this matter.

Sincerely,

REFERENCES (SAMPLE LETTER 3)

1. Kribbs NB, Pack AI, Kline LR, et al. (1993) Objective measurement of patterns of nasal CPAP use by patients with obstructive sleep apnea. Am Rev Respir Dis 147:887–895.
2. Massie CA, Hart RW, Peralez K, et al. (1999) Effects of humidification on nasal symptoms and compliance in sleep apnea patients using continuous positive airway pressure. Chest 116:403–408.
3. Weist GH, Lehnert G, Bruck WM, et al. (1999) A heated humidifier reduces upper airway dryness during continuous positive airway pressure therapy. Respir Med 93:21–26.

Sample Policy and Procedure for Split-Night Study

Samaritan hospital
Policy and procedure
Title/description: Split-night study

Policy no.
Page 1 of 1

Policy type: ( ) Administrative ( ) Human Resources ( ) Collaborative Patient Care
( ) Nursing (x) Departmental

Effective date: 03/22/02 Reviewed/revised dates:

Departments involved: Sleep Apnea Center and Cardiopulmonary Department

Replaces policy: DPP no. 19.0.0
Approval by and date:

Protocol:
A split-night study is intended to both diagnose sleep apnea and to determine effective CPAP/BIPAP pressure levels. Split-night studies are performed under the CMS guidelines for continuous positive airway pressure therapy used in the treatment of obstructive sleep apnea. Application and titration of positive airway pressure in split-night studies is done by protocol, by physician's order.
Policy:

1. The AHI is equal to the average number of apneas and hypopneas per hour of sleep and must be based on a minimum of 2 hours of sleep recorded by PSG using actual recorded hours of sleep.
2. Definitions are as follows:
   a. Apnea is defined as a cessation of airflow for at least 10 seconds.
   b. Hypopnea in the adult is defined as an abnormal respiratory event lasting at least 10 seconds, with at least a 30% reduction in thorocoabdominal movement or airflow as compared with baseline, and at least 4% O_2 desaturation.
3. A split-night study can be initiated if the patient has an average AHI of ≥15 events/hour of sleep at any point after the first 2 hours of testing.

Procedure:

1. Explain the procedure to the patient at the beginning of the study and at the time of CPAP initiation.
2. Fit the patient with the mask and attach the circuit. Set the CPAP remote at the lowest pressure setting, and let the patient fall asleep.
3. Increase the CPAP in 1 cm increments until apneas, snoring, hypopneas, snore arousals, and oxygen desaturations stop.
4. For snoring, increase the CPAP in 0.5-cm increments, until snoring stops.
5. If at all possible, attempt recording during REM sleep supine to reach an optimal CPAP pressure.

6. When the apnea, hypopneas, and snoring stop, note the final setting, and record this pressure as the critical breaking point.
7. If patients cannot tolerate CPAP, attempt use of BiPAP.
8. If the patient continues to have frequent arousals after reaching the critical breathing point, adjust the pressure up or down in 0.5 cm increments, until the arousals stop.
9. Check the patient, and mask for air leaks.
10. If the patient remains hypoxic ($SaO_2 \leq 87$) after the snoring, apneas, and hypopneas have stopped, add supplemental oxygen, starting at 1 L/minute.

Index

N

T

FSC
www.fsc.org
MIX
Papier | Fördert
gute Waldnutzung
FSC® C083411

Zeitfracht Medien GmbH
Ferdinand-Jühlke-Straße 7
99095 Erfurt, Deutschland
produktsicherheit@kolibri360.de